VACCINATION
AND ITS CRITICS

RECENT TITLES IN
DOCUMENTARY AND REFERENCE GUIDES

Immigration: A Documentary and Reference Guide
Thomas Cieslik, David Felsen, Akis Kalaitzidis

Gun Control: A Documentary and Reference Guide
Robert J. Spitzer

Culture Wars in America: A Documentary and Reference Guide
Glenn H. Utter

Civil Liberties and the State: A Documentary and Reference Guide
Christopher Peter Latimer

The Politics of Sexuality: A Documentary and Reference Guide
Raymond A. Smith

U.S. Election Campaigns: A Documentary and Reference Guide
Thomas J. Baldino and Kyle L. Kreider

U.S. Foreign Policy: A Documentary and Reference Guide
Akis Kalaitzidis and Gregory W. Streich

White-Collar and Corporate Crime: A Documentary and Reference Guide
Gilbert Geis

Homelessness: A Documentary and Reference Guide
Neil Larry Shumsky

Victims' Rights: A Documentary and Reference Guide
Douglas E. Beloof

Substance Abuse in America: A Documentary and Reference Guide
James A. Swartz

The Iraq War: A Documentary and Reference Guide
Thomas R. Mockaitis

Animal Rights and Welfare: A Documentary and Reference Guide
Lawrence W. Baker

Water Rights and the Environment in the United States: A Documentary and Reference Guide
John R. Burch Jr.

Endangered Species: A Documentary and Reference Guide
Edward P. Weber

9/11 and the War on Terror: A Documentary and Reference Guide
Paul J. Springer

VACCINATION AND ITS CRITICS

A Documentary and Reference Guide

Lisa Rosner

Documentary and Reference Guides

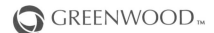
GREENWOOD™

An Imprint of ABC-CLIO, LLC
Santa Barbara, California • Denver, Colorado

Copyright © 2017 by ABC-CLIO, LLC

Library of Congress Cataloging-in-Publication Data

Names: Rosner, Lisa, author.
Title: Vaccination and its critics : a documentary and reference guide / Lisa Rosner.
Description: Santa Barbara, California : Greenwood, [2017] | Series: Documentary and
   reference guides | Includes bibliographical references and index.
Identifiers: LCCN 2016033601 (print) | LCCN 2016038544 (ebook) | ISBN 9781440841835
   (pbk. : alk. paper) | ISBN 9781440841842 (ebook)
Subjects: LCSH: Vaccination—History. | Immunization. | Health attitudes.
Classification: LCC RA638 .R68 2017 (print) | LCC RA638 (ebook) | DDC 614.4/7—dc23
LC record available at https://lccn.loc.gov/2016033601

ISBN: 978–1–4408–4183–5
EISBN: 978–1–4408–4184–2

21 20 19 18 17   1 2 3 4 5

This book is also available as an eBook.

Greenwood
An Imprint of ABC-CLIO, LLC

ABC-CLIO, LLC
130 Cremona Drive, P.O. Box 1911
Santa Barbara, California 93116-1911
www.abc-clio.com

This book is printed on acid-free paper ∞

Manufactured in the United States of America

CONTENTS

READER'S GUIDE
TO RELATED DOCUMENTS

PREFACE

Vaccination is one of the miracles of modern public health and safety. Together with those two other miracles, clean water and pure food, it has shaped modern expectations that we can live safe from deadly infectious diseases, have children and watch them grow, and live ourselves to see their children and even their grand-children.

Why, then, would this book be called *Vaccination and Its Critics*? It is hard to imagine a book called *Clean Water and Its Critics* or *Pure Unadulterated Food and the People Who Oppose It*. What makes vaccination different?

To many, in the modern world, there is no difference: the vaccination that pro-tects them is as much a part of their understanding of health and well-being as clean water and food. But there is a basic biological difference: people or societies who have a choice will never choose tainted or polluted water over clear, fresh water. Even if we seem to have no choice, our stomach and intestines will take over and try to rid us of the bad water or spoiled food.

Vaccines are radically different, because we must decide to use them. Our body gives us no clear indication of whether they are good or harmful for us. We must trust to other mechanisms besides biology: to family members, to doctors, to scien-tists, to communities, to governments.

Above all, we must trust to our own understanding of what it means to decide. We must understand that a decision made when children are three months old may affect whether they live or die at the age of 23. We must understand that a deci-sion made to keep vaccination in the hands of physicians may radically affect how many patients will have access to it. We must understand that a decision to spend millions of dollars on vaccination instead of clean water will dilute the public health miracle. And we must understand the need of patients to be in charge of their own health care, to be persuaded, not ordered, to help protect their families and their community.

In Chapter 1, "How Vaccines Work," we will look at how vaccines work. What that means has changed from the earliest accounts of processes that prevented children from getting a specific disease, smallpox, to modern accounts of the biology of our immune system. All have the same purpose—to educate people as to why they should make the decision to vaccinate.

Chapter 2, "Nature's Way and the Beginning of Immunization," will explore the experience of infectious diseases such as smallpox, diphtheria, and yellow fever from the 1500s through the 1790s. Most devastating of all were the childhood diseases, like measles, mumps, and whooping cough, which meant that only one in five children survived to adulthood. And it will trace the controversies surrounding a new practice, originally known as *engrafting* or *variolation*, that offered hope in protecting some communities from smallpox.

Chapter 3, "Vaccination by Design: Smallpox," describes the rise of the first man-made technology to confer immunity against a specific disease: inoculation with cowpox to prevent smallpox. Later known as *vaccination*, from the Latin word for cowpox (*variolae vaccinae*, "pox of cows"), this technique was pioneered by Edward Jenner and endorsed by the Parliament of Great Britain. Between 1790 and 1830, it was adopted by medical practitioners around the globe and formed the scientific basis for all modern vaccination research and practice.

The rise of vaccination coincided with the development of both professional medical journals and newspapers and journals that used sensational subjects to attract a wide audience. While vaccination was praised throughout the professional press, books and illustrations intended for a lay audience sold copy by criticizing it as an "unnatural" scientific practice that would harm children and create monsters. A more serious impediment to vaccination in many communities was the medical profession's insistence that only licensed physicians could administer vaccination. Only in the wealthiest communities in Europe and the United States would a physician be the primary care practitioner for young children; for everyone else, health care of children was in the hands of midwives. For that reason, countries like Sweden that licensed ministers and midwives to administer vaccination had the lowest rates of endemic smallpox.

Where people go, so go the microorganisms that cause disease. That is the subject of Chapter 4, "Epidemics in the Industrial Age." The period of the Industrial Revolution saw the development of trade, communication, and military networks that stretched around the world. These networks are responsible for many positive aspects of the modern world; they are also responsible for epidemic diseases that can travel thousands of miles and kill hundreds of thousands of people. Quarantine regulations, public health measures, and the application of scientific and statistical methods to medicine were the techniques used to combat the threats to human life, but these techniques engendered their own controversies.

In Chapter 5, "The Germ Theory and Vaccination," we can see how the development of the germ theory transformed modern medical theory and practice. The works of Louis Pasteur and Robert Koch provided the first scientific understanding of how vaccination protects the body against disease, and the methods they pioneered led to numerous vaccines against once-deadly epidemic diseases. The medical profession, previously divided in many countries between "allopathic" and "homeopathic" physicians, rallied behind the germ theory and promoted the new vaccines. Many countries passed vaccination laws and called for increased government regulation. But legislation opened the issues up for public debate. As some diseases, like smallpox, became less virulent, public opposition to vaccination regulations increased.

Chapter 6, "Vaccination and Everyday Life," examines how vaccination expanded from an emergency treatment to part of ordinary childhood experience as the number and supply of vaccines increased. Yet large-scale production and marketing of vaccines brought its own problems, especially quality control. In order to produce high-quality, consistently safe vaccines, industrial processes had to carefully monitor every aspect of production; failure to do so led to high-profile cases of contaminants introduced in the production process. The role of government increased in all industrialized countries in this period, and legislation requiring vaccination was one aspect of that increase.

Due to the new vaccines, World War I has the distinction of being the first war in history in which more soldiers died from armaments than from disease. That tradition of vaccination in wartime continued through World War II, as vaccines combined with other medical breakthroughs made it possible to keep more troops deployed on a global scale than ever before.

In the 1930s and 1940s, the question posed by Chapter 7, "Do We Trust Our Doctors? Vaccination, Patients' Rights, and Consumer Advocacy," would have made little sense to most middle-class Americans. Vaccinations had become a standard, accepted part of well-child medical practice. When the Salk vaccine for polio was announced in 1954, it was proclaimed one of the crowning achievements of American medical research. Together with penicillin and other antibiotics, the prescribed vaccination regimen created widespread herd immunity for children who had access to it and transformed childhood illnesses from deadly threats to routine rites of passage on the way to adulthood.

The social and political turmoil of the 1960s, though, posed new challenges for the medical establishment. Anesthesiologist Henry Beecher raised serious questions about the ethics of medical research carried out with no attention to informed concern; patient advocacy groups challenged the lack of transparency in medical decision making characterized by the phrases "doctor knows best" and "take two pills and call me in the morning." The thalidomide scandal of the early 1960s led to lawsuits and deep distrust of the connections forged between physicians and pharmaceutical companies.

The efficacy of medical and public health measures ensured that more children in First World countries were healthier than ever before. That, combined with concerns about vaccination, old and new, led a new generation of parents to question why they should give their own healthy child something that might make him/her sick. Parent groups raised concerns over the lack of transparency in vaccination research studies, leading to additional federal oversight. In the 1990s, Andrew Wakefield published a study in the *Lancet* allegedly linking Measles Mumps Rubella (MMR) vaccine to autism. Though thoroughly refuted, the study has been linked to rising rates of whooping cough in the United Kingdom. Similarly, the January 2015 outbreak of measles associated with Disneyland shows clearly how a parent's individual decision to withhold vaccination from his/her children can prevent herd immunity. The United States is currently the only country where vaccination rates are declining, making children and adults again vulnerable to infectious diseases.

In the modern world, as the website *VaccinateYourBaby.org* proclaims, "Vaccine-preventable diseases are only a plane ride away." The documents in Chapter 8, "Global Vaccination Ideals and Reality," show that fast-paced, global transportation networks mean that any local outbreak can become a global health-care problem. Since the 1960s, international vaccination efforts have focused on two main areas: addressing health-care inequities by making already-existing vaccines accessible to people around the globe and promoting scientific research to find new vaccines for emerging infectious diseases.

Taken together, the documents in this book show how vaccination has become such an effective public health measure and how its beneficiaries have become some of its sternest critics.

INTRODUCTION

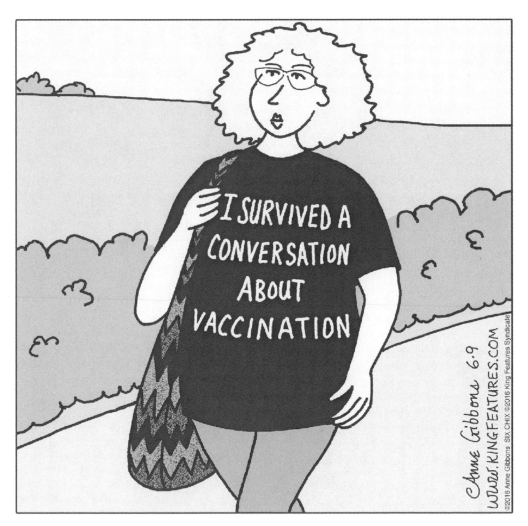

(© 2016 Anne Gibbons. Distributed by King Features Syndicate, Inc.)

Anne Gibbons's comic is intended as a wry joke about the contested status of vaccination in 21st-century America. However, it also conveys a profound truth about the history of vaccination and its critics for the past 300 years: we are all survivors of an ongoing conversation about the efficacy, safety, cost, policies, practices, values, and beliefs surrounding immunization.

For most of us, the term *survivor* may seem overblown, because we have not, ourselves, undergone any particular trauma beyond a series of injections when we were very young. Perhaps we may remember the pain caused by the syringe or the sore arm and slight fever. But the real trauma took place years before we were born, before the vaccine was available to the 21,000 children and their families in the United States who contracted diphtheria between 1936 and 1945 and the 1,800 who died, to the 530,000 who contracted measles between 1953 and 1962 and the 440 who died, to the 16,000 who contracted polio between 1951 and 1954 and the 1800 who died (Rousch, Murphy, and Vaccine-Preventative Table Working Group, 2007, Table 1). The immunizations we get as children or adults mean that we are not at risk from those diseases. More children live to grow up and to lead healthy lives free from epidemic diseases than at any previous time in the world's history.

We are also survivors of the historical conversation about vaccination if the only adverse effect we encountered was a little pain and fever, instead of something worse. The history of immunization preceded the science of how vaccines work and what risks this new scientific achievement carried. Before government regulation and quality control, the practice of vaccination carried risks to individuals and to public health. Even now, with all our scientific knowledge, medical professionals and prospective patients—or their parents—must weigh the risks of an adverse reaction against the benefits of immunization.

The U.S. National Vaccine Injury Compensation Program (NVICP) statistics from 2006 to 2014 gives some measure of the risks. The NICP process was set up to provide a mechanism for compensating patients or their families for adverse reactions related to vaccination. For diphtheria, 198 million doses of vaccine were administered throughout the country. Only 323 patients came forward claiming adverse reactions—an average of about 35 per year—with a total of 180 cases awarded compensation. For measles, 80 million doses were administered in the same period; 178 cases were brought forward, and 96 were awarded compensation. For polio, 62 million doses were administered. Six cases were brought forward, and four were awarded compensation. Those cases, and indeed the NVICP itself, can be considered survivors of the conversation on vaccination.

There is another kind of trauma associated with the history of vaccination and that is when people over the world die from vaccine-preventable diseases. This is especially heartrending when children die, since their young lives hold so much promise. Historically, the most common reasons for deaths from vaccine-preventable diseases had been poverty and lack of access. Often, of course, the two go together. Even in the modern world, those two conditions hinder the progress of vaccination. Only smallpox, of all the major vaccine-preventable diseases, has been completely eradicated worldwide. Polio is very close, with only 359 cases reported in 2014.

In order to further explore the dynamics of the historical conversation on vaccination, we can take a close look at one of the most important settings in which it has recently taken place, the June 2015 meeting of the Advisory Committee on Immunization Practices (ACIP) at the Centers for Disease Control and Prevention (CDC) in Atlanta, Georgia. The ACIP is, in its quiet way, one of the most influential committees in the United States. Once the Food and Drug Administration (FDA) has approved a specific vaccine for manufacture, the ACIP is charged with formulating official recommendations for its use. If the CDC director approves those recommendations—as generally happens—they become official federal policies.

ACIP recommendations, therefore, carry enormous weight. By statute, they must be incorporated into the recommended vaccination schedule, the schedule that determines doses and timing of all those childhood and young adult injections. ACIP recommendations have the power to compel insurance companies to cover specific kinds of immunizations for all Americans of a specific age or at-risk group. Since 1993, they have had the power to require the federal government to pay for vaccination under the Vaccines for Children (VFC) program. Since 2010, that power has been expanded, since the Affordable Care Act (ACA) requires all vaccinations to be provided free of charge, with no co-payment. If the ACIP decides a particular vaccine belongs on the vaccination schedule, it means, in effect, that every American has the right to receive it.

Many people present at the June meeting, however, would have a much more succinct statement of the power of the ACIP: the power of life and death. One of the key items on the meeting's agenda concerned recommendations for the MenB vaccine, the only protection against the potentially deadly B strain of meningitis (formally known as "serogroup B meningococcal disease") that had unexpectedly attacked college-age men and women in 2013 and 2014. High-profile cases at Princeton University, the University of California at Santa Barbara, Georgetown University, and San Diego State University had led the FDA to facilitate an accelerated process for licensing two potential vaccines, previously approved in other countries, in order to protect at-risk students. Now it was up to the ACIP to decide whether this would remain an emergency measure or whether the MenB vaccine would be added to the vaccination schedule, joining the existing vaccines against other strains of meningitis.

The conversation about vaccination at the ACIP meetings proceeds in a deliberate, formal manner. At this June meeting, the Meningococcal Work Group charged with examining the MenB vaccine had formulated a recommendation. They were tasked with presenting it, not just to the full committee but also to members of the public. There was a public comments section, and anyone could register to present a comment, limited to six minutes. ACIP meetings are also open to any other members of the public who wish to attend, whether or not they wish to speak. Nowadays the meetings are also live-streamed, and the minutes of every meeting since the 1990s are available to anyone who contacts the ACIP, with minutes, presentations, and videos available on the webpage. As Jonathan Temte, the ACIP chair during the June 2015 session, reminded everyone, the ACIP was a federal advisory committee and was therefore obligated to take public comments into account. "During this meeting's meningococcal session," he noted, "there would be an unprecedented number of public comments." The committee had also received over 40 letters, including one "with approximately 1200 co-signatures and a petition with 601 co-signatures." It is ACIP's duty, he said, "not only to review all the [scientific] evidence, but also to consider other issues such as values and preferences" as expressed in public comments (ACIP, 2015a, 17).

The ensuing interaction between the committee and the public showcased many of the key issues in the history of vaccination and its critics: efficacy, safety, cost-effectiveness, access, and equity. The ACIP had three recommendation options with respect to the new MenB vaccines. It could choose a Category A recommendation, so the new vaccine would become a mandatory part of the vaccination schedule, like vaccines against diphtheria, measles, polio, and other strains of meningitis (strains A, C, W, and Y). All insurance companies as well as the VFC program and ACA would have to pay for it. A majority of primary care physicians and clinics would keep it in stock so that it would be readily available to all prospective patients. A Category A recommendation would also require the ACIP to decide just where in the schedule to fit the new, required vaccine.

A Category B recommendation, sometimes called a "permissive" recommendation, would still require all insurance companies, the VFC program, and the ACA to pay for the new vaccine. The ACIP would still have to decide where the new vaccine fit in the existing schedule. However, it would leave the decision about recommending the vaccine up to the individual physician in consultation with the patient or parent. Although the ACIP does not make any recommendation to individual physicians about whether they should or should not stock any particular vaccine, a Category B recommendation might well mean the MenB vaccine would be less available. Patients or their parents might have to advocate to ensure they could get it.

The third option open to the ACIP was no recommendation for use of the vaccine, but that was not the anticipated outcome for the June 2015 meeting. Both MenB vaccines had evidence to support some sort of recommendation. The question was, which one was best for the American people?

It may seem puzzling and distressing that anyone, let alone a committee made up of physicians, researchers, and public health professionals, would even think twice about providing the widest possible protection for a potentially deadly disease, and that point of view was clearly expressed during the public comments. As Frankie Milley, founder of the national advocacy group Meningitis Angels put it, a Category B recommendation "to me, is like having a ship that's sinking. You have 100 passengers, 100 life vests, and you only give out 50, and the other 50 people on that boat drown as they watch their life vest hanging in the closet" (ACIP, 2015a, 43). But ACIP members are bound, by charter, to consider "disease epidemiology and burden of disease, vaccine efficacy and effectiveness, vaccine safety, economic analyses and implementation issues. The committee may revise or withdraw their recommendation(s) regarding a particular vaccine as new information on disease epidemiology, vaccine effectiveness or safety, economic considerations or other data become available." They must carefully consider all the evidence available for a particular vaccine, what is known about it and what is unknown. They must also be aware that the science of immunization is fast-moving and constantly evolving, and therefore, as Temte put it, they must pay particular attention to the "known unknowns and unknown unknowns" that might arise in the course of their deliberations (ACIP, 2015a, 37).

In order to assess the complex data concerning "safety, efficacy, and burden of illness" with respect to vaccines, ACIP members use a framework for evidence-based decision making called GRADE, short for Grades of Recommendation Assessment, Development, and Evaluation. Health-care professionals throughout the world use the GRADE framework to make recommendations and decisions. The framework is designed for "transparency; use of evidence of varying strengths; considering of individual and community health" (ACIP, 2010, 93). ACIP working groups tasked with evaluating a particular vaccine use GRADE to assess all the knowns and unknowns in order to decide whether there is enough hard data to make a recommendation, either for or against its use.

Although there are a number of steps to the GRADE process, the overall structure is very simple. First, the working group must look at all the scientific evidence available for a particular vaccine and decide whether the evidence is complete enough, and good enough, to provide solid answers to their questions. Do they have confidence, from the existing data, that the vaccine will work as expected? Do they have confidence, from the existing data, that the vaccine is safe? If the answer is no, then they stop. They do not have enough evidence to make a recommendation. If the answer is yes, then they continue. They can make a firm recommendation, either that the vaccine should become part of federal immunization policy or that it should not. In effect, the evidence-based framework codifies an enormous amount of complex decision making that, in the 18th through late 20th centuries, would have taken place through trial and error, only after new vaccines had been used on patients.

On June 24, 2015, members of the Meningococcal Work Group presented an overview of the committee's work that highlighted the complexities of assessing and recommending new vaccines. Vaccines for other strains of meningitis had been recommended and administered for years; indeed, many colleges and universities in the United States require proof of the meningitis vaccine before allowing a student to live on campus. But the two existing MenB vaccines had only been licensed following the outbreaks on college campuses: by Pfizer, on October 29, 2014, and by Novartis, on January 23, 2015, respectively. They had been licensed under an accelerated pathway with very careful CDC oversight so that they could be made available to patients and reduce the risk that this especially virulent strain would spread. But that also meant the evidence was more limited and so required the most careful assessment. As Rubin put it, "MenB vaccines certainly are challenging for ACIP. Of course, the goal is to prevent the largest proportion of cases of meningococcal disease possible. The recently licensed MenB vaccines are an important step forward. However, data for making policy decisions for vaccine use are not complete in terms of effectiveness, strain coverage in the US, duration of protection, effect on carriage and herd immunity, and expanded safety. In addition, the burden of serogroup B meningococcal disease in adolescents and young adults is currently low" (ACIP, 2015a, 23).

Several members of the working group presented their overall assessment. The process began with a study question, a specific question that can be answered based on available evidence. Choosing the right study question is key to the ensuing analysis: the more precise the question, the more precise the assessment of the available evidence. The MenB study question was, "Should MenB vaccines be routinely administered to all adolescents and young adults (including college students)?" The answers had addressed the evidence for making the decision. The two options were: 1) There was strong evidence for saying yes or no to the question; and 2) There was not strong evidence for saying yes or no, and therefore, no recommendation could be made.

The next step was "to select outcomes that the WG [working group] believed to be important and critical to answer this question." The first had to do with burden of disease. How many cases were there? How likely was the disease to kill patients who contracted it? Did the disease carry with it any long-term effects? The second had to do with how well the existing MenB vaccines worked against the known strains of meningitis B. There was not just one "B strain" of meningitis. Indeed, there were thousands. It was important for the working group to assess whether the existing vaccines would be useful against all the MenB strains out there or only a subset.

These outcomes were essential to the assessment process. The incidences of all cases of meningococcal disease were reported to be at "historic lows" in the United States: there were only 564 cases in 2013. For meningitis B, there were only 55–65 cases each year among young adults, with 10%–15% ending in death. As reported, it was not only a life-threatening but also a rare disease: to put it into perspective, as one ACIP participant pointed out, "There are 20,000 to 30,000 deaths a year in this country from mental health-related diseases in the same age category" (ACIP, 2015a, 40).

It was, therefore, the first task of the working group to decide how confident they were in that data: did they think it was accurate? Did they feel they needed additional research to improve its accuracy? Or did they believe that no additional research was necessary for them to accurately characterize the burden of disease?

After carefully reviewing the data, the working group felt very confident in the evidence on burden of illness. As one of its members noted, "Meningitis is one of the better reported diseases in the US" (ACIP, 2015a, 56). That is, the disease was not overreported or underreported: there was no evidence to suggest that there might be much higher, or much lower, numbers of MenB disease now or in the foreseeable future.

Breadth of coverage was a different matter. The existing vaccines had been introduced to save the lives of at-risk young people, and there simply was not much data available on all possible meningitis B strains. The vaccine manufactures had provided estimates, but they had used different methods. Additional scientific studies were still in progress and had not yet published any results. That meant further research was certainly necessary to fully assess how well either vaccine would work against the many strains of serogroup B. The working group was not confident that they had enough scientific evidence to answer this question.

The working group also identified additional five outcomes for their formal, evidence-based assessment:

1. Efficacy in producing short-term immunity, defined as one month after the patient receives the vaccine. This would ensure that a patient who received the vaccine was protected for the duration of a meningitis B outbreak.

2. Efficacy in producing long-term immunity, defined as 11–24 months for one vaccine or 48 months in the other. This was essential if the vaccine was to become part of a routine vaccination schedule. Patients—and their parents—would have to be informed whether they might need one injection at age 16 or one at age 16 and another at 18. And they would have to be certain that an injection at, say, 18 would provide protection for two or four years of college.

3. Efficacy when administered with other vaccines. Nowadays, no routine immunization is given in isolation. Existing recommendations for other meningitis vaccines stated that one dose was to be given around age 11 and a booster at age 16. As one of the ACIP members pointed out, it was hard enough getting adolescents back to their pediatricians to get the currently recommended meningitis booster shot. If the ACIP recommended the new MenB vaccines for the same age group, it would have to be effective when administered at the same time as the existing meningitis vaccines.

4. Serious adverse effects caused by the vaccine. Vaccines have to be safe as well as effective.

5. Safety when administered with other vaccines. Would the new vaccines add to the existing adverse effects of currently administered vaccines?

Again, the point of the GRADE assessment process was to assess the quality of the evidence. Working group members used published and unpublished data in their assessment. They divided the existing scientific studies into two groups, randomized control trials (RCTs) and observational studies. RCTs were usually taken as the gold standard for clinical research, so they are assigned an initial number of "1" as the highest ranking, while observational studies are ranked lower, at "3." But studies could move up or down on the table, based on a number of factors: risk of bias or other methodological limitations, inconsistency, indirectness, imprecision, publication bias. They could also be moved up in the table, though only if they have not previously been moved down.

The working group examined each vaccine in turn. The first was Bexsero (MenB-4C), produced by Novartis. There were only five studies, one noncontrolled study and four RCTs. None of them dealt with efficacy or safety when administered with other vaccines. The second was Pfizer's Trumenba (MenB-FHbp). Again, the evidence was limited, two noncontrolled studies and five RCTs. For Trumenba, there was some evidence on its impact with other vaccines. This question was especially important for its administration to young adults. Young adults are not an easy population to vaccinate. If young adults did not go to their pediatrician for the current vaccine, which was strongly recommended for their age group, it was unlikely they would go for this new vaccine. The best way to get patients to take it would be to incorporate it into the existing MenB vaccine—but to recommend that, the working group would need more data.

Modern reporting data have changed the nature of vaccine evidence, particularly when it comes to reporting severe adverse effects (SAEs). Of the approximately 70,000 patients who received the vaccines, fewer than 300 reported any SAEs. The deaths that occurred were caused by car accidents and intoxication, unrelated to the vaccine and unfortunately often linked to the age group who had received the vaccines.

The working group found it could not assign a "1" type to any of the evidence. The evidence for benefits seemed strongest in the short term but less certain in the long term. For short-term efficacy of both vaccines, the working group designated the evidence type 2, "further research may change the estimate of effect." For long-term efficacy, the evidence type was designated type 3 and 4, indicating that more research would be necessary for them to have confidence in the results. When it came to safety, the evidence seemed clearer, as the evidence for SAEs for both vaccines was assessed as evidence type 2. But there were significant gaps: the evidence for the MenB-4C vaccine with other vaccines could not be assessed at all.

What this meant was that the working group did not have enough confidence in the existing scientific evidence to make a Category A recommendation, one that would require the routine use of the new MenB vaccines for all children. This decision was bolstered by a cost-effectiveness analysis carried out by the CDC. The ACIP is not charged to consider the cost, in dollars, of their recommendations. As Temte had noted in a previous meeting, "ACIP has always been asked specifically to make recommendations based on safety and efficacy first. Other considerations follow that. ACIP has never been asked to make a recommendation based solely on the cost of a vaccine. In fact, ACIP should be fairly neutral to that based upon its charge" (ACIP, 2010, 40).

But ACIP members are able to include consideration of what is known as Number Needed to Vaccinate (NNV) when making their recommendations. This is the number of patients who would need to be vaccinated in order to prevent a case of or a death from a disease. In the case of meningitis B, the CDC's analysis found that, assuming a population of 4 million adolescents and young adults, between 100,000 and 400,000 would have to be vaccinated to prevent even a single case of the disease. Between 1 million and 3 million adolescents and young adults would have to be vaccinated in order to prevent a single death. The NNVs are thus very high compared to the number of cases and deaths they would prevent. They also have a wide range: there is clearly a very great practical difference between vaccinating 100,000, 400,000, 1 million, or 3 million people. Currently, only 30% of adolescents and young adults routinely get their recommended booster shot for the existing meningitis vaccine—that is, what would be 1.33 million of the hypothetical 4 million people in the CDC analysis. If "1 million" was the correct NNV, then adding the MenB vaccine to the routine schedule would be effective in preventing that one death. But what if "3 million" was the correct number? Clearly—again—more evidence on cost-effectiveness would be necessary before the working group could agree on a Category A recommendation (ACIP, 2015a, 31).

The Meningococcal Work Group concluded their report by acknowledging "that meningococcal disease is a rare but serious illness and each case is life-threatening." There was "a strong desire" within the working group "to ensure access to MenB vaccines." However, they felt "important data for making policy recommendations for MenB vaccines are not yet available." For that reason, they favored "a Category B rather than a Category A recommendation." The key reasons were "First, the current burden of diseases is low. This means that the [Number Needed to Vaccinate] to prevent a case and death is high, and the number of cases prevented may be comparable to the number of [serious adverse effects] to vaccine. Second, additional data are still needed to consider a routine recommendation. Most importantly, a better understanding is needed of the true proportion of serogroup B cases that could be prevented with MenB vaccine." They were aware that "it is difficult to accept that, in the absence of a vaccination program, there may be cases that are preventable. However, even with a fully implemented vaccination program," the evidence indicated that "the MenB vaccines will not prevent all cases" (ACIP, 2015a, 32).

The Meningococcal Work Group had provided an exemplary analysis, fully living up to the standards of "transparency; use of evidence of varying strengths; considering of individual and community health." It was clear, scientific, and evidence-based: as one ACIP member put it, it was "one of the best presentations of the data she had ever heard" (ACIP, 2015a, 40).

But it is part of the historical conversation on vaccination as well as part of the charge of the ACIP that good science must form the basis for any recommendation but cannot be the only consideration. Values and preferences, from professional colleagues and from the public, must be incorporated into the ACIP's deliberations. In the June 2015 meeting, criticism of the working group's recommendations stemmed from the historical success of the United States' vaccination program and the enormous power of the ACIP to influence that success in the case of individual diseases and individual patients. Routine vaccination saved millions of lives every day and billions of dollars in health-care costs every year. The data showed, time and again, that Category A recommendations worked better than Category B recommendations to make vaccines available to American citizens. By the early 21st century, governments worldwide were working to end vaccine-preventable diseases. When it came to MenB, as the working group itself said, "It is difficult to accept that … there may be cases that are preventable." But Frankie Milley was more forceful: "How many tears do we have to cry and how many children and young adults have to be debilitated or die before … we do the right thing and just stop this disease?" (ACIP, 2015a, 44).

While the working group's recommendations recapitulated techniques promoted by vaccine advocates over the previous three centuries, the questions and comments from ACIP members and the public distilled many of the concerns of their critics. One medical professor pointed out the problem of translating the recommendation in its current form into actual practice. As "the parent of one college-aged child," she said, "and one child who just finished college, she was completely unclear about what the [ACIP] expected parents to do. If she or her daughter goes to the doctor and indicates that they have heard there is a vaccine that will protect her daughter from a deadly disease, they would have to rely on the doctor to make a value-based judgment about whether she should receive this vaccine. This kicks it back to the 19-year-old who is going to call her mother, who is just as confused." They already knew, from their professional experience, that it can be very hard to get a healthy young adult to go to a doctor. Another physician pointed out that "unlike huge health maintenance organizations (HMOs), it has been her experience with permissive recommendations in the past that smaller practices may not even carry Category B vaccines in their offices. While practitioners can council patients, the patients may have to go elsewhere to be vaccinated" (ACIP, 2015a, 40).

That, of course, assumed that practitioners were knowledgeable about the dangers of meningitis. ACIP members "emphasized that it is the responsibility of physicians to educate themselves on the risks and benefits of vaccines. Physicians must understand the risk of the disease and make recommendations as appropriate for the child. If there is a vaccine that works, it should be ACIP's job to educate their colleagues and promote its use if a Category B recommendation is made." A representative from the National Association of Nurse Practitioners "acknowledged the importance of the use of the vaccines for outbreak management and that local public health and colleges have to be prepared in advance to use the vaccine. Education of clinicians, adolescents, and parents about the signs and symptoms of meningococcal disease and early recognition, early treatment, and prompt community response may be one of the most important efforts they could make with regard to this disease" (ACIP, 2015a, 41).

If only it were that simple, argued Steven Black, a pediatric infectious disease specialist, during the six minutes he was allocated as part of the public comments. "I've been a Pediatric Infectious Disease Specialist and Vaccinologist for more than 30 years," he said, going on to make "two disclosures. [First,] I'm a consultant for GSK, Protein Sciences, Takeda, and WHO. And secondly, I really hate this disease . . ." The problem with a Category B recommendation, which made the MenB vaccine optional, is that the disease "evolves too rapidly . . . I became a doctor to save lives, and I think that it's difficult to save lives one on one, especially with meningococcal B disease . . . One . . . of the greatest fears of pediatricians and parents is to miss a case of this disease because, once it commences, the risk of sequelae and mortality is so high. So, I think the committee has an opportunity today to prevent these deaths, to prevent the suffering and loss of life potential in dozens of children each year." He, therefore, urged "the committee members to seize that opportunity and to routinely recommend this vaccine for children" (ACIP, 2015a, 42).

Those ideas—the rapid spread of the disease among otherwise healthy young adults who had no reason to go to a doctor, the difficulty of diagnosis on the ground, the devastating effect of even a few hours' delay—were repeated over and over by family members and meningitis survivors during the public comments. Ryan Milley, Frankie Milley's son, developed a fever on the Father's Day after his high school graduation. Like any concerned parents, the Milleys put Ryan to bed and called his doctor Monday morning to make an appointment. Within a few hours it was clear he was very sick, and they rushed him to the emergency room. He died at 10:15 that night. Since that time, Frankie Milley has worked tirelessly to advocate for meningitis vaccines. As she said, "I've been coming to these ACIP meetings for 12 years. I've testified at almost all of them, almost 36 times. For a total of 108 minutes, I've been allowed to speak about my son and the importance of immunizing kids. In those 12 years, the working groups, the ACIP voting committee, and us old warriors that are here every time have come very far. We've left here celebrating, and we've left here crying. One of the worst was when we had a vaccine to prevent meningococcal B in infants and we didn't get a recommendation for it." We know from past experience, she said, "that permissive recommendations don't allow for education of the disease and the vaccine. We know, in many cases, there's no affordability or accessibility. We know that there's a hesitancy of physicians and healthcare providers to give it because [they feel] it's really not recommended . . . We know that there [are] provider reimbursement problems" with the Category B recommendation (ACIP, 2015a, 42–43).

Scott Parkhurst told a similar story of his son Jacob, a 17-year-old high school junior who died within 36 hours of falling ill. Once again, he felt sick on Sunday and by Monday morning, "he was in the emergency room. The ER doctor pulled Jake's mom and I aside and informed us that Jake may not survive and appeared to have bacterial meningitis. I told Jake to fight for his life and he yelled back to me, "Okay" as he was taken off to intensive care and put into a medically induced coma. That was the last contact I ever had with Jake" (ACIP, 2015a, 44). Alicia Stillman, founder and director of the Emily Stillman Foundation, got a call from her daughter Emily, a college sophomore, reporting, "I have a headache." I said, "Why do you think you have a headache? I bet you're coming down with the flu." She said, "No, mom, I was up all night studying for two big tests. But don't worry. I did good." I said, "Great, so take a couple of MOTRIN® and we'll see how you feel in the morning." "The morning never came. By the time I was called back to the hospital the next day and told to get en route immediately, Emily was in a coma" from which she never awoke (ACIP, 2015a, 45).

Nor was it only parents sharing the heartbreak seeing their healthy child move inexorably from a headache to a life-threatening disease, from a rare "case," in the ACIP's clinical language to a "fatality." ACIP members had talked about the need to educated colleges and universities, but those same colleges and universities begged the ACIP for help. Dozens of colleges, universities, and professional associations wrote letters to the ACIP, pointing out, time and again, that though all adolescents and young adults were at risk for meningitis B, the conditions of college living were particularly conducive to its spread. They pointed out the potentially devastating effects on college and university communities, whatever the outcome of a specific case. And they pointed out the historical evidence of two centuries of vaccine-related public health measures that routine immunization is the most efficacious and most cost-effective way of eliminating vaccine-preventable diseases (ACIP, 2015a, 185–254).

The public comments hammered home the limitations to the most scientific analyses of burden of illness. As Scott Parkhurst said, "I understand this disease only affects a small percentage of the population. But when it's your son, daughter, grandchild, cousin, niece, or friend, it's 100%. I don't think anyone here who has children would want to lose their child to something that is preventable" (ACIP, 2015a, 45). Mike Barnes described how his family "lost our 20-year old son, Jimmy, to serogroup B meningococcal disease this March. He went to the ER on a Monday with a terrible headache, neck pain, and high fever. He was told it was the flu and sent home. He was gone in 28 hours. He was not a college student living in a dorm, and his story was not covered by the media, so I'm here to share it with you today. He was, however, we thought, fully vaccinated, including with the meningitis vaccine . . . In my family, among my two children, the incidence of men B was 50%. For Jimmy, it was 100%" (ACIP, 2015a, 46).

Andy Marso, meningitis survivor, brought up the question of cost-effectiveness when it came to the shouldering the burden of illness. "I know there's concerns about the cost of these vaccines, but I hope you're accounting for all of the costs of not vaccinating and you're also accounting for the cost burden and who bears the cost burden. Is it society at large, or is it just families like mine?" As he explained, "Unfortunately, most people don't know how afraid of this disease they should be. I know because 11 years ago, I went from a perfectly healthy college student to almost dead within 24 hours. Then I spent four months in the hospital having my skin debrided and parts of my limbs amputated. As I told you all a few months ago, the first year of my medical bills were almost $2 million. That's just for the initial year. $2 million. That would've bought a lot of vaccines, right? And that doesn't even account for the year of work that my parents missed and that I missed as I was recovering, nor for the ongoing medical costs that I've had every year since. I've been fortunate to have health insurance, but I've basically maxed out my out-of-pocket every single year and I probably will for most of my life ..." (ACIP, 2015a, 49–50).

ACIP members had pointed out that a Category B recommendation could be seen as "fairly neutral" on cost, since it would place the MenB vaccines on the list of vaccines paid for through the VFC program and ACA. But as public presenters responded, there still might be enormous inequities in who actually could afford to get the vaccines. Before the FDA licensed the vaccine, Alicia Stillman had driven "busloads to Canada and I protected whole families in Canada with this vaccine. Now we have it here and I field phone calls and emails all day long from parents all over the country who can't get their hands on this vaccine" (ACIP, 2015a, 45). Jacqueline Ross, sister of a Drexel University student who had died of meningitis B, described how "since December, my parents have worked to get me the serogroup B vaccine. This was no easy task. It took many phone calls and e-mails between them, the vaccine manufacturers, my pediatrician, various pharmacies, and even the Department of Public Health. I was finally able to get vaccinated just last week, but the process took nearly six months and it only occurred because our pediatrician finally thought to recommend that we look into a travel vaccination clinic. My parents also tried to get the vaccine through several pharmacies. Most did not have the access to it, and those that could get it did not have anyone on staff that could administer it, so ordering it would not have mattered. Parents should not have to work this hard to get an FDA-approved vaccine to protect their children" (ACIP, 2015a, 48). If the vaccine was that inaccessible for families of advocacy groups, how accessible would it be for less privileged or informed families?

The public comments also raised the issue of vaccination as a human right and a right of all American citizens, which the ACIP, like other federal agencies, had a responsibility to protect and serve. Neil Raisman, who lost his son Isaac to meningitis, concluded "that informed people with the money to pay for the vaccine have lived and those who can't afford it or don't even know about it have been infected. This is counter to everything the ACIP, the CDC, the FDA, and the NIH stand for. Your endorsement vote for the FDA recommendation would realign this committee with its mission ... We expect the government to tell us when the health of our children is in danger, and then help us decide what to do" (ACIP, 2015a, 55). Kamay Lafalaise, from the National Consumers League, pointed out that healthcare advocacy is part of consumer advocacy and that "making safe and effective medications and healthcare widely available to all Americans has been a longstanding priority to NCL . . . 84% of parents cite protecting a child from disease as the top reason to vaccinate . . . and of all childhood diseases, parents are most concerned about meningitis. Not only do these findings highlight that there is an ongoing need for vaccine education, but that Americans see vaccines as a way to protect our children and community from disease, and they take very seriously the threat of meningitis." A Category A recommendation would be much more effective in creating opportunities for consumer education and would make that education available to the largest number of potential patients, "not just those who are aware of the vaccine and specifically request it or those who can pay out-of-pocket costs." Lafalaise concluded, in words that echoed the "values and preferences" expressed by so many others, "You have heard powerful testimony today from several people afflicted by this frightening disease. If we wait, it could be too late. How many lives need to be lost before we take preventative action?" (ACIP, 2015a, 54).

Of all the advocacy groups, the only one that supported a Category B recommendation came from the National Vaccine Information Center (NVIC), described in its own statement as "advocates for the institution of vaccine safety and informed consent protections and public health policy and laws." ACIP members may have been disconcerted to find themselves on the same side as the NVIC, which has promoted anti-vaccination campaigns since the 1990s. As a consumer education group, however, the NVIC has been consistent in "supporting the availability of all preventive healthcare options, including vaccines, and the right of consumers to make educated, voluntary healthcare choices." Like many other anti-vaccination advocates in the past 200 years, they have insisted that vaccination must be voluntary, not required by law. For that reason, while agreeing that "parents have a right to know about the benefits and risks and availability of meningococcal vaccines so they can make an informed decision for their children," they did not recommend what they termed a "universal-use recommendation." Instead, they encouraged "ACIP and the CDC to revisit stakeholder support and need for greater flexibility in the ACIP recommendations" (ACIP, 2015a, 46).

Though there have been times when the NVIC and other anti-vaccination advocacy groups have seemed like the strongest voices, it was not true in the June 2015 meeting. Instead, a representative from the Immunization Action Coalition, a pro-vaccine advocacy group, opposed to the NVIC in this as in so many other arenas and summarized the overwhelming public opinion when she noted, "As public health professionals, we are all dedicated to prevention. I know that you as ACIP members are charged with making recommendations that balance difficult and seemingly competing objectives. But to me, the answer is clear. I choose prevention, and I ask you to choose a routine recommendation to protect all teens with MenB vaccine. You have the power to prevent a deadly and devastating disease that can have an overwhelming impact on young people and all the people who love them, as we have just heard. A routine recommendation is quite simply the right thing to do" (ACIP, 2015a, 53).

At the end of the public session, Temte thanked all of the participants "for sharing what must be very difficult stories, and expressed ACIP's appreciation for their heartfelt and very thoughtful comments" (ACIP, 2015a, 55). ACIP members had additional discussion to address, at least in part, some of the public comments. One committee member "stressed that members considering support of a Category B recommendation were not doing so because they were wildly enthusiastic that it would be exactly the right recommendation long-term for this vaccine. There simply was not adequate information at this point to support a Category A recommendation. In that context, she urged the manufacturers to provide those data as quickly as possible." She as well as others explained that they did not consider burden of disease solely in terms of statistics and that they recognized how important it was "to understand the long-term consequences and the cost of medical expenses to survivors and families out-of-pocket. Survivors are dealing with profound lifelong consequences, which should be factored in."

In order to address concerns about practitioner and patient education, ACIP members on the Childhood Vaccination Schedule working group agreed to put information about the MenB vaccines on the official U.S. Childhood Vaccination Schedule and to make it available on all other information outlets. There was some discussion of the need for revising the color-coding on the family-friendly vaccination schedule charts. In response to the many letters from colleges and universities, a representative from the American College Health Association noted, "They are pleased to have reached a point of making some recommendations, which offers a springboard before the fall semester" (ACIP, 2015a, 57).

The final point of discussion was the recognition that a Category B recommendation, if approved, was not set in stone. As more evidence became available or as new vaccines were approved, the ACIP could move quickly to review and, if appropriate, revise the recommendation to a Category A. One promising possibility for the future was a combined vaccine that could combine protection against meningitis B with the other meningococcal vaccines already available for routine use.

Having completed the discussion, the ACIP prepared to vote on the Meningococcal Work Group's proposed recommendation for use of MenB vaccines in adolescents:

A serogroup B meningococcal (MenB) vaccine series may be administered to adolescents and young adults 16 through 23 years of age to provide short term protection against most strains of serogroup B meningococcal disease. The preferred age for MenB vaccination is 16 through 18 years of age. (Category B)

In addition, the following language would be provided as guidance for use:

- MenB should be administered as either a 2-dose series of MenB-4C or a 3-dose series of MenB-FHbp
- The same vaccine product should be used for all doses
- Based on available data and expert opinion, MenB-4C and MenB-FHbp may be administered concomitantly with other vaccines indicated for this age, but at a different anatomic site, if feasible
- No product preference to be stated

The ACIP approved the working group's recommendation by a vote of 14-1. It was subsequently approved by the director of the CDC and thereby became federal policy. In October 2015, the ACIP and CDC approved a new system of color-coding to emphasize the importance of MenB vaccines in protecting the health of the nation's adolescents and young adults.

At the conclusion of the June 2015 meeting, ACIP members, public participants, and the entire country had survived yet another of the historical conversations about vaccination. The rest of this book will show how that conversation began and how it has grown, added significant features, and engaged global participants, through to the present day.

FURTHER READING

Advisory Committee on Immunization Practices (ACIP). (2010, October 27–28). *Summary Report*. Atlanta, GA. http://www.cdc.gov/vaccines/acip/meetings/downloads/min-archive/min-oct10.pdf.

Advisory Committee on Immunization Practices (ACIP). (2015a, June 24–25). *Summary Report*. Atlanta, GA. http://www.cdc.gov/vaccines/acip/meetings/downloads/min-archive/min-2015-06.pdf.

Advisory Committee on Immunization Practices (ACIP). (2015b, October 21). *Summary Report*. Atlanta, GA. http://www.cdc.gov/vaccines/acip/meetings/downloads/min-archive/min-2015-10.pdf.

Centers for Disease Control and Prevention. (2016a). "ACIP Charter." http://www.cdc.gov/vaccines/acip/committee/charter.html.

Centers for Disease Control and Prevention. (2016b). "ACIP Meeting Information." http://www.cdc.gov/vaccines/acip/meetings/meetings-info.html.

Centers for Disease Control and Prevention. (2016c). "Immunization Schedules for Preteens and Teens." http://www.cdc.gov/vaccines/schedules/easy-to-read/preteen-teen.html.

Chatterjee, Archana, ed. (2013). *Vaccinophobia and Vaccine Controversies of the 21st Century*. New York: Springer.

"Data and Statistics." (2016). National Vaccine Injury Compensation Program. *Health Resources and Services Administration*. http://www.hrsa.gov/vaccinecompensation/data/statisticsreport.pdf.

"Poliomyelitis Fact Sheet." (2014). *World Health Organization*. http://www.who.int/mediacentre/factsheets/fs114/en/.

Rousch, Sandra, Trudy Murphy, and the Vaccine-Preventative Table Working Group. (2007). "Historical Comparisons of Morbidity and Mortality for Vaccine-Preventable Disease in the United States." *Journal of the American Medical Association* 298: 2155–2163.

"The Vaccine Wars." Teacher Resources. *Frontline, WHYY*. http://www.pbs.org/wgbh/pages/frontline/teach/vaccine/related.html.

1

HOW VACCINES WORK

A MOTHER'S VIEW OF VACCINATION

- **Document:** Lady Mary Wortley Montagu, Letter written to a friend in Great Britain. Though this letter was not published until after her death in 1762, it probably circulated in manuscript form.
- **Date:** 1717
- **Where:** Written in Constantinople, modern Istanbul, Turkey
- **Significance:** Lady Mary Wortley Montagu's letter states as clearly as any modern account how vaccination works, from the point of view of a mother who wishes to protect her children from the deadly disease, smallpox. Lady Mary herself had been a celebrated beauty whose appearance, in her own eyes and those of her contemporaries, had been ruined when she caught smallpox. As she knew, she was lucky to have survived, smallpox scars and all.

DOCUMENT

A propos of distempers, I am going to tell you a thing, that will make you wish yourself here. The small-pox, so fatal, and so general amongst us, is here entirely harmless, by the invention of engrafting, which is the term they give it. There is a set of old women, who make it their business to perform the operation, every autumn, in the month of September, when the great heat is abated. People send to one another to know if any of their family has a mind to have the small-pox; they make parties for this purpose, and when they are met (commonly fifteen or sixteen together) the old woman comes with a nut-shell full of the matter of the best sort of small-pox, and asks what vein you please to have opened. She immediately rips open that you offer to her, with a large needle (which gives you no more pain than a common scratch) and puts into the vein as much matter as can lie upon the head of her needle, and after that, binds up the little wound with a hollow bit of shell, and in this manner opens four or five veins.

The Grecians have commonly the superstition of opening one in the middle of the forehead, one in each arm, and one on the breast, to mark the sign of the Cross; but this has a very ill effect, all these wounds leaving little scars, and is not done by those that are not superstitious, who chuse to have them in the legs, or that part of the arm that is concealed.

The children or young patients play together all the rest of the day, and are in perfect health to the eighth. Then the fever begins to seize them, and they keep their beds two days, very seldom three. They have very rarely above twenty or thirty in their faces, which never mark, and in eight days time they are as well as before their illness. Where they are wounded, there remains running sores during the distemper, which I don't doubt is a great relief to it. Every year, thousands undergo this operation, and the French Ambassador says pleasantly, that they take the small-pox here by way of diversion, as they take the waters in other countries. There is no example of any one that has died in it, and you may believe I am well satisfied of the safety of this experiment, since I intend to try it on my dear little son.

I am patriot enough to take the pains to bring this useful invention into fashion in England, and I should not fail to write to some of our doctors very particularly about it, if I knew any one of them that I thought had virtue enough to destroy such a considerable branch of their revenue, for the good of mankind. But that distemper is too beneficial to them, not to expose to all their resentment, the hardy wight that should undertake to put an end to it. Perhaps if I live to return, I may, however, have courage to war with them. Upon this occasion, admire the heroism in the heart of your friend, etc. etc.

Source: Montagu, Lady Mary Wortley. (1822). *Letters of Lady Mary Wortley Montague, Written during Her Travels in Europe, Asia, and Africa.* Paris: Firman Didot.

ANALYSIS

Lady Mary Wortley Montagu (1689–1762) heard about "engrafting" to prevent smallpox when she accompanied her husband, the British ambassador to Turkey, to Constantinople. Inoculation had been a part of Turkish medical practice for centuries, and the Royal Society of London, the leading scientific society in Great Britain, had published accounts of it by Dr. Emanuel Timoni (also known as Timonius, the Latinized version of his name) in 1713. Dr. Timoni was the Montagu family physician in Constantinople, and his professional opinion may well have influenced Lady Mary's decision. But it was Lady Mary's letter and her subsequent advocacy for inoculation when she returned to Great Britain that caught the attention of the wealthy, literate public. We will meet advocates of her type very frequently in the history of vaccination and its critics: celebrities whose personal and family experience lead them to champion one or another side of the debate.

DID YOU KNOW?

Lady Mary and Domestic Health

Lady Mary Wortley Montagu's *Turkish Embassy Letters* are famous, not just for their advocacy of smallpox inoculation but also for detailed observations on the countries through which she travelled. She was particularly interested in innovations and cultural attitudes toward hygiene and domestic health, especially as they affected women's lives.

Her enthusiasm for light, clean, airy environments comes through in her very first letter, written from Rotterdam, in the Netherlands. "All the streets are paved with broad stones," she wrote, "and before many of the meanest artificers doors are placed seats of various coloured marbles, so neatly kept, that, I assure you, I walked almost all over the town yesterday, *incognito*, in my slippers without receiving one spot of dirt; and you may see the Dutch maids washing the pavement of the street, with more application than ours do our bed-chambers." While in The Hague, she noted, "Nothing can be more agreeable than travelling in Holland. The whole country appears a large garden; the roads are well paved, shaded on each side with rows of trees." She was much less pleased with Vienna, for though there were certainly many magnificent sights, the city itself was dark and crowded. "As the town is too little for the number of the people that desire to live in it," she complained, "the builders seem to have projected to repair that misfortune, by clapping one town on the top of another, most of the houses being of five, and some of them six stories . . . The streets being so narrow, the rooms are extremely dark; and, what is an inconveniency much more intolerable . . . there is no house has so few as five or six families in it."

Yet what Vienna lacked in space and light, it made up for by its treatment of older women. Lady Mary had a keen sense of the respect owed to women and was all too aware that it was often lacking in her own country. On hearing from a correspondent that a friend, owing to her age, had been badly treated at a gathering in London, she wrote, "I pity her much more, since I know, that they are only owing to the barbarous customs of our country." In Vienna, a woman, "till five and thirty, is only looked upon as a raw girl, and can possibly make no noise in the world, till about forty. I don't know what your ladyship may think of this matter; but 'tis a considerable comfort to me, to know there is upon earth such a paradise for old women."

As her travels continued throughout the fall and winter, another custom, neglected in England, caught her attention: the stove, valuable for warmth and for lengthening the growing season. At one of the formal dinners she attended, she was offered oranges and bananas and wondered how they could possibly be grown in Austria. "Upon inquiry," she wrote, "I learnt that they have brought their stoves to such perfection, they lengthen their summer as long as they please, giving to every plant the degree of heat it would receive from the sun in its native soil. The effect is very near the same; I am surprised we do not practise [*sic*] in England so useful an invention. This reflection leads me to consider our obstinacy in shaking with cold, five months in the year rather than make use of stoves, which are certainly one of the greatest conveniencies [*sic*] of life."

From her ongoing interest in domestic health and technological improvements, it isLR no wonder that Turkish inoculation caught her attention. You can read her complete letters online at Project Gutenberg, http://www.gutenberg.org/ebooks/author/7433.

After she returned to London, her advocacy was triggered by a smallpox epidemic that broke out in 1722. Only Lady Mary's son had been inoculated in Turkey; her daughter was still at risk. She therefore decided to inoculate her daughter, and the operation was performed with great success. Physicians who visited her found "Miss Wortley playing about the Room, cheerful and well," with a few slight marks of smallpox. Those soon healed, and the child recovered completely. The visiting physicians were impressed, and they began to incorporate inoculation into their own practices.

As the epidemic raged, one of Lady Mary's most prominent friends, Caroline, Princess of Wales, also became interested in the technique for her own children. As the wife of the heir to the British throne, she carried out her own experiment: she requested that six condemned criminals be allowed to volunteer to be inoculated, with the promise of full pardon if they survived. From a modern standpoint, this was not a very ethical or scientific experiment, but in contemporary terms, it worked beautifully: five of the six had slight cases of smallpox, which then healed, while the sixth, who had had smallpox before, had no effect from the inoculation. All six were pardoned. Princess Caroline then extended the experiment to poor children, six orphans and five babies born in a public hospital. Though again, unethical in modern terms, this experiment, too, was successful according to 1700s standards, in that all 11 children survived unscathed. Finally, after a year of these clinical trials, the two royal princesses, Amelia and Caroline, were successfully inoculated. Having received the royal seal of approval, smallpox inoculation became fashionable practice among British elites.

Lady Mary's letter was not published until after her death, but it is likely that it circulated in manuscript. Though, as she said, she was "patriot enough to bring this useful invention into fashion in England," she had to pay attention to what was considered appropriate behavior for a lady of rank and fortune. When a medical opponent to inoculation criticized the "ignorant women" who supported it, she wrote a rebuttal and published it in a London newspaper. She did so, however, under an assumed persona, an anonymous "Turkey merchant" providing "A Plain Account of the Inoculating of the Small Pox." In it, she repeated and sharpened her criticism of physicians who make money from other people's suffering, opposing inoculation in order to "receive two guineas a day as before, of the wretches that send for them" when sick with smallpox.

Lady Mary's 1717 letter seems like a simple description, but it is actually a masterful piece of persuasive writing. The "old women" who perform the technique are presented as careful, skilled medical technicians; the operation is presented as hardly more than a pinprick; the young patients are barely affected by subsequent disease, and all make a perfect recovery. The Turkish manner of performing the operation is contrasted with a harsher Grecian system and compared to the pleasant French pastime of "taking the waters," that is, going to a spa. Lady Mary presents herself as a loving mother protecting her son from harm, in sharp distinction to money-grubbing physicians for whom the distemper is "beneficial." This collection of rhetorical strategies proved so useful that we will encounter them frequently in documents throughout this book.

FURTHER READING

Glynn, Ian and Jenifer Glynn. (2004). *The Life and Death of Smallpox*. New York: Cambridge University Press.

Grundy, Isobel. (2001). *Lady Mary Wortley Montagu, Comet of the Enlightenment*. Oxford, England: Oxford University Press.

Guerrini, Anita. (2003). *Experimenting with Humans and Animals: From Galen to Animal Rights*. Baltimore, MD: The Johns Hopkins University Press.

Halsband, Robert. (1953). "New Light on Lady Mary Wortley Montagu's Contribution to Inoculation." *Journal of the History of Medicine and Allied Sciences* 8: 390–405.

Montagu, Lady Mary Wortley. (1722). "Plain Account of the Inoculating of the Small Pox by a Turkey Merchant." *Oxford Scholarly Editions Online*. http://www.oxford scholarlyeditions.com/view/10.1093/actrade/9780198124443.book.1/actrade-978019812 4443-div1-8.

A SCIENTIST'S VIEW OF VACCINATION

- **Document:** Edward Jenner, first published in *An Inquiry into the Causes and Effects of the Variolae Vaccinae, or Cowpox*
- **Date:** 1798
- **Where:** London, United Kingdom
- **Significance:** Jenner's *Inquiry* is considered the foundation of modern vaccination practice as well as a classic of scientific investigation. Written about 80 years after Lady Mary's letter, it proposed substituting inoculation with a common, minor skin disease—cowpox—as a preventative for the deadly smallpox. Cowpox was such an ordinary disease that it did not have a formal Latin name, so Jenner invented one. He took the Latin name for smallpox, *variola*—which merely means "pox"—and added the Latin form for "cows," *vaccinae*. The resulting term, *variolae vaccinae*, or "pox of cows," ultimately gave rise to vaccination as a general term for a technique that could be used to prevent a wide range of diseases.

DOCUMENT

What renders the cow-pox virus so extremely singular is that the person who has been thus affected is forever after secure from the infection of the small-pox; neither exposure to [smallpox], nor the insertion of the matter into the skin, producing this distemper.

In support of so extraordinary a fact, I shall lay before my reader a great number of instances.

Mrs. H——, a respectable gentlewoman of this town, had the cow-pox when very young. She received the infection in rather an uncommon manner: it was given by means of her handling some of the same utensils which were in use among the servants of the family, who had the disease from milking infected cows. Her hands had many of the cow-pox sores upon them, and they were communicated to her nose, which became inflamed and very much swollen. Soon after this event Mrs. H—— was exposed to the contagion of the smallpox, where it was scarcely possible for her to have escaped, had she been susceptible of it, as she regularly attended a relative who had the disease in so violent a degree that it proved fatal to him.

In the year 1778 the smallpox prevailed very much at Berkeley, and Mrs. H——, not feeling perfectly satisfied respecting her safety (no indisposition having followed her exposure to the smallpox), I inoculated her with active [smallpox] matter. The same appearance followed as in the preceding cases—an efflorescence on the arm without any effect on the constitution.

... In the month of May, 1796, the cow-pox broke out at Mr. Baker's, a farmer who lives near this place. [One of the dairymaids], Sarah Wynne, who never had the smallpox ... caught the complaint from the cows, and was affected with the symptoms ... in so violent a degree that she was confined to her bed, and rendered incapable for several days of pursuing her ordinary vocations in the farm. [On] March 28th, 1797, I inoculated this girl and carefully rubbed the [smallpox] matter into two slight incisions made upon the left arm. A little inflammation appeared in the usual manner around the parts where the matter was inserted, but so early as the fifth day it vanished entirely without producing any effect on the system.

Source: Jenner, Edward. (1909). "An Inquiry into the Causes and Effects of the Variolae Vaccinae, or Cowpox. 1798." *The Three Original Publications on Vaccination against Smallpox. The Harvard Classics, 1909–1914.* New York: P.F. Collier and Son Company.

ANALYSIS

Edward Jenner (1749–1823) is best known as a scientist, but, in this extract, he, like Lady Mary, was writing to persuade a general audience. By the 1790s, both the value of the usual form of smallpox inoculation and its dangers were well known. Inoculation could certainly save lives, as it did with Princess Caroline's experimental subjects, the convicted criminals and London orphans. But its effects were not predictable, and a small percentage of those inoculated developed the virulent form of the disease and suffered disfigurement or death. Not only that, even a mild case of smallpox was contagious. Children who formed part of an inoculation party had to be kept isolated so that they did not pass the disease on to others. This was only possible in wealthy households, and smallpox inoculation remained a medical practice most favored by elites.

Jenner's use of cowpox, rather than smallpox, transformed the practice. Cowpox was a skin disease,

DID YOU KNOW?

Who Really Invented Cowpox Vaccination?

In 1802, when Parliament awarded Edward Jenner £10,000 for the discovery of the process of cowpox inoculation, his status as the inventor of the process seemed assured. But some of his contemporaries and historians have claimed that two other innovators have priority, Benjamin Jesty (1736–1816) and John Fewster (1738–1824).

Jesty was a dairy farmer, who, like many others, was aware of the commonplace assumption that dairymaids who had had cowpox could not get smallpox. Two of his dairymaids, Anne Notley and Mary Reade, had nursed their relatives with smallpox without being infected. In 1774, when smallpox broke out in his own neighborhood, he took some cowpox from a neighbor's cow on the head of a needle and then pricked his wife and two sons on the arm. The sons recovered with no problems, but his wife's arm became infected, and Jesty called the local doctor. "You have done a bold thing," the doctor is reported as saying, "but I will get you through if I can." Jesty's wife recovered, but, according to his contemporaries, the neighborhood disapproved so strongly of his "bold thing" that the family moved away.

John Fewster was a surgeon-apothecary who practiced inoculation—immunization with the live smallpox virus—in a town about 7 miles away from Jenner's own practice. The two men were professional friends, and they could have discussed the nature of smallpox and its connection to cowpox. By the 1760s, Fewster had noted that his patients who had had cowpox seemed to be immune to smallpox. In 1765, he presented a paper to the London Medical Society entitled "Cowpox and Its Ability to Prevent Smallpox," but he never followed up with any experiments or with any additional scientific papers.

Though by modern standards, either Jesty or Fewster could claim priority over Jenner, neither man was interested in doing so at the time. Fewster consistently refused any credit for inventing vaccination. Jesty's contribution was only brought to light after Jenner published his own experiments. A clergyman in his community, interested in encouraging the practice of vaccination, brought his 1774 experiment to the attention of a London physician, George Pearson. Pearson was one of Jenner's professional rivals, and when he heard what Jesty had done, he realized the opportunity this could provide to undercut Jenner's achievements. He invited Jesty and his son to London for a special ceremony honoring him as the true founder of vaccination and presented him with gold-mounted lancets, a testimonial scroll, and 15 guineas—a very substantial sum of money for the time. Jesty and his family seemed to have been pleased with the recognition, and he subsequently returned to his peaceful life as a dairy farmer. When he died in 1818, his wife wrote his epitaph: "He was born at Yetminster in this County, and was an upright and honest Man: particularly noted for having been the first Person (known) that introduced the Cowpox by Inoculation, and who from his great strength of mind made the Experiment from the (Cow) on his Wife and two Sons in the year of 1774." Her scrupulous precision in describing her husband's accomplishments is a worthy match for Jenner's careful scientific depiction of a similar subject.

Source: Williams, Gareth. (2011). "Who Invented Vaccination?" *Malta Medical Journal* 23: 29–32.

itchy and uncomfortable, perhaps, but never fatal. Even more important, while smallpox was spread from person to person through simple contact, cowpox could only be spread by actual physical contact with the cowpox matter. Dairymaids got it through direct contact of their bare hands with cows, and, in unusual cases, as with Mrs. H in Jenner's case history, it could be spread through secondary contact with dairymaids. But outbreaks of cowpox were purely local, and afflicted cows and people recovered rapidly.

Throughout this section, Jenner contrasts the simple, ordinary disease, common to English farms, with the dangerous intruder, smallpox. His patients are gentlewomen and dairymaids, who have been exposed to cowpox while going about their daily lives. They are "affected by symptoms," certainly; sometimes, even violently so. But when epidemics of smallpox rage, those symptoms turn out to be their best defense against a disease that so often "proved fatal." So strong, in Jenner's account, is the protective force field created by cowpox that even after direct injection of smallpox virus, the disease "vanished entirely without producing any effect on the system."

Within 10 years, Jenner's cowpox "vaccine" had been widely adopted by medical practitioners around the world.

FURTHER READING

Davies, Hugh. (2007). "Ethical Reflections on Edward Jenner's Experimental Treatment." *Journal of Medical Ethics* 33: 174–176.

Dr. Jenner's House and Garden. http://www.jennermuseum.com/.

History of Vaccines. An Educational Resource by the College of Physicians of Philadelphia. http://www.historyofvaccines.org/.

Jenner, Edward. (1983). *Letters of Edward Jenner, and Other Documents Concerning the Early History of Vaccination.* Edited by Genevieve Miller. Baltimore, MD: Johns Hopkins University Press.

"Jenner, Edward." *Science Museum Brought to Life.* http://www.sciencemuseum.org.uk/broughttolife/people/edwardjenner.aspx.

VACCINATION AND THE PUBLIC HEALTH

- **Document:** *Memorial of Joseph G. Nancrede, Vaccine Physician, Philadelphia*, presented to Congress
- **Date:** January 14, 1828
- **Where:** House of Representatives, 20th Congress, Washington, DC
- **Significance:** Though Nancrede's call for a national vaccination law was not successful, his appeal to Congress raised many of the points that public health advocates would reprise over the next two centuries. In early 19th-century America, well-to-do individuals and families readily adopted the new vaccination techniques. Having seen firsthand the ravages of smallpox, they readily chose to protect themselves and their loved ones, especially when an outbreak threatened. But many physicians believed it made little sense to wait for the death toll to rise before providing the vaccine. Instead, they turned to public authorities, from city, state, and federal governments, to make the case for the value of vaccination as a public health measure.

DOCUMENT

To the Senate and House of Representatives of the United States in Congress assembles:

The memorial of the subscriber, Vaccine Physician, under an ordinance of the Select and Common Councils of the City of Philadelphia,

Respectfully representeth:

That, anxious to promote the extermination of the small-pox, by diffusing the blessings of vaccination to the People of the United States, and, more especially, to secure its advantage to those citizens who inhabit our remote and newly settled frontiers; and, believing that he possesses ample means to facilitate the extension of vaccination, he humbly requests leave to call the attention of Congress to this important subject.

On the acknowledged utility of vaccination, it is deemed useless here to comment. Every member of this House is aware of the blessings it imparts, and its influence on the population of a young and growing nation. At a moment when our country is ravaged by small-pox, no subject is better calculated to attract the attention of a wise Legislature, than the encouragement of a remedy which saves from the ravages of a loathsome and fatal disease, the fairest portion of the human family.

In 1813, a vaccine agency was established by Congress, and located in Baltimore; but, in consequence of an error having unfortunately occurred in that institution, whereby the small-pox, instead of cow-pock, was communicated to a number of individuals in Tarboro, North Carolina, that agency was, in 1822, annulled by a vote of this House.

It is not the intention of your memorialist to point out to Congress any of its duties; but, he will be permitted to suggest, that the protection, or rather the legislative sanction, of Congress, in favor of vaccination, will be hailed, by the People of the United States, as one of the most useful measures your body can adopt during its present session. As a further incentive, it may not be amiss to inquire, how far it comports with the dignity of our free Government, to be anticipated in the career of public usefulness, by the monarchical Governments of Germany, Prussia, Russia, Sweden, Denmark, France, Italy, and Spain; in all which countries, vaccination is enforced by the strong hand of power.

Your memorialist is aware, that it is contrary to the spirit of our Constitution to employ force in favor of vaccination; and, consequently, that it is by encouraging the diffusion of the [cowpox] virus, that Congress can most effectually extend the remedy, and exterminate the small-pox.

As a motive for locating, for the present, a Vaccine Institution here, your memorialist will not lay before your honorable body, the reasons which render Philadelphia a suitable situation. Independent of its central situation, and large population, its literary and charitable institutions, which, on a fair comparison, will give it a due share of importance, and, without wishing to claim precedence over other cities of the Union, in point of rank, your subscriber will state that the lofty pre-eminence of the Medical School, decidedly the first in reputation, as in the number of its pupils, the constant influx of medical practitioners from every section of our country, towards this their alma mater, and the immense intercourse thus established between medical men, will, it is believed, be powerful reasons for locating here a National Vaccine Institution. But the strongest claim which this city possesses, perhaps, on the justice of Congress, in this respect, is the fact that it is the only city in the Union, it is believed, where vaccination is performed under a uniform, legal system. It is the duty of the Vaccine Physician, to vaccinate, at all seasons, all indigent persons belonging to the city, who may require it. He is, by law, obliged, therefore, to be in constant readiness, and vaccinates, annually, about one thousand persons. With a population such as this, it will always be an easy matter to obtain a supply of virus for all exigencies.

Possessed of means peculiar to his situation as Vaccine Physician, which he confidently believes are amply sufficient for the purposes mentioned in this memorial, and desirous of extending his sphere of usefulness, your memorialist respectfully requests of the wisdom of Congress, the enactment of such a law, in relation to vaccination, as the importance of the subject may require.

Source: Nancrede, Joseph. (1828). *Memorial of Joseph G. Nancrede, Vaccine Physician, Philadelphia.* Washington, DC: Gales and Seaton.

ANALYSIS

Dr. Joseph Nancrede's *Memorial* was presented to Congress in 1828 at the height of a smallpox epidemic that attacked major American port cities. As Nancrede noted, Congress had previously enacted the Vaccine Act of 1813, which empowered the president to appoint a National Vaccine Agent to "preserve supplies of genuine vaccine matter and furnish the same to any citizen of the United States, whenever it might be applied for." Dr. James Smith, the first agent, faced challenges that many later reformers would recognize: he had a federal position but no funding, and he had to recruit—and pay for—his own medical staff. State governments challenged the legality of the new position, claiming the federal government had no constitutional authority over state public health practices. In 1822, a smallpox epidemic broke out in Tarboro, North Carolina, because Smith accidentally sent smallpox matter, instead of cowpox, to the physician acting there on the agency's behalf. Ten people died, and Smith's critics in Congress, led by the representative from North Carolina, successfully argued for his dismissal and the repeal of the 1813 act. Congress refused to consider any other piece of vaccination legislation for the rest of the 19th century.

Nancrede clearly hoped to use the 1828 outbreak to get Congress to reconsider. His reference to "the blessings of vaccination" invokes the famous Preamble to the U.S. Constitution: "We the People of the United States, in Order to form a more perfect Union, establish Justice, insure domestic Tranquility, provide for the common defence, promote the general Welfare, and secure the Blessings of Liberty to ourselves and our Posterity, do ordain and establish this Constitution for the United States of America." In effect, Nancrede was arguing that it was perfectly constitutional for Congress to appoint a National Vaccine Agent, no matter what state governments might say. His focus on the "population of a young and growing nation" and on "the fairest portion of the human family" also refers to the Preamble's regard, not only for "ourselves" but also "our Posterity," that is, our children. In 1828, the constitution was less than 50 years old; Nancrede could certainly expect his audience to recognize his rhetoric.

He might also expect his audience to be moved by his claim that Congress, the "free Government" of the United States, was falling behind the despotic monarchies of Europe. The United States had fought against Great Britain in the War of 1812 and against the Barbary pirates in northern Africa between 1803 and 1815. Patriotism, then as now, was often a successful strategy when addressing Congress. But Nancrede was careful to note that he was not advocating compulsory vaccination. Instead, he argued for a new vaccination agency that would be better located, with a larger population and better-educated medical staff than the old one.

Yet, however convincing Nancrede's argument was to its writer, it is easy to see why his memorial was unsuccessful. The Tarboro scandal, six years ago, had led to contentious debate inside and outside of Congress: why would any politician want to reopen the controversy? And Nancrede's advocacy for Philadelphia as the obvious place to put a national vaccine center—with Dr. Nancrede himself as the new national director —must have seemed self-serving. Physicians from New York or Boston could well have made the same arguments. If Philadelphia wanted to become the vaccination center for the "young and growing nation," Congress might have said, let Philadelphia pay for it.

Within 25 years, the Civil War broke out, highlighting even more pointedly than the Vaccine Act the conflict between states' rights and the federal government. Philadelphia became one of the major vaccination centers for northern troops, and

Nancrede's successors did, in fact, do much to secure the "blessings of vaccination" to posterity.

FURTHER READING

America's Second Revolution. Civil War Philadelphia and Its Countryside. http://www. civilwarphilly.net/.

DeLancey, Dayle. (2010). "Vaccinating Freedom: Smallpox Prevention and the Discourses of African American Citizenship in Antebellum Philadelphia." *Journal of African American History* 95: 296–321.

Finger, Simon. (2010). "An Indissoluble Union: How the American War for Independence Transformed Philadelphia's Medical Community and Created a Public Health Establishment."*Pennsylvania History* 77: 37–72.

Newton, David. (2013). *Vaccination Controversies.* Santa Barbara, CA: ABC-CLIO.

Singla, Rohit. (1998). "Missed Opportunities. The Vaccine Act of 1813." http://dash .harvard.edu/bitstream/handle/1/10015266/rsingla.html?sequence=2.

A CENTURY OF VACCINATION PROGRESS

- **Document:** William Osler, *A Lay Sermon*, presented to the University of Edinburgh in conjunction with the Edinburgh meeting of the National Association for the Prevention of Tuberculosis
- **Date:** 1910
- **Where:** Edinburgh, United Kingdom
- **Significance:** By the beginning of the 20th century, there was little doubt that vaccination had worked wonders as a public health measure in industrialized countries like Great Britain and the United States. It worked so well, in fact, that even individuals who were not vaccinated might be protected by those who were. This concept, known as herd immunity, carried its own challenge: the less likely it was that any individual or family would contract a disease, the harder it was to convince that individual or family to be vaccinated. In this document, eminent physician Dr. William Osler speaks to that challenge.

DOCUMENT

Man's redemption of man is nowhere so well known as in the abolition and prevention of the group of diseases which we speak of as the fevers, or the acute infections. This is the glory of the science of medicine, and nowhere in the world have its lessons been so thoroughly carried out as in this country. It is too old a story to retell in detail, but I may remind you that in this city within fifty years there has been an annual saving of from four to five thousand lives, by measures which have directly prevented and limited the spread of infectious diseases. The man is still alive, Sir Henry Little-John, who made the first sanitary survey of the city. When one reads the account of the condition of the densely crowded districts on the south side of the High Street, one is not surprised that the rate of mortality was 40 and over per thousand. That you now enjoy one of the lowest death rates in Europe—15.3 per thousand for last year—is due to the thoroughness with which measures of recognized efficiency have been carried out. When we learn that last year there were no deaths from smallpox, not one from typhus, and only 21 from fevers of the zymotic group, it is scarcely credible that all this has been brought about within the memory of living men. It is not too much to say that the abolition of small-pox, typhus and typhoid fevers have changed the character of the medical practice in our hospitals. In this country typhoid fever is in its last ditch, and though a more subtle and difficult enemy to conquer than typhus, we may confidently hope that before long it will be as rare.

Here I would like to say a word or two upon one of the most terrible of all acute infections, the one of which we first learned the control through the work of Jenner.

A great deal of literature has been distributed, casting discredit upon the value of vaccination in the prevention of small-pox. I do not see how any one who has gone through epidemics as I have, or who is familiar with the history of the subject, and who has any capacity left for clear judgment, can doubt its value. Some months ago I was twitted by the Editor of the Journal of the Anti-Vaccination League for maintaining a curious silence on the subject. I would like to issue a Mount Carmel-like challenge to any ten unvaccinated priests of Baal. I will take ten selected vaccinated persons, and help in the next severe epidemic, with ten selected unvaccinated persons (if available!). I should choose three members of Parliament, three anti-vaccination doctors, if they could be found, and four anti-vaccination propagandists. And I will make this promise—neither to jeer nor to jibe when they catch the disease, but to look after them as brothers; and for the three or four who are certain to die I will try to arrange the funerals with all the pomp and ceremony of an anti-vaccination demonstration.

Source: Osler, William. (1913). *Man's Redemption of Man A Lay Sermon.* London: Constable and Co, Ltd.

ANALYSIS

Sir William Osler, MD (1849–1919), was one of the most prominent physicians of his time. He had been a founding member of the Johns Hopkins Medical School, and, in 1910, when he gave this address, he was professor of medicine at Oxford University. He was a noted medical reformer, responsible for introducing hands-on clinical residency as a key component of medical education.

Osler's audience, consisting of University of Edinburgh's medical students and members of the National Association for the Prevention of Tuberculosis, would have agreed with him that "man's redemption of man" was most clearly shown through modern medicine. The germ theory of disease, modern sanitation, and improved nutrition had extended life expectancy and protected children and adults against many of the deadliest diseases in human history. As Osler notes, it hardly seemed possible that "all this had been carried out within the memory of living men." Many of those in the audience would have lived to see the extension of this grand promise to vaccines against tuberculosis and polio, the development of antibiotics, and further increase in life expectancy.

But that rapid change brought with it a new challenge. Vaccination, once hailed as a medical triumph, seemed much less necessary in a world where smallpox, typhus, and yellow fever were exotic, rare diseases, and not ever-present threats. As fear of infectious disease decreased, physicians found it harder to convince their patients to be vaccinated, and, as the numbers of vaccinations decreased, so did the protection of herd immunity. For physicians of Osler's generation, who had spent their lives and professional careers fighting against the deadliest diseases, it was inconceivable that "anyone with the capacity for clear judgment" could oppose vaccination. The fewer the vaccinations, the greater the risk that deadly epidemics could recur.

Osler's pointed challenge to the anti-vaccinators that they put their principles into practice and themselves at risk is a playful rhetorical strategy to make a grim point. Anti-vaccine advocates, like the editors of the journal of the Anti-Vaccination League, could afford to maintain their opinions because of the principle of herd immunity. In effect, they were protected by their medical opponents like Osler, who promoted vaccination. If the editor of the journal ever succeeded in convincing everyone to join his Anti-Vaccination League, herd immunity would vanish and the epidemics would return. The league would find themselves facing a much more deadly opponent: the killer diseases that ravaged human society.

FURTHER READING

Bliss, Michael. (1999). *William Osler. A Life in Medicine*. New York: Oxford University Press.

Brunton, Deborah. (2008). *The Politics of Vaccination: Practice and Policy in England, Wales, Ireland, and Scotland, 1800–1874*. Rochester, NY: University of Rochester Press.

Bynum, William. (1994). *Science and the Practice of Medicine in the Nineteenth Century*. New York: Cambridge University Press.

Colgrove, James. (2005). " 'Science in a Democracy': The Contested Status of Vaccination in the Progressive Era and the 1920s." *Isis* 96: 167–191.

"History of Anti-Vaccination Movements." *History of Vaccines. An Educational Resource by the College of Physicians of Philadelphia*. http://www.historyofvaccines.org/content/articles/history-anti-vaccination-movements.

A MICROSCOPIC VIEW OF IMMUNITY

- **Document:** Eula Biss, *On Immunity: An Inoculation*
- **Date:** 2014
- **Where:** Chicago, IL
- **Significance:** In this section, American writer Eula Biss describes the science of the immune system.

DOCUMENT

[The immune system] begins at the skin, a barrier capable of synthesizing bio-chemical that inhibit the growth of certain bacteria and containing, in its deeper layers, cells that can induce inflammation and ingest pathogens. Then there are the membranes of the digestive, respiratory, and urogenital systems with their pathogen-ensnaring mucous and their pathogen-expelling cilia and their high concentration of cells equipped to produce the antibodies responsible for lasting immunity. Beyond those barriers, the circulatory system transports pathogens in the blood to the spleen, where the blood is filtered and antibodies are generated, and the lymphatic system flushes pathogens from body tissues to the lymph nodes, where the same process ensues—pathogens are surrounded by an assortment of cells that ingest them, eliminate them, and remember them for a more efficient response in the future.

Deep in the body, the bone marrow and the thymus generate a dizzying array of cells specialized for immunity. These include cells that can destroy infected cells, cells that swallow pathogens and then display pieces of them for other cells to see, cells that monitor other cells for signs of cancer or infection, cells that make antibodies, and cells that carry antibodies. All of these cells, falling into an intricate arrangement of types and subtypes, interact in a series of baroque dances, their communication depending in part on the action of free-floating molecules. Chemical signals travel through the blood from sites of injury or infection, activated cells release substances to trigger inflammation, and helpful molecules poke holes in the membranes of microbes to deflate them.

Infants have all the components of this system at birth. There are certain things the infant immune system does not do well—it has trouble penetrating the sticky coating of the Hib bacteria, for example. But the immune system of a full-term infant is not incomplete or undeveloped. It is what immunologists call "naive." It has not yet had the opportunity to produce antibodies in response to infection. Infants are born with some antibodies from their mothers already circulating in their systems, and breast milk supplies them with more antibodies, but this "passive immunity" fades as an infant grows, no matter now long it is breast-fed. A vaccine tutors the infant immune system, making it capable of remembering pathogens it has not yet seen. With or without vaccination, the first years of a child's life are a time of rapid education on immunity—all the runny noses and fevers of those years are the symptoms of a system learning the microbial lexicon.

Source: Biss, Eula. (2014). *On Immunity: An Inoculation.* Minneapolis, MN: Graywolf Press, 57–59. Copyright © 2013 by Eula Biss. Reprinted with the permission of The Permissions Company, Inc., on behalf of Graywolf Press, www .graywolfpress.org.

ANALYSIS

As Eula Biss explains in her best-selling book, *On Immunity*, she only started to pay attention to vaccination when she became a mother. Her first step—like every other mother of her age—was to search the Internet for information. The bewildering array of contradictory information first puzzled and then frightened her, and she decided to research her own pathway through the complex history of people, vaccines, and vaccination controversies.

As she learned when she attended lectures by a professor of immunology, "our bodies and the viruses were two competing intelligences locked in a mortal game of chess" (Biss, 60). The rest of *Vaccination and Its Critics* will trace the efforts people have made to make sure they stayed on the winning side.

FURTHER READING

"How Vaccines Work." *The History of Vaccines. An Educational Resource by the College of Physicians of Philadelphia.* http://www.historyofvaccines.org/content/how-vaccines -work.

"The Human Immune System and Infectious Disease." *The History of Vaccines. An Educational Resource by the College of Physicians of Philadelphia.* http://www .historyofvaccines.org/content/articles/human-immune-system-and-infectious-disease.

Martin, Emily. (1994). *Flexible Bodies. Tracking Immunity in American Culture from the Days of Polio to the Age of AIDS.* Boston, MA: Beacon Press.

Oldstone, Michael. (1998). *Viruses, Plagues, & History.* New York: Oxford University Press.

Sompayrac, Lauren. (2015). *How the Immune System Works.* New York: Wiley.

2

NATURE'S WAY AND THE BEGINNING OF IMMUNIZATION (1500s–1790s)

SMALLPOX AS CHILDHOOD DISEASE

- **Document:** Abu Bakr Muhammad Ibn Zakariya al-Razi, known as Rhazes, *A Treatise on the Smallpox and Measles*
- **Date:** ca. 900 CE
- **Where:** Baghdad, Persia
- **Significance:** al-Razi was the first to provide a clinical examination of smallpox and measles and to differentiate between them. He was also the first to note that survivors of smallpox develop immunity to the disease.

DOCUMENT

AUTHOR'S PREFACE

In the name of GOD, the Compassionate, the Merciful.

It happened on a certain night at a meeting in the house of a nobleman, of great goodness and excellence, and very anxious for the explanation and facilitating of useful sciences for the good of mankind, that, mention having been made of the Small-Pox, I then spoke what came into my mind on that subject. Whereupon our host (may GOD favour men by prolonging the remainder of his life) wished me to compose a suitable, solid, and complete discourse on this disease, because there has not appeared up to this present time either among the ancients or the moderns an accurate and satisfactory account of it. And therefore I composed this discourse, hoping to receive my reward from the Almighty and Glorious GOD, and awaiting His good pleasure.

On the symptoms which indicate the approaching eruption of the Small-Pox and Measles

The eruption of the Small-Pox is preceded by a continued fever, pain in the back, itching in the nose, and terrors in sleep. These are the more peculiar symptoms of its approach, especially a pain in the back, with fever; then also a pricking which the patient feels all over his body; a fullness of the face, which at times goes and comes; an inflamed colour, and vehement redness in both the cheeks; a redness of both the eyes; a heaviness of the whole body; great uneasiness, the symptoms of which are stretching and yawning; a pain in the throat and chest, with a slight difficulty in breathing, and cough; a dryness of the mouth, thick spittle, and hoarseness of the voice; pain and heaviness of the head; inquietude, distress of mind, nausea, and anxiety; (with this difference, that the inquietude, nausea, and anxiety are more frequent in the Measles than in the Small-Pox; while, on the other hand, the pain in the back is more peculiar to the Small-Pox than to the Measles;) heat of the whole body, an inflamed colour, and shining redness, and especially an intense redness of the gums.

When, therefore, you see these symptoms, or some of the worst of them, (such as the pain of the back, and the terrors in sleep, with the continued fever,) then you may be assured that the eruption of one or other of these diseases in the patient is nigh at hand . . .

Of the fatal and the mild species of Small-Pox and Measles

The Small-Pox and Measles are of the number of acute and hot diseases, and therefore they have many things in common with them, with respect to the symptoms which indicate the disease to be mild or fatal. Now the chief prognostic signs in those who recover are, a freedom of respiration, soundness of mind, appetite for food, lightness of motion, a good state of the pulse, the patient's confident opinion respecting the event of his own illness, a convenient posture in bed, and but little tossing about and inquietude of body. Hence a judgment may be formed of the bad signs . . .

The circumstances which peculiarly regard the Small-Pox and Measles are the following. When the pustules of the Small-Pox are white, large, distinct, few in number, and easy in coming out, and the fever is without much violence and heat, or distress and anxiety; and when the patient's heat and distress and anxiety diminish upon the very first eruption, and entirely cease after the eruption is completed; that sort is the most curable and least dangerous. To these the next in goodness are those that are white and large, though they may be very numerous and close together, if the eruption has been easy, and has relieved the patient from his anxiety and heat, as we have already mentioned.

But when the appearance of the pustules is brought about with difficulty, and the patient is not relieved upon their eruption, they are a bad sort; although there is not so much reason to be afraid if the patient's condition be unfavorable during their appearance, as if it continues so afterwards. But there is a bad and fatal sort of the white and large pustules, viz. those which become confluent and spread, so that many of them unite and occupy large spaces of the body, or become like broad circles, and in colour resemble fat.

As to those white pustules which are very small, close to each other, hard, warty, and containing no

DID YOU KNOW?

Global Medical Knowledge

We tend to think of the global expansion of medical knowledge as a characteristic of the modern world, but we can trace it back to the ancient and medieval periods as well. The famous English poet Geoffrey Chaucer (1340–1400) provided a roll call of prominent physicians from around the world, including al-Razi, in his poem *The Canterbury Tales*. The poem tells the story of a set of pilgrims going to Canterbury. To pass the time, they each tell a story, which Chaucer cleverly sets up to be fascinating in its own right while providing insight into the character of each pilgrim. One of the characters is a physician, "a Doctor of Medicine":

In all the world there was none like him
    To speak of medicine and surgery.

He was in fact so learned that he had read all the great physicians of the past and present, in Europe and beyond:

Well he knew the old Esculapius,
    And Deiscorides, and also Rufus,
    Old Hippocrates, Hali, and Galen,
    Serapion, Rhazes, and Avicen,
    Averroes, Gilbertus, and Constantine,
    Bernard and Gatisden, and John Damascene.

Aesculapius was the Greek god of medicine, but the rest of the names belonged to real historical figures. Hippocrates (c. 360—c. 470 BCE), Dioscorides (c. 40–90 CE), Rufus of Ephesus (fl. 1st century CE), and Galen (129–c. 216 CE) were known to Chaucer as great physicians of the Greek and Roman era. 'Ali ibn al-'Abbas al-Majusi, known in the West as Haly Abbas, (died c. 982), Serapion the Younger (no known dates), Abū Alī al-usayn ibn Abd Allāh ibn Al-Hasan ibn Ali ibn Sīnā (Avicenna, c. 980–1037), and Abū l-Walīd Muammad Ibn Aḥmad Ibn Rušd (Averroes, 1126–1198) were famous physicians from the Arabic world. Early Christianity is represented by St. John Damascene (c. 675–749), a father of the Eastern Orthodox Church, and Constantine the African (died before 1098), who compiled wide-ranging medical textbooks, still in use in Chaucer's day. Chaucer brought his catalog of global medical authorities back to contemporary Europe with his last set of names. Gilbert of England (c. 1180–1250) wrote an influential compendium of medicine, while Bernard de Gordon (fl. 1270–1330) and John of Gaddesden (c. 1280–1361) were prominent physicians and scholars.

Thus, while highlighting his physician's—and his own—medical erudition, Chaucer was also making a claim for the universality of medical knowledge.

You can read the Physician's introduction in Chaucer's Prologue, in its 14th-century and modern form, online here: http://www.librarius.com/canttran/genpro/genpro413-446.htm.

Source: Pūyān, Nāsir. (2014). "Al-Razi (Rhazes), an Independent Medical Thinker Who Gave the First Description of Measles and Smallpox and Distinguished between Them." *Journal of Microbiology Research* 4: 183–186.

fluid, they are of a bad kind, and their badness is in proportion to the degree of difficulty in their ripening. And if the patient be not relieved upon their eruption, but his condition continues unfavorable after it is finished, it is a mortal sign.

And as to those which are of a greenish, or violet, or black colour, they are all of a bad and fatal kind; and when, besides, a swooning and palpitation of the heart come on, they are worse and still more fatal. And when the fever increases after the appearance of the pustules, it is a bad sign; but if it is lessened on their appearance, that is a good sign. Doubled pustules indicate an abundance of the matter of the disease, and if they are of the curable sort, they portend recovery, but if they are of the mortal kind, they portend death.

The safest kind of Measles is that where the redness is not very deep; but the pale or tawny coloured are bad; and the green and violet coloured are both mortal.

When either the Small-Pox or Measles sink in suddenly after they have begun to come out, and then the patient is seized with anxiety, and a swooning comes on, it is a sign of speedy death, unless they break out afresh ...

When the pustules begin to be confluent and to spread, and the anxiety is very great, and the abdomen is inflated, then death is near at hand.

When the smaller sort of pustules, which contain no fluid, break, and at the same time a delirium comes on, then the patient is near his end ...

When towards the end of the Small-Pox there is a great perturbation of the humours, and the patient is seized with a very violent pain in the leg, or hand, or any other limb, or the pustules turn to a green or black colour, and thereupon he becomes weaker than he was before, and the weakness still increases with the increase of the pain, or the limb is deeply coloured; these are signs of death.

But if, nevertheless, the patient's strength increases, he will recover, but the limb will mortify ...

Now, therefore, as we have gone over all the articles which were proposed concerning the mode of treating this disease, and of preservation from it, we will here break off the thread of our discourse; and to HIM Who hath given us understanding to accomplish the work be praise and glory without end, even as HE is most worthy and deserving thereof.

Source: al-Razi [Rhazes], Abu Bakr Muhammad Ibn Zakariya. (1848). *A Treatise on the Smallpox and Measles*, trans. William Greenhill. London: Sydenham Society.

ANALYSIS

Abu Bakr Muhammad Ibn Zakariya al-Razi (865?–925?) was a court physician and director of a large hospital in Baghdad, a major center of medieval Islamic science and medicine. The classics of Greek and Roman medicine, including that of Hippocrates and Galen, had been translated into Arabic and became the basis for medical theory and practice. Astute observers like al-Razi and Ibn Sina (ca. 980–1037) built on this legacy, augmenting the literature with contemporary clinical observations and their own discoveries. The works of Rhazes and Ibn Sina (known as Avicenna), as they became known in Latin-speaking countries, were incorporated into medical schools throughout Europe.

al-Razi's *Treatise* shows his careful attention to clinical observation. His focus is the appearance of the two diseases within the patient. In the early part of the *Treatise*, he describes the causes of smallpox, but what he means by that is the reason why smallpox is more likely to appear in one kind of patient rather than another: in children and young men, for example, rather than in old men. He asserts that it is because children and young men have hotter, wetter blood than old men, referring to medieval medical theories linked to characteristics of heat, cold, wet, and dry. Though those theories are not used today, al-Razi's observation introduced into the medical literature one of the most striking characteristics of smallpox and measles: young people are much susceptible than adults. The reason, as we now know, is that both convey immunity to those who have had them. The idea that these, and other diseases, were "childhood diseases," led ultimately to the scientific research behind the development of vaccines.

In the 9th century, there was not much al-Razi could do to prevent either disease. Instead, he concentrated on providing as much detailed description as possible, so the physicians would know what to do once the diseases had arrived. He began by identifying their onset, so physicians and patients could see the danger coming. He provided differential diagnosis so that they could understand which of the virulent diseases they were dealing with. Many of the chapters deal with treatment, some systemic—that is, affecting the entire body—and some local. Systemic treatment included bed rest and cooling drinks to reduce the fever; local treatment included rosewater for cleaning the eyes and ears when encrusted with pustules. And he provided indications for prognosis, showing under what circumstances it was reasonable for the patients and the physicians to hope for recovery and under what conditions, sadly, the disease would prove fatal.

Though al-Razi must have seen many patients dying of smallpox, he appears to have written his *Treatise* with every expectation that many would recover. His belief in the power of scientific medicine to cure disease, together with his careful clinical description, explains why his works were so often reprinted and translated throughout the 19th century.

FURTHER READING

Carmichael, Ann and Arthur Silverstein. (1987). "Smallpox in Europe before the Seventeenth Century: Virulent Killer or Benign Disease?" *Journal of the History of Medicine* 42: 147–168.

Clendening, Logan, ed. (1942). *Source Book of Medical History*. New York: Dover.

Harmaneh, Sami. (1974). "Ecology and Therapeutics in Medieval Arabic Medicine." *Sudhoffs Archiv* 58: 165–185.

Pormann, Peter and Emilie Savage-Smith. (2007). *Medieval Islamic Medicine*. Washington DC: Georgetown University Press.

Wallis, Faith. (2010). *Medieval Medicine: A Reader*. Toronto: University of Toronto Press.

MEASLES IN CHILDREN

- **Document:** Thomas Sydenham, "Of the Measles of 1670"
- **Date:** 1670
- **Where:** London, United Kingdom
- **Significance:** Thomas Sydenham was a prominent clinician who believed that diseases, like plants, had a set of characteristics that could allow them to be precisely identified and treated. His description of measles clearly differentiated it from other skin diseases and as clearly marked it as a disease of children. He notes that measles can lead to pneumonia, often a fatal disease in his day. The Centers for Disease Control (CDC) confirm that this is still a health hazard for children who are not vaccinated against measles.

DOCUMENT

In the beginning of January, 1670, the measles appeared as is usual, and increased daily till the approach of the vernal equinox, when it came to its height; after which it abated in the same gradual manner, and went quite off in July following. I intend to deliver an accurate history of this sort, so far as I was then enabled to observe it, because it seemed to be the most perfect in its kind of all those I have hitherto met with.

This disease arises and terminates at the times above specified. It chiefly attacks children, and especially all those who live under the same roof. 1. It comes on with a chillness, shivering, and on inequality of heat and cold, which succeeded alternately during the first day; 2. the second day these terminate in a perfect fever, attended with 3. vehement sickness; 4. thirst; 5. loss of appetite; 6. the tongue white, but not dry; 7. a slight cough; 8. heaviness of the head and eyes, with continual drowsiness; 9. an humour also generally distils from the nose and eyes, and this effusion of tears is a most certain sign of the approach of the measles; whereto must be added, as a no less certain sign, 10. that though this disease mostly shews itself in the face, by a kind of eruptions, yet, instead of these, large red spots, not rising above the surface of the skin, rather appear in the breast; 11. the patient sneezes as if he had taken cold; 12. the eyelids swell a little before the eruption; 13. he vomits; 14. but is more frequently affected with a looseness, attended with greenish stools: but this happens chiefly in children during dentition, who are also more fretful in this distemper than ordinary.

The symptoms usually grow more violent till the fourth day at which time generally little red spots, like flea bites, begin to appear in the forehead and other parts of the face, which being increased in number and bigness, run together, and form large red spots in the face, of different figures; but sometimes the eruption is deferred till the fifth day. These red spots are composed of small red pimples, seated near each other, and rising a little higher than the surface of the skin, so that they may be felt upon pressing them lightly with the finger, though they can scarce be seen. From the face, where only they first appear, these spots extend by degrees to the breast, belly, thighs, and legs; but they affect the trunk and limbs with a redness only, without perceptibly rising above the skin.

The symptoms do not abate here upon the eruptions, as in the small pox; yet I never found the vomiting continue afterwards, but the cough and fever grow more violent, the difficulty of breathing, the weakness of, and defluxion upon the eyes, constant drowsiness, and loss of appetite, persisting in their former state. On the sixth day, or thereabouts, the eruptions begin to dry, and the skin separates, whence the forehead and face grow rough, but in the other parts of the body the spots appear very large and red. About the eighth day those in the face vanish, and very few appear in the rest of the body; but on the ninth day they disappear entirely, and the face, limbs, and sometimes the whole body, seem as if they were sprinkled over with bran, the particles of the broken skin being raised up a little, and scarce cohering, so that as the disease is going off, they fall from all parts of the body like scales.

The measles therefore generally disappear on the eighth day, when the vulgar, deceived by the term of the duration of the small pox, affirm, that the eruptions are struck in; though in reality they have run through the course assigned them by nature, and they suspect that the symptoms which succeed upon their going off, are occasioned by their striking in too soon. For it is observable that the fever and difficulty of breathing increase at this time, and the cough becomes more troublesome, so that the patient can get no rest in the day, and very little in the night. Children chiefly are subject to this bad symptom, which comes on at the declension of the disease especially if an heating regime, or hot medicines have been used to promote the eruption; whence a peripneumony, which destroys greater numbers than small pox or any of its concomitant symptoms; yet notwithstanding, if this disease be skillfully treated, it is in no ways dangerous.

These bad symptoms are likewise often followed by a looseness, which either immediately succeeds the disease, or continues several weeks after the disease and all its symptoms are gone off, with greater danger to the patient, by reason of the continual waste of spirits hence arising.

Source: Sydenham, Thomas. (1809). *The Works of Thomas Sydenham, M.D., on Acute and Chronic Diseases, with Their Histories and Modes of Cure,* with notes . . . by Benjamin Rush. Philadelphia, PA: Benjamin and Thomas Kite.

ANALYSIS

Thomas Sydenham (1624–1689) was hailed by his contemporaries as the "English Hippocrates" for his emphasis on clinical observation. He lived during the period of European history known as the Scientific Revolution, and his precursors included the English physician William Harvey (1578–1657), who discovered the circulation of blood and was the first to identify the human ova. His contemporaries included Robert Hooke (1635–1703), who published a groundbreaking work on microscopy, Edmond Halley (1656–1742), who first identified Halley's Comet, and Isaac Newton (1643–1727), the most famous scientist of his day, who developed the mathematical principles of gravity.

Sydenham's goal was to strike a balance in medicine between the science and the art of medicine. The science consisted of attention to the exact sciences like anatomy and botany, where it was possible to take the subject apart and see how all the pieces fit together. Diseases could be studied in the same analytical way: they could be linked to specific times of the year, identified precisely by their symptoms, and charted day by day to mark their progress and termination. But medicine was also an art, because diseases did not always follow the same course in different patients. The skill of the physician consisted in his ability to chart the course of a specific disease in a specific patient, to ameliorate symptoms, and to promote, wherever possible, a cure. Sydenham, like al-Razi, was a therapeutic optimist: as the excerpt shows, he believed that under the treatment of a knowledgeable practitioner, even "bad symptoms" could be treated successfully.

Sydenham's approach was all the more valuable in that he looked at the social conditions of the disease. He noted that children who lived in the same household were apt to catch measles together. He also noted that measles had a "course assigned them by nature," and that once they had run that course, children were susceptible to other diseases, such as pneumonia and diarrhea. Modern pediatricians have confirmed the validity of these observations.

Sydenham's works were very influential and frequently reprinted. The edition from which the excerpt was taken was edited by Benjamin Rush, a prominent medical professor at the newly founded University of Pennsylvania and a signatory of the Declaration of Independence. Rush was probably drawn to Sydenham for his optimistic approach to medicine, an approach that fit well with the confident style of the new United States.

FURTHER READING

Dear, Peter. (2001). *Revolutionizing the Sciences: European Knowledge and Its Ambitions, 1500–1700*. Princeton, NJ: Princeton University Press.

O'Malley, Charles and Allen Debus, eds. (1974). *Medicine in Seventeenth Century England*. Berkeley, CA: University of California Press.

Sydenham, Thomas. (1979). *The Works of Thomas Sydenham, MD*. Birmingham, AL: The Classics of Medicine Library.

Wear, Andrew. (2000). *Knowledge and Practice in English Medicine, 1550–1680*. Cambridge, England: Cambridge University Press.

Yost, R. M. (1950). "Sydenham's Philosophy of Science." *Osiris* 9: 84–105.

A DOCTOR DESCRIBES SMALLPOX INOCULATION

- **Document:** Emanuel Timonius, "An Account, or History, of the Procuring the Small Pox by Incision, or Inoculation; As It Has for Some Time Been Practised at Constantinople," communicated by John Woodward
- **Date:** 1713
- **Where:** London, United Kingdom
- **Significance:** This is the first published account of the Turkish practice of inoculation for smallpox. Published in the *Philosophical Transactions*, the official publication of the Royal Society of London, it provided a legitimately scientific pedigree for the process, for physicians who preferred not to cite lay women advocates like Lady Mary or Princess Caroline.

DOCUMENT

The Writer of this ingenious Discourse observes, in the first place, that the Circassians, Georgians, and other Asiaticks, have introduc'd this Practice of procuring the Small-Pox by a sort of Inoculation, for about the space of forty Years, among the Turks and others at Constantinople.

That altho' at first the more prudent were very cautious in the use of this Practice; yet the happy Success it has been found to have in thousands of Subjects for these eight Years past, has not put it out of all suspicion and doubt; since the Operation having been perform'd on Persons of all Ages, Sexes, and different Temperments, and even in the worst Constitution of the Air, yet none have been found to die of the Small-Pox; when at the same time it was very mortal when it seized the Patient the common way, of which half the affected dy'd. This he attests upon his own Observation.

Next he observes, they that have this Inoculation practised upon them, are subject to very slight Symptoms, some being scarce sensible they are ill or sick; and what is valued by the Fair, it never leaves any Scars or Pits in the Face.

The Method of the Operation is thus. Choice being made of a proper Contagion, the Matter of the Pustules is to be communicated to the Person proposed to take the Infection; whence it has, metaphorically, the name of Incision or Inoculation. For this purpose they make choice of some Boy, or young Lad, of a sound healthy Temperament, that is seized with the common Small-Pox (of the distinct, not Flux sort) on the twelfth or thirteenth day from the beginning of his Sickness: they with a Needle prick the Tubercles (chiefly those on the Shins and Hams) and press out the Matter coming from them into some convenient Vessel of Glass, or the like, to receive it; it is convenient to wash and clean the Vessel first with warm Water:

A convenient quantity of this Matter being thus collected, is to be stop'd close, and kept warm in the Bosom of the Person that carries it, and, as soon as may be, brought to the place of the expecting future Patient.

The Patient therefore being in a warm Chamber, the Operator is to make several little Wounds with a Needle, in one, two, or more places of the Skin, till some drops of Blood follow, and immediately drop out some drops of the Matter in the Glass, and mix it well with the Blood issuing out; one drop of the Matter is sufficient for each place prick'd. These Punctures are made indifferently in any of the fleshy parts, but succeed best in the Muscles of the Arm ... The Needle is to be a three-edg'd Surgeon's Needle; it may likewise be perform'd with a Lancet: The custom is to run the Needle transverse, and rip up the Skin a little, that there may be a convenient dividing of the Part, and the mixing of the Matter with the Blood more easily perform'd; which is done, either with a blunt Stile, or an Ear-picker: The Wound is cover'd with half a Walnut shell, or the like Concave Vessel, and bound over, that the Matter be not rub'd off by the Garments; which is all removed in a few Hours ...

The Small-Pox begins to appear sooner in some than in others, in some with greater, on others with lesser Symptoms; but with happy Success in all.

Source: Timonius, Emanuel and John Woodward. (1714). "An Account, or History, of the Procuring the Small Pox by Incision, or Inoculation; As It Has for Some Time Been Practised in Constantinople." *Philosophical Transactions* 29: 72–82.

ANALYSIS

We understand the term *inoculation* as meaning "preventing a disease," but here Dr. Emanuel Timonius gives it the meaning current in the early 18th century, of grafting, as in the agricultural process of grafting a limb from one fruit tree onto another. In account, the "graft" comes from the leg of an otherwise healthy child, who is on his way to recovery from smallpox. It is then inserted onto the arm of another healthy child or adult. The smallpox is thus "procured," or grafted, in the patient.

The inoculation process, wherein physicians "rip up the skin a little" with a needle or lancet, cannot have been very comfortable for young patients, and Timonius reports the case of one boy who "prevented the insertion of the Matter, for he struggled very much under the Operation," and the physician had no one there "to hold him still." The smallpox was not, in his case, successfully grafted at that time, but Timonius reported that when the boy caught smallpox the regular way, "he did very well."

Later reports of the process would show that Timonius was entirely too optimistic in predicting "happy Success in all" cases of smallpox inoculation. Usually, the "engrafted" cases of smallpox were mild, but, occasionally, it proved fatal; it could still cause some scarring; worst of all, the inoculated smallpox was still contagious.

FURTHER READING

Bazin, Hervé. (2011). *Vaccination: A History from Lady Montagu to Genetic Engineering.* Esher, England: John Libbey Eurotext.

Cunningham, Andrew and Roger French, eds. (1990). *The Medical Enlightenment of the Eighteen Century.* New York: Cambridge University Press.

Miller, Genevieve. (1957). *The Adoption of Inoculation for Smallpox in England and France.* Philadelphia, PA: University of Pennsylvania Press.

Rusnock, Andrea. (2002). *Vital Accounts: Quantifying Health and Population in Eighteenth-Century England and France.* Cambridge, England: Cambridge University Press.

Shapin, Steven. (1994). *A Social History of Truth: Civility and Science in 17th Century England.* Chicago, IL: University of Chicago Press.

RASH INNOVATION OR NEW DISCOVERY?

- **Document:** William Wagstaffe, *A Letter to Dr. Friend, Shewing the Danger and Uncertainty in Inoculating the Smallpox*
- **Date:** 1722
- **Where:** London, United Kingdom
- **Significance:** The smallpox epidemic of 1721–1722 led to the introduction of inoculation in both London and Boston and to heated medical controversy. In many ways, these early conflicts were precursors of those that followed for the next 300 years. Opponents of inoculation argued that the practice was new and untried; that no one understood exactly why it worked; that it violated God's judgment over who deserved to live or die; that it spread contagion. Proponents of inoculation argued for its efficacy and safety; they argued, too, that inoculation was one of God's blessings for mankind, like other forms of preventative medicine. They soon found, though, that they could not dismiss their opponents' arguments out of hand. Inoculation was not completely safe: some patients died, and all were capable of spreading the disease.

  Ironically, though both sides of the controversy wished to uphold the authority of the physician, its end result was to leave the decision about whether or not to inoculate in the hands of the patient or his/her parent. Physicians soon found they could attract and keep more patients by offering the new treatment than by opposing it.

DOCUMENT

Tho' the Fashion of Inoculating the Small Pox has so far prevail'd, as to be admitted into the greatest Families, yet I entirely concur with you in Opinion, that, till we have fuller Evidence of the Success of it, both with regard to the Security of the Operation, and the Certainty of preventing the like Distemper from any other Cause, Physicians at least, who of all Men ought to be guided in their Judgments chiefly by Experience, shou'd not be over hasty in encouraging a Practice, which does not seem as yet sufficiently supported either by Reason, or by Fact. Nor is it only necessary to enquire into the Manner of the several repeated Tryals on Persons of different Ages, Sexes, and Constitutions, in different Seasons of the Year, and in different Climates, but to examine the Nature of Infusing such a Fluid into the Blood, as is the Matter contain'd in the Pustules of the Small Pox, and what Consequences it may produce. Other People may be satisfied with being told, that the Operation is Successful; but Physicians, I shou'd think, cannot with Pruence give into any thing which is the peculiar Subject of their Profession, merely because it has been cry'd up by those who are no Physicians, and have not the least Knowledge of Distempers.

The Country from whence we have deriv'd this Experiment, will have but very little Influence on our Faith, if we consider either the Nature of the Climate, or the Capacity of the Inhabitants; and Posterity perhaps will scarcely be brought to believe, that an Experiment practiced only by a few Ignorant Women, amongst an Illiterate and unthinking People, shou'd on a sudden, and upon a slender Experience, so far obtain in one of the Politest Nations in the World, as to be receiv'd into the Royal Palace . . .

It is, sir, another of their [pro-inoculation physicians'] Aphorisms, that there was no contagion from the inoculated sort; and an Inoculator confesses, he was surprised in the Family of Mr. Batt near Hertford, to see six Persons, of whom one died, catch the Infection in this manner. And I am well informed by Persons of unquestionable Reputation, that the Town of Hertford is a lamentable Evidence of the Danger of this Practice, where the Distemper was spread by it to that degree, as not only to make an havock of the Inhabitants, but to hinder the Commerce of the place. Thus the Operator has it in his Power to convey the Small Pox to distant Places and Persons, who neither avow his practice, or desire his Experiment: And if 'tis possible that the ingrafted Pox can be so poisonous as to communicate certain Death to all around, by this method, they may Ingraft as violent a Plague, as has been known among us.

How far the Legislature may think fit to interpose, in order to prevent such an artificial way of depopulating a Country, is not my Province to determine; but if any one should willfully set an House on Fire, and from thence lay the Neighbourhood in Ashes; tho' in the first House it should be happily extinguished, he would unquestionably be accounted guilty of burning down the whole, and receive Punishment suitable to so general a destruction.

Source: Wagstaffe, William. (1722). A Letter to Dr. Friend, Shewing the Danger and Uncertainty in Inoculating the Smallpox. London: Samuel Butler.

- **Document:** Charles Maitland, *Maitland's Account of Inoculating the Smallpox Vindicated, from Dr. Wagstaffe's Misrepresentations of That Practice*
- **Date:** 1722
- **Where:** London, United Kingdom
- **Significance:** Charles Maitland uses the polite language of debate to refute Wagstaffe's arguments, but his key point is anything but polite: he repeatedly compares Wagstaffe to other members of the "faculty"—that is, the medical profession—who have opposed worthwhile discoveries because of their own self-interest.

DOCUMENT

I am very Sensible of the Respect that is due to the Profession, and Character of the Author of the Letter against Inoculating the Small Pox; but am no less sensible of the Obligation I lye under to vindicate my own Reputation, which a violent Fit of Sickness hath hitherto hinder'd me from doing. And I can do it with the more Freedom, because I am conscious to my self, that I began this Practice in England with the same View to the Publick Good, with which, I hope, the Learned Author condemns it. I must take the Liberty to say, that allowing the Doctor's Abilities to be as great as possible in his own Profession, he seems not quite so well qualify'd to write upon this Subject; because of the Narrowness of his Experience (as far as appears by his Letter) and his partial Credulity, or Incredulity in Matters of Fact, which he takes from others; and lastly, because of strong Prejudices, which impose upon his most excellent Understanding; and draw him into Reasonings, which either are inconsequential, or conclude strongly for the Practice of Inoculation, which they are brought to overturn . . .

The Letter pretends to be an Admonition to Physicians not to meddle in this Practice of Inoculation, 'till they are better ascertain'd by Experience, of the Success of it. At the same Time, it is a most warm Dissuasive, not only to Physicians, but to all Sorts of People, not to practise it at all; and consequently, to deprive them of all Possibility of coming by Experience. Would it not sound somewhat absurd, if any one should say to a young Physician, Pray, Sir, don't Practise 'till you have Experience? But it is still more so in this Case, because in a Practice that is entirely to be laid aside, you can neither have the Benefit of your own, nor other Peoples Experience.

. . . Physicians cannot ingraft People against their own, or their Parents Consent; and a Physician would be out of his Duty, who should persuade them to it contrary to their Inclinations: On the other Hand, If a Person, from the Experience of the Fatality of the Small Pox in general, or in his own Family in particular, should resolve to ingraft his Child, any Physician, who should dissuade him from it, might in great measure, be chargeable with the fatal Consequences of the Neglect of a Method, which the Parent had propos'd, as the only Means to save his Child's Life: And he would be still as much to blame, if when the Parent had resolv'd to ingraft his Child, he should refuse to attend him. It is very common with Parents, not only to leave their Children in Houses infected with the Small Pox, but to bring them into the Room, where their Brethren or Sisters lye ill of them; and a Parent who does so, conveys the Infection to his Child as deliberately, and according to the Doctor, certainly more than he, who orders him to be Inoculated. Would it not then be equally impertinent in the Physician to deny his Attendance in either Case?

I must put the Doctor in Mind, that there are very few of the most useful Discoveries in Physick, that have not been strenuously oppos'd by many of the Faculty upon their first Appearance . . .

[Wagstaffe stated that in Hertford], the Inoculated Small Pox propagated the Mortality of the natural Sort . . . I think it is hard to exclude Men from the Means of securing themselves from a great Pestilence, upon a meer Suggestion.

The Influence of the natural Small Pox upon Mankind, in any Place, in a Circle of Years, may be affirm'd to be uniform with strong Probability; ... it is [therefore] a strong Motive for People to take the Advantage of a good Season, and secure themselves in Time from a plague, which is so likely to destroy them: And if Prudence only were to be consulted, it would perhaps be much more the Duty of the Legislature to order, than to forbid this Practice.

Source: Maitland, Charles. (1722). *Mr. Maitland's Account of Inoculating the Small Pox Vindicated, from Dr. Wagstaffe's Misrepresentations of That Practice.* London: J. Peele.

ANALYSIS

Although today we speak of one unified medical profession, in the early 18th century, it makes more sense to think of medical practitioners as being divided into several different groups. The first consisted of university-trained physicians, who were the best educated and also charged the highest fees. The second consisted of surgeons, generally trained through apprenticeship and organized into guilds. The third consisted of apothecaries, also typically trained through apprenticeship and organized into guilds. In cities like London, they were organized into professional associations, which claimed the legal privilege of regulating medical practices within the city. The three professions did not make common cause. Instead, the Royal College of Physicians, the Royal College of Surgeons, and the Worshipful Society of Apothecaries often fought amongst themselves over the control of medical practices within the city limits. Lawsuits were fierce and frequently accompanied by pamphlet wars. A persistent source of conflict had to do with foreign physicians who settled in London. The Royal College of Physicians extended special privileges to graduates of the English universities of Oxford and Cambridge; graduates from other medical schools, even British ones, felt that they were treated as second-class citizens.

Charles Maitland (1668–1748) introduced inoculation practices in London by vaccinating Lady Mary Wortley Montagu's daughter and subsequently received a royal license to vaccinate Newgate prisoners and orphans as part of Princess Caroline's experiment. He then vaccinated the royal children. His success brought him acclaim from some of his professional colleagues, but it also brought him notoriety. Maitland was an outsider, a surgeon from Scotland, not one of the London's elite physicians. Many of the physicians who supported him were also from Scotland. When, in this excerpt, William Wagstaffe (1685–1725) stated that a civilized country like Great Britain should not adopt the medical teachings of "illiterate and unthinking people"; he may have been referring to Scotland as well as Turkey. He was certainly implying that Maitland and his fellow inoculators were spreading a plague, rather than preventing it. His juxtaposition of plague and fire were guaranteed to catch the attention and heighten the fears of London readers.

Maitland, in his response, kept his tone "polite" and reasonable. He was acting only at the request of parents in order to save their children from certain diseases.

The decision was really up to the parents, and a physician who believed he could save a child's life and refused to do so would be culpable. He was acting in the public good, based on his own experience—which was, as he pointed out, more extensive than that of Wagstaffe.

By the early 18th century, new scientific methods were widely accepted, and every educated person knew the story of Galileo, who had been punished for maintaining that the earth moves around the sun. Maitland invoked this story when he noted, "that there are very few of the most useful Discoveries in Physick, that have not been strenuously oppos'd by many of the Faculty upon their first Appearance." In this he is equating the discovery of inoculation with Galileo's discovery of the telescope and Wagstaffe with Galileo's opponents. This remained a successful rhetorical strategy as long as science itself was considered to be a "publick good."

FURTHER READING

Carrell, Jennifer. (2004). *The Speckled Monster. A Historical Tale of Battling Smallpox*. New York: Penguin Group.

Cook, Harold. (1994). "Good Advice and Little Medicine: The Professional Authority of Early Modern English Physicians." *Journal of British Studies* 33: 1–31.

Dobson, Mary. (1997). *Contours of Death and Disease in Early Modern England*. Cambridge, England: Cambridge University Press.

Duncan, S. R., Susan Scott, and C. J. Duncan. (1994). "Smallpox Epidemics in Cities in Britain." *Journal of Interdisciplinary History* 25: 255–271.

Porter, Dorothy. (1989). *Health for Sale. Doctors and Doctoring in Eighteenth-Century England*. Stanford, CA: Stanford University Press.

GOD'S JUDGMENT OR GOD'S BLESSING?

- **Document:** Samuel Grainger, *The Imposition of Inoculation as a Duty Religiously Considered*
- **Date:** 1721
- **Where:** Boston, MA
- **Significance:** Cotton Mather, a prominent Boston minister and prolific writer, championed inoculation for smallpox during a 1721 epidemic that killed 800 people out of a population of 12,000. Mather claimed to have heard of the practice first from an African slave, Onesimus, and then from Timonius's account in the Philosophical Transactions. Convinced it could save lives, he enlisted the aid of Boston practitioner Zabdiel Boylston. They may have inoculated as many as 300 patients. Though they had supporters among Boston's medical profession, they were attacked on both religious and medical grounds. In this excerpt, Grainger gives reasons for his strong religious objections to inoculation.

DOCUMENT

[We are told that] the strange and wonderful discovery of Inoculation . . . [is] a great Blessing to Mankind, and should be thankfully received, as being a Way to defend our selves against a Dreadful and Deadly Disease, by Over-Ruling (notwithstanding it is to belook'd upon as a Judgment) the way of its coming at us when we see 'tis a coming. What a horrid sound it here . . .

Another, whom I suppose to have been a great Traveller tells us, that none ever died this way; and that 'tis probably, nay more than probably which is a pretty kind of Certainty, they never will.

. . . The Strong, the Weak; the Holy and the Profane? If they will but come into the late and easie practice of Inoculation . . . he dares with an unparallel'd assurance, almost warrant their Lives will be secure against the Malignity and Danger of this Worst of Plagues. Is this the Spirit and Language of David, crying out, My Flesh trembleth for fear of Thee, and I am afraid of Thy judgments.

It is not amiss to observe, The Evils which befall us, may be the Moral and Natural Effects of Sin; as when we suffer in our Estates by Prodigality, Excess or Mismanagements and want of fore-cast. In our Health, by Lust and Intemperance. It may extend even to Life itself, when men by the willful breach of a known Law, forfeit their Lives by the Transgressing of it. These are the Natural and Moral Consequences of Sin . . .

But there are other Evils which befall us, that more immediately proceed from the Volition of God, and may be properly said to be his Doings, as be in a more especial manner National Judgments, and though they are inflected upon a Land for the Sin thereof ... And as these Designs of Providence are part of the secret and hidden Will. So are we to yield a passive Obedience of Submission, Resignation and Dependent thereunto. It is the Lord, let him do what seemeth him good ... We are no where directed to Humane Means to over-rule them, in the say of their coming at us, when we see them coming; for such means cannot any ways deliver us from, but rather encrease our Punishment, and make our Condemnation the greater, because it is too apparent that we Distrust Gods Promise, throw off Resignation and Submission to the Divine Will, and proclaim our selves Rebels ...

It is impossible that any Humane Means, or preventive Physick should defend us from, or Over-rule a Judicial National Sickness ...

Source: Grainger, Samuel. (1721). *The Imposition of Inoculation as a Duty Religiously Considered.* Boston, MA: Nicholas Boone.

- **Document:** William Douglass, *Inoculation of the Smallpox as Practised in Boston*
- **Date:** 1721
- **Where:** Boston, MA
- **Significance:** Dr. William Douglass spoke for Boston's elite physicians in his objections to Mather and Boylston. He argued that they had simply rushed into inoculating patients, without considering the costs either to those they treated or to those around them. His opinion on "bold experiments" in medicine, that they put early patients at risk even if they lead to public, remained true until the modern era of carefully regulated clinical trials.

DOCUMENT

My humble Opinion of *Inoculation* is as of all bold Experiments of Consequence in the Practice of Physick. That whatever the Success or Consequences may be, (and the more Tryals the more Light) they may be of a publick Advantage, tho' at the *Risque* of the first patients. If it answer, after Generations will reap the benefit of it; if otherways, the miserable Sufferers will be recorded as bold, rash, infatuated *Fools*, the Practice for everafter abhor'd, and the Promoters thereof stigmatized as *Murderers*.

All solid and sound *Phylosophy,* that is *Natural History,* is founded on *Observations* made, and *Experiments* taken of the various Actions and Influences of *Natural Bodys* on one another. I was always fond of this kind of Knowledge, especially as it related to *Humane Bodies* in a *Healthy* or *Morbid* state; and if these two dear Characters of a

Good Citizen and a Good *Christian* could be dispensed with, I should have been pleased to see some Thousands inoculated with several other *Distempers* as well as the *Small Pox*; but for the following *Reasons* I could not at present comply with this novel . . . and *dubious* practice.

Poysoning and spreading infection, are by the penal Law of England *Felony.* Inoculation falls in with the first without any Contradiction, and if a Person of so *weak a Constitution*, that any the least Illness may prove fatal to him; should be inoculated, and suffer but the tenth part of what several of the *Inoculated* have done, he must unavoidably perish, and his *Inoculator* deem'd guilty of wilful *Poysoning* . . . If the Inoculators had designed a publick Good, why did they run headlong into it, without observing the *Circumstances* and *Cautions* which might have made it useful; to begin in the Heart of the Town, where was no Infection; to inoculate all *Ages* and *Constitutions* from the very Beginning, without being first assur'd of it's Success on the *Young and Healthy*. Why did they not *petition the Government*, that [none] should be inoculated till his Name was recorded, that for the publick Good *in times to come*, it might be known who dy'd, and what *state of Health* they afterwards enjoy'd who surviv'd; say also have contriv'd some Method, that none might take the Infection from the *Inoculated*; This Neglect has occasioned the Death of many . . .

Instead of contriving Methods to secure the *Inoculated* from taking the Infection the common Way, and their Neighbours from being infected by them, they inoculate indifferently in all Corners, and set the Town all in a Flame in one Moment as it were . . .

Source: Douglass, William. (1722). *Inoculation of the Small Pox as Practised in Boston, Consider'D in a Letter to A—S—M.D. & F.R.S. in London.* Boston, MA: J. Franklin.

- **Document:** Zabdiel Boylston, *Some Account of What Is Said of Inoculating or Transplanting the Small Pox*
- **Date:** 1721
- **Where:** Boston, MA
- **Significance:** In this pamphlet, Boylston addressed the religious and medical arguments against inoculation.

DOCUMENT

It might be easy for me to make Answers to the Scurrilous things lately Published against me, and satisfy the Publick of the Falsehood and Baseness in them. But I think it rather becomes a considerate Man to decline foolish Contentions, especially at a time, when there is a grievous Calamity upon us, that calls us (instead of railing at one another) to Unite in Prayers to Almighty God, for his Mercies to us.

The Case of Conscience distresses many worthy Good People. The Case in short we take to be this. 'Almighty God in His great mercy to Mankind, has taught us a Remedy, to be used when the dangers of the Small Pox distress us; upon the use of which Medicine, they shall in an ordinary way be sure not to have it so severely as in the other way, and consequently not to be in such danger from this dreadful Distemper, and also to be delivered from the terrible Circumstances which many of them who recover of the Distemper do suffer for it.

Whether a Christian may not employ this Medicine (let the matter of it be what it will) and humbly give Thanks to God for His good Providence in discovering of it to a miserable World; and humbly look up to His Good Providence (as we do in the use of any other Medicine) for the success of it? It may seem strange, that any wise Christian cannot answer it . . .

It is objected, That you Presume upon Providence in this Essay for the Prevention of the Small Pox; for you don't know whether you shall ever have the Small Pox, or no. I Answer, But what if it be as likely that I shall have it, as it is that my House will take Fire, when my Neighbours an Inch and a half off, is in Flames. Pray, sit still, my Neighbour, your House is not yet on Fire: The Almighty can preserve it. But I Enquire, whether this Objection will not lie against all the Preventive Physick in the World? I don't Infallibly know, that I shall ever suffer the Disease I am going to prevent . . .

The Objection here is, I make my self Sick, when I am well. But I again say, Will any Man decry all Preventing Physick, as Unlawful? . . . To say that our Saviour's words, The whole need not a Physician, forbid all preventing Physick, is a gross abuse of them . . .

But an Anxious Fear of the Small Pox; is not this an Evil Disease? Especially, when I have it so near me, that 'tis next to a Miracle if I escape it? If I take Physick only to Remove and Prevent this Fear, it can't be said, that I make my self Sick before I have any Disease . . .

There is a silly cavil, we pray that the Small Pox may not spread; and yet we do our selves by Transplantation spread it. But I Enquire whether People know what they Pray for? Our Prayers are that a Dangerous and Destructive Small Pox may not Spread. We do not Pray, that the use of an Effectual means to save our Lives from the Danger of Destruction by the Small Pox, may not be Revealed, Practiced & Prospered . . .

It is Cavilled (for to say, Objected, would be too easy a word for such Impertinence) that this new Way comes to us from the Heathen, and we Christians must not Learn the Way of the Heathen. I Enquire, whether our Hippocrates were not an Heathen? And whether our Galen were not an Heathen? . . . And whether we have not learnt some of our very Good Medicines from our Indians? . . . And, Gentlemen Smoakers, I pray, whom did you learn to smoke of?

Source: Boylston, Zabdiel and Cotton Mather. (1721). *Some Account of What Is Said of Inoculating or Transplanting the Small Pox.* Boston, MA: S. Gerrish.

ANALYSIS

In colonial Boston, medical authority was not vested in professional associations, as it was in London. Particularly, during epidemics, patients were as likely to turn to their ministers as to their doctors. While all medical practitioners would have agreed that prayer and religious observance were necessary in sickness as in health, they did not want to see religious authorities treating the sick. Many religious leaders agreed, arguing, as Samuel Grainger (ca. 1686–1738) did in the first excerpt, that it was the role of religious authorities to use disease as a way of inculcating moral lessons. This struck a responsive chord in a community that believed itself established for a divine purpose, where all public assemblies, from meals to meetings of the legislature to criminal executions, began with prayers and often a sermon. If Divine Providence had sent smallpox, surely it was tempting Providence to prevent it?

As one of Boston's leading physicians, William Douglass (ca. 1691–1752) was no fatalist in the face of disease; he would later become known for his detailed clinical description of childhood epidemics. In this excerpt, Douglass objects to Mather's and Boylston's inoculation practices on public health grounds: when introducing any new method, he argues that practitioners should keep careful records and not spread the disease they were trying to contain. He also had a long-standing objection to ministers, like Mather, acting outside of their own religious sphere. Like Wagstaffe in London, he compares the Boston inoculators to criminals who spread poison and arson. Though he later admitted, in print, that the inoculations had probably done more good than harm, Mather never forgave him for the attack.

Like many on the pro-inoculation side, Zabdiel Boylston (1679–1766) was so convinced of its value that he used the technique on his own family. He faced enormous opposition; according to his biographer: "His house was attacked with so much violence that he and his family could not feel themselves safe in it. He was assaulted in the streets, loaded with every species of abuse, and execrated as a murderer. Indeed many sober pious people were deliberately of opinion, when he commended the practice of inoculation, that if any of his patients should die, he ought to be capitally punished" (Thatcher, 1:21).

As the excerpt shows, though, Boylston remained certain that he was serving the public good. He took the metaphor of a house on fire and turned it against his opponents: so far from causing destruction, he says, are we not preventing our neighbor's fire from spreading to ours, if we prevent the disease? If we see the house next door in flames, would we really do nothing to stop it or to protect our own? "As to the spiteful and scurrilous things written against me and this Practice," he concluded, "at present I shall take no further Notice of them, but remind the Writers of the ill natur'd Dog in the Fable, that would neither eat the Oats himself, nor let the Horse eat them: So neither will these use a true and certain way to save the Peoples Lives, nor are they willing to let any one else use it to save them."

FURTHER READING

Blake, John. (1952). "The Inoculation Controversy in Boston: 1721–1722." *New England Quarterly* 25: 489–506.

Burton, John. (2001). " 'The Awful Judgments of God upon the Land': Smallpox in Colonial Cambridge, Massachusetts." *New England Quarterly* 74: 495–506.

Herbert, Eugenia. (1975). "Smallpox Inoculation in Africa." *Journal of African History* 16: 539–559.

Minardi, Margot. (2004). "The Boston Inoculation Controversy of 1721–1722: An Incident in the History of Race." *William and Mary Quarterly* 61: 47–76.

Thatcher, James. (1828). *American Medical Biography*, 2 vols. Boston, MA: Richardson and Lord, 1: 1–21.

DISTURBING THE PEACE AND QUIET
OF HIS MAJESTY'S SUBJECTS

- **Document:** "An Act to Regulate the Inoculation of the Small-Pox within This Colony"
- **Date:** 1769
- **Where:** Virginia
- **Significance:** In 1768–1769, a determined group of anti-inoculation householders in Norfolk, Virginia, decided on a course of legal and physical harassment against anyone who requested inoculation. Both sides took each other to court, with the pro-inoculation families represented by the young Thomas Jefferson. While the legal arguments wound their way through the judicial system, the Virginia Legislature took the part of the anti-inoculation side, passing the following act. It made inoculating for the smallpox an offense unless two conditions held: first, a family had to be in immediate danger from smallpox and second, the practitioner had to be issued a special license by municipal or county authorities. Since the act made it almost impossible for anyone to obtain inoculation in advance of a serious epidemic, many Virginians, like Jefferson, traveled to Philadelphia, where inoculation could be performed without fear of harassment or litigation.

DOCUMENT

I. WHEREAS the wanton introduction of the Small-Pox into this colony by inoculation, when the same was not necessary, hath, of late years, proved a nuisance to several neighbourhoods, by disturbing the peace and quietness of many of his majesty's subjects, and exposing their lives to the infection of that mortal distemper, which, from the situation and circumstances of the colony, they would otherwise have little reason to dread: To prevent which for the future, *Be it enacted, by the Governor, Council, and Burgesses, of this present General Assembly, and it is hereby enacted, by the authority of the same,* That if any person or persons whatsoever, shall wilfully, or designedly, after the first day of September next ensuing, presume to import or bring into this colony, from any country or place whatever, the small-pox, or any variolous or infectious matter of the said distemper, with a purpose to inoculate any person or persons whatever, or by any means whatever, to propagate the said distemper within this colony, he or she, so offending, shall forfeit and pay the sum of one thousand pounds, for every offence so committed; one moiety whereof shall be to the informer, and the other moiety to the churchwardens of the parish where the offence shall be committed, for the use of the poor of the said parish; to be recovered, with costs, by action of debt, bill, plaint, or information, in any court of record within this dominion.

II. But forasmuch as the inoculation of the smallpox may, under peculiar circumstances, be not only a prudent but necessary means of securing those who are unavoidably exposed to the danger of taking the distemper in the natural way, and for this reason it is judged proper to tolerate it, under reasonable restrictions and regulations:

III. *Be it therefore enacted, by the authority aforesaid,* That from and after the said first day of September next, if any person shall think him or herself, his or her family, exposed to the immediate danger of catching the said distemper, such person may give notice thereof to the sheriff of any county, or to the mayor or chief magistrate of any city or corporation and the said sheriff, mayor, or chief magistrate, shall, immediately, and without loss of time, summon all the acting magistrates of the said county, city, or borough, to meet at the most convenient time and place in the said county, city, or borough, and the said magistrates, or such of them as shall be present, being assembled, shall consider whether, upon the whole circumstances of the case, inoculation may be prudent or necessary, or dangerous to the health and safety of the neighbourhood, and thereupon either grant a licence for such inoculation, under such restrictions and regulations as they shall judge necessary and proper, or prohibit the same, as to them, or a majority of them, shall seem expedient.

IV. *And be it further enacted, by the authority aforesaid,* That if any person or persons shall inoculate, or procure inoculation of the small-pox to be performed within this colony, without obtaining a licence in the manner before directed, or shall not conform to the rules and regulations prescribed by such justices, he, she, or they, shall forfeit and pay respectively, for every such offence, the sum of one hundred pounds; one moiety whereof shall be to the informer, and the other moiety to the churchwardens of the parish wherein such offence shall be committed, for the use of the poor of the said parish; to be recovered, with costs, by action of debt, bill, plaint, or information, in any court of record within this dominion. And moreover it shall and may be lawful for any justice of the peace, upon information given to him, upon oath, to issue his warrant against any person so offending, and upon sufficient proof, before him made, to cause such offender to give security, in such reasonable penalty as such justice shall think fit, for his or her good behaviour, and upon failure to give such security, to commit him or her to the gaol of his county, there to be confined until such security is given.

V. And whereas checking of the progress of the said distemper, where it may accidentally break out, or the regulations which may be established for carrying on inoculation, may be attended with some expence: *Be it therefore enacted, by the authority aforesaid,* That it shall and may be lawful for the justices of the court of every county, at the time of laying their levy, and for the mayor, recorder, aldermen, and common council, of any city or borough, at such time as they shall judge most convenient, to levy on the tithable persons in their said county, city, or borough, so much tobacco or money as will be sufficient to defray the expences necessarily incurred for the purposes aforesaid, in any such county, city, or borough.

VI. *And be it further enacted, by the authority aforesaid,* That if any sheriff, mayor, or chief magistrate, shall, upon application to him made, in manner aforesaid, refuse, or unreasonably delay, to summon the magistrates of any county, city, or borough, for the purpose aforesaid, or if any magistrate so summoned, shall refuse or neglect to attend according to such summon, every such sheriff, mayor, or chief magistrate, shall forfeit the sum of one hundred pounds, upon his refusing or neglecting to give such notice, without reasonable excuse; and every other magistrate so refusing or neglecting, without reasonable excuse, shall forfeit and pay the sum of five pounds, to the person aggrieved; to be recovered, with costs, by action of debt, in any court of record within this dominion.

Source: "An Act to Regulate the Inoculation of the Small-Pox within This Colony." (1821). In *The Statutes at Large: Being a Collection of All the Laws of Virginia,* edited by William Waller Hening. Richmond, VA: George Cochran, 371–374.

ANALYSIS

By the 1760s, smallpox had become endemic throughout the Atlantic world, facilitated by busy transportation networks linking New World colonies with their respective European mother countries. Frequent movements of troops and civilians led to frequent outbreaks, and though inoculation was an established method of prevention, inoculation without strict attention to quarantine only spread the disease further. Local political elites were increasingly divided into factions over the value of inoculation, and Norfolk was only one of the cities where attempts at inoculation led to harassment and violence.

Much of the problem had to do with the difficulty of controlling either doctors' or patients' behavior. When John Smith set up practice as an inoculator in Yorktown, Virginia, in 1767, no regulation existed against it. Though neighbors complained, there was nothing they could do to stop it. But inoculation, to be safe, required that patients be isolated for a complete course of the disease, until each and every scab had fully healed. This could take up to 30 days, and many families found it impossible—or simply refused—to remain in isolation for that period. Complete isolation during illness in any case went against the usual practices for looking after the sick, especially during convalescence, when neighbors or religious leaders would drop by. A few college students, treated by Smith, left town early and transmitted the disease to Williamsburg, causing a deadly outbreak.

No wonder, then, that there was violent opposition in Norfolk when Dr. Alexander Campbell invited a colleague, Dr. Dalgleish, to inoculate his wife and family at his plantation three miles away. Campbell had originally invited some other families, but after local protests, he agreed to keep to the group already invited. That did not satisfy the anti-inoculation faction, and they insisted that the families be moved to the Norfolk pesthouse. Campbell resisted, but a mob surrounded the house, and he and his family fled in fear of their lives. Two days later, the Campbells' house was burned down. No one was ever indicted for arson.

Generally, anti-inoculation legislation followed geographic lines. The New England and southern colonies agreed with the Virginia legislators that inoculation could be carried out only in cases of a virulent outbreak, while the mid-Atlantic colonies allowed inoculation at the patient's request. That means that wealthy patients in New York, Philadelphia, and Baltimore had ready access to inoculation, while their counterparts in Virginia and Vermont did not. By the 1770s, the Philadelphia Almshouse even offered free inoculation to their poor patients. In contrast, a similar establishment at Salem, Massachusetts, was set on fire by angry residents.

As political tensions increased between the American colonies and Great Britain, the danger of this patchwork of anti-inoculation policies became clear. Whenever warfare broke out in the 18th century, it always brought pestilence in its wake. If American troops were mustered, which would be the more dangerous foe? British armies? Or smallpox?

FURTHER READING

Dewey, Frank. (1983). "Thomas Jefferson's Law Practice: The Norfolk Anti-Inoculation Riots." *Virginia Magazine of History and Biography* 91: 39–53.

Gilje, Paul. (1996). *Rioting in America*. Bloomington, IN: Indiana University Press.

Henderson, Patrick. (1965). "Smallpox and Patriotism. The Norfolk Riots, 1768–1769." *Virginia Magazine of History and Biography* 73: 413–424.

"Inoculation." *Thomas Jefferson's Montecello*. https://www.monticello.org/site/research-and-collections/inoculation.

Tannenbaum, Rebecca. (2012). *Health and Wellness in Colonial America*. Santa Barbara, CA: ABC-CLIO.

GEORGE WASHINGTON ORDERS COMPULSORY INOCULATION OF THE CONTINENTAL ARMY

- **Document:** Letter from George Washington to Dr. William Shippen
- **Date:** 1777
- **Where:** New Jersey
- **Significance:** By the Revolutionary War, the practice of smallpox inoculation was widespread in Great Britain but much less so in the American colonies. Repeated outbreaks of smallpox among his troops convinced George Washington that inoculation was necessary to win the war. Aware of the need to keep inoculated soldiers isolated, the army set up special military smallpox hospitals. Members of the Continental Congress, meeting in Philadelphia, were also inoculated as part of the war effort.

DOCUMENT

To DOCTOR WILLIAM SHIPPEN, JUNIOR
Head Quarters, Morristown, January 6, 1777.

Dear Sir: Finding the small pox to be spreading much and fearing that no precaution can prevent it from running thro' the whole of our Army, I have determined that the Troops shall be inoculated. This Expedient may be attended with some inconveniences and some disadvantages, but yet I trust, in its consequences will have the most happy effects. Necessity not only authorizes but seems to require the measure, for should the disorder infect the Army, in the natural way, and rage with its usual Virulence, we should have more to dread from it, than from the Sword of the Enemy. Under these Circumstances, I have directed Doctr. [Nathaniel] Bond, to prepare immediately for inoculating in this Quarter, keeping the matter as secret as possible, and request, that you will without delay inoculate all the Continental Troops that are in Philadelphia and those that shall come in, as fast as they arrive. You will spare no pains to carry them thro' the disorder with the utmost expedition, and to have them cleansed from the infection when recovered, that they may proceed to Camp, with as little injury as possible, to the Country thro'

DID YOU KNOW?

Women of the Revolutionary Army

There are romantic folk songs from the 18th century about women dressing up as soldiers to be with their sweethearts, but not many people know that women really could join the Revolutionary Army. Generally they were wives of enlisted soldiers, and the army hired them to perform essential services, including working in military hospitals. They were supposed to be paid, but the Continental Congress often ran out of money to pay soldiers or officers, so the women of the army had to forego pay as well. They were, however, given a ration allowance for themselves and their children. As George Washington himself explained, "I was obliged to give provisions to the extra women of these regiments, or lose to desertion, perhaps to the Enemy, some of the oldest and best soldiers in the service" (cited in DePauw, 1981, 212). In exchange, the women were expected to follow military discipline, march with the baggage train, follow orders, and stay out of the way during the fighting. They could be court-martialed, just like any other military personnel.

Women were also employed in hospitals. From 1777, Congress authorized one matron and 10 nurses for every 100 wounded. Matrons supervised hospital arrangements and staff and were paid $.50 per day plus one food ration.

Nurses were paid $.24 per day plus food ration, roughly the same rate as an army sergeant. Using women, instead of male soldiers, as hospital staff meant that more soldiers could be deployed in battle. But dependable women were in short supply, despite the high rate of pay: army hospitals could be as dangerous to their staff as to their patients, since they were breeding grounds for infectious diseases.

We do not have records indicating whether women of the army participated in the army-mandated inoculation against smallpox, but it seems likely that many would have done so. In spring 1778, as Washington prepared to lead his reorganized, rebuilt army from Valley Forge through New Jersey, he had to consider what to do with the nearly 3,800 sick, including those suffering or contagious after smallpox inoculation. He arranged for them to stay behind in Valley Forge until they recovered, provided with food, camp kettles, and "as many Women of the Army as can be prevailed on to serve as nurses" at "the usual price" (cited in Fenn, 2001, 102) It seems reasonable to assume that women who stayed would have had the same protection as the soldiers they cared for.

By June, only 900 remained in the hospitals in Valley Forge; the rest of the newly inoculated had recovered and were able to join the army. They may well have made the difference during the Battle of Monmouth on June 28, 1778, the first prolonged engagement in which Washington and the Continental Army held their ground against enemy forces.

Sources:

DePauw, Linda Grant. (1981). "Women in Combat. The Revolutionary War Experience." *Armed Forces and Society* 7: 209–226.

Fenn, Elizabeth. (2001). *Pox Americana: The Great Smallpox Epidemic of 1775–82.* New York: Hill and Wang.

which they pass. If the business is immediately begun and favoured with the common success, I would fain hope they will be soon fit for duty, and that in a short space of time we shall have an Army not subject to this, the greatest of all calamities that can befall it, when taken in the natural way.

Source: Washington, George. (1932). Letter of January 6, 1777, to Doctor William Shippen. In *The Writings of George Washington*, Volume 6, edited by John C. Fitzpatrick. Washington, DC: Government Printing Office, pp. 473–474.

ANALYSIS

George Washington's decision to carry out mass inoculation has been called one of his most important strategic decisions of the War of Independence. The mustering of the Continental Army brought together thousands of young men vulnerable to smallpox; not surprisingly, deadly smallpox outbreaks were a feature of the early years of the war, from 1775 to 1778. Washington and his staff also believed that the British army would employ a deliberate strategy of germ warfare: since inoculation was much more frequent in Great Britain than in the colonies, their own troops would be much less vulnerable to the disease.

In order to protect the troops, Washington relied on Dr. William Shippen (1736–1808), director general of hospitals. Shippen and his staff faced an extremely complicated administrative task. Wherever new recruits joined the army, up and down the eastern seaboard, they had to be interviewed to find out if they ever had smallpox. If they were not judged immune, they were sent to inoculation hospitals in Virginia, Maryland, Pennsylvania, New York, and Connecticut, to be inoculated and quarantined until they were no longer contagious. All these had to be carried out secretly so that the British would never learn that the Continental Army was vulnerable. The locations of some of the inoculation hospitals remain unknown to this day.

Washington defeated smallpox for his troops: the mass inoculations of soldiers between 1777 and 1778 did much to keep the Continental Army at full strength for the rest of the war. But smallpox itself was far from defeated, as both the British and American armies helped carry it to vulnerable communities of civilians and Native Americans. By the 1780s, smallpox had spread across the New World, following trade and military networks overland south to the Gulf of Mexico, north to the Arctic Circle, and west to the Pacific Ocean.

FURTHER READING

Becker, Ann. (2004). "Smallpox in Washington's Army: Strategic Implications of the Disease during the American Revolutionary War." *The Journal of Military History* 68: 381–430.

Black, Francis. (1994). "An Explanation of High Death Rates among New World Peoples When in Contact with Old World Diseases." *Perspectives in Biology and Medicine* 37: 292–307.

Fenn, Elizabeth. (2001). *Pox Americana. The Great Smallpox Epidemic of 1775–1782*. New York: Hill and Wang.

Gillette, Mary. (1981). *The Army Medical Department 1775–1818*. Washington, DC: Government Printing Office. http://history.amedd.army.mil/booksdocs/rev/gillett1/default.html.

Thacher, James. (1854). *Military Journal, during the American Revolutionary War, from 1775–1783*. Hartford, CT: Silas Andrus and Son.

3

VACCINATION BY DESIGN: SMALLPOX (1790s–1830s)

DR. JENNER'S VACCINATION REWARDED BY PARLIAMENT

- **Document:** George C. Jenner, *Evidence at Large, as Laid before the Committee of the House of Commons, Respecting Dr. Jenner's Discovery of Vaccine Inoculation*
- **Date:** 1805
- **Where:** London, United Kingdom
- **Significance:** Edward Jenner's experiments showed it was scientifically feasible to artificially stimulate an immune response in people, using a biological agent other than the disease organism. He did this by using a mild disease, cowpox, to create an immune response to a deadly disease, smallpox. His insight, followed by careful experimentation, created the science of vaccines. In 1805, the British Parliament passed a resolution awarding him £10,000, because he had made the new technique available to everyone, rather than treating it as a trade secret and patenting it for his own profit. This was, in effect, the beginning of government support for vaccination research.

DID YOU KNOW?

Napoleon and Jenner

Napoleon Bonaparte (1769–1821) was a towering figure in late18th- and early 19th-century history. A brilliant general, he rose to power in France in the aftermath of the French Revolution, becoming consul in 1799 and declaring himself emperor in 1804. During the first eight years of his government, he led French armies to victory against all the great powers of Europe while carrying out legal and political reforms at home.

Napoleon had great admiration for Edward Jenner's work on vaccination as well as an excellent eye for self-promotion. He made a practice of issuing medals to commemorate important public events, including battles, peace treaties, and founding of universities and museums. In 1804, to commemorate the newly instituted French commission on vaccination, he issued a medal with his own bust on one side and a tribute to vaccine (*La Vaccine* in French) on the other. The medal shows Aesculapius, Greek god of medicine, next to the Venus de Medici,

DOCUMENT

[No. 1] The Committee having met, Dr. Jenner was called upon for his evidence, which he delivered in the form of a printed paper as follows:

My inquiry into the nature of the cow-pox commenced upwards of twenty-five years ago. My attention to this singular disease was first excited by observing, that among those whom in the country I was frequently called upon to inoculate, many resisted every effort to give them the smallpox. These patients I found had undergone a disease they called the cow-pox, contracted by milking cows affected with a peculiar eruption on their teats. On inquiry, it appeared that it had been known among the dairies time immemorial, and that a vague opinion prevailed that it was a preventive of the small-pox ...

During the investigation of the casual cow-pox, I was struck with the idea that it might be practicable to propagate the disease by Inoculation, *after the manner of the small-pox, first from the cow, and finally from one human being to another.* I anxiously waited some time for an opportunity of putting this theory to the test. At length the period arrived. The first experiment was made upon a lad of the name of Phipps, in the spring of the year 1796, in whose arm a little vaccine virus was inserted, taken from the hand of a young woman who had been accidentally infected by a cow. Notwithstanding the resemblance which the pustule, thus excited on the boy's arm, bore to variolous inoculation, yet as the indisposition attending it was barely perceptible, I could scarcely persuade myself the patient was secure from the smallpox. However, on his being inoculated some months afterwards, it was proved he was secure.

This case inspired me with confidence, and as soon as I could again furnish myself with virus from the cow, I made an arrangement for a series of inoculations. A number of children were inoculated in succession, one from the other; and after several months had elapsed, they were exposed to the infection of the small-pox; some by inoculation, others by variolous effluvia, and some in both ways; but they all resisted it. The result of these trials gradually led me into a wider field of experiment, which I went over not only with great attention, but with painful solicitude. This became universally known through a Treatise published in June 1798. The result of my further experience was also brought forward in subsequent publications in the two succeeding years, 1799 and 1800. The distrust and scepticism which naturally arose in the minds of medical men, on my first announcing so unexpected a discovery, has now nearly disappeared. Many hundreds of them, from actual experience, have given their attestations that the inoculated cow-pox proves a perfect security

which Napoleon had looted from Florence the previous year. Venus's arm is bandaged, as if she had just been vaccinated. A cow is depicted on the left of the two figures and a lancet on the right. The message was clear: Emperor Napoleon, as patron of the arts and sciences, protected the the health and well-being of all citizens through this new medical innovation.

Since Napoleon had made such a strong public statement, Jenner was approached on a number of occasions to intercede for British citizens who were held captive by the French while the two countries were at war. In one famous interchange, Jenner wrote directly to Napoleon, asking that two of his friends, scientists and writers, be released. According to a later account, the letter was brought to Napoleon when "the Emperor was in his carriage and the horses were being changed. The petition was then presented to him ..."

Napoleon "exclaimed 'Away, Away!' The Empress Josephine who accompanied him said, 'But Emperor, do you see who this comes from? Jenner.' He changed his tone of voice that instant and said 'What that man asks is not to be refused' and the petition was immediately granted" (cited in Nixon, 1939, 50).

Jenner interceded on a number of other occasions on behalf of British detainees, and his petitions seem to have been generally successful, though there were some occasions when release orders were lost in transit. Napoleon had every reason to be grateful to Jenner. Under his authority, vaccination became routine practice in the French armies and contributed to preserving the health of soldiers and their fighting strength, for years to come.

Sources:

Nixon, J. A. (1939). "British Prisoners Released by Napoleon at Jenner's Request." *Proceedings of the Royal Society of Medicine* 32: 877–883.

"Peace." *Commemorative Medals Relating to Napoleon.* http://fortiter.napoleonicmedals.org/medals/history/peace.htm.

against the small-pox; and I shall probably be within compass if I say, thousands are ready to follow their example; for the scope that this inoculation has now taken is immense. An hundred thousand persons, upon the smallest computation, have been inoculated in these realms. The numbers who have partaken of its benefits throughout Europe and other parts of the globe are incalculable: and it now becomes too manifest to admit of controversy, that the annihilation of the small-pox, the most dreadful scourge of the human species, must be the final result of this practice ...

No. 3. Dr. Bradley, *Fellow of the Royal College of Physicians, called in and examined.*

Q. Are you in the habit of receiving communications from the faculty on the continent, and in this kingdom?

A. Constantly.

Q. What is their opinion of the vaccine inoculation?

A. I have received accounts from Cambridge near New York, and Philadelphia in America, and Germany, in all which the experience of the English practitioners is entirely confirmed; and I have strong grounds to believe it is also introduced into Turkey . . .

Q. Whom do you look upon as the original discoverer of this mode of treatment?

A. Certainly Dr. Jenner; and I believe no medical man in the world doubts it, and that in my extensive correspondence no person has put in a claim to priority . . .

[No. 4] Mr. Home, *Surgeon, called in and examined.*

Q. At what period were you first made acquainted with the vaccine inoculation?

A. In some part of the year 1788 Dr. Jenner presented to Mr. Hunter a drawing of a finger, on which there was a pustule formed by the vaccine matter, and at that time Dr. Jenner proposed to Mr. Hunter the vaccine inoculation as a mode of preventing the small-pox; which drawing Mr. Hunter at the time shewed to me, mentioning Dr. Jenner's proposition. At that time Mr. Hunter's opinion was, that Dr. Jenner should prosecute the inquiry, as it was too new for him to form an opinion upon. My own opinion is best stated by saying, I have inoculated one of my own children with it, and am satisfied with its being perfectly secure. When I have been called upon to inoculate children of delicate constitutions for the small-pox I have objected to it, and used my influence in favour of the vaccine inoculation, in which I have always succeeded, considering that in such children the risk of the small-pox was too great to be hazarded.

Q. Can the vaccine inoculation excite or create a predisposition to any other disease?

A. In my judgment I can form no idea how it should, as it disturbs the constitution less than almost any other disease. The great advantage of the vaccine inoculation over that of the small-pox is, that the constitution is less liable to be impaired by it, and therefore less liable to fall into any subsequent diseases . . .

No. 5. *Sir* Walter Farquhar *called in and examined.*

Q. Did you ever hear of the vaccine inoculation prior to its introduction by Dr. Jenner?

A. Never.

Q. Have you ever seen any cases which prove that a person who has undergone this mode of treatment is rendered unsusceptible of the smallpox?

A. I certainly have, and in my own family particularly. I had two grandchildren that had not had the small-pox; the eldest was inoculated in the usual manner, the youngest was sent out of the house to an aunt's and was inoculated with the vaccine matter. The eldest had the disease with every favourable appearance at first, but at last very violently, with a considerable eruption, and accompanied with convulsive fits. The youngest went through the vaccine inoculation in the easiest manner possible, and upon the twelfth day from the inoculation was brought home, and lived with his brother with the small-pox eruption then out, without any symptom of catching any complaint . . .

Q. Do you conceive that any very great advantage will be derived from this discovery of Dr. Jenner's?

A. I think it the greatest discovery that has been made for many years.

Q. Do you think that Dr. Jenner, by making this discovery public, suffered his own private advantage to give way to the public benefit?

A. I certainly do; and beg leave to relate what passed between Mr. Cline and myself on the subject. When it was first communicated to me by Mr. Cline, I entertained doubts respecting it, and said, if Dr. Jenner is confident of its success, and would come to town and reside in Grosvenor Square, I would insure him £10,000; but if he allowed the secret to be divulged, every practitioner would get hold of it, as it was so easily done, and he would lose all chance of emolument. Dr. Jenner's answer was, that *he would prosecute the discovery to perfection before he would quit his present situation*; by which I am of opinion he has actually lost the opportunity of making his fortune ...

No. 9. *Dr. Woodville, Physician of the Small-fox Hospital, called in and examined.*

Q. Are you conversant with the practice of vaccine inoculation?

A. Yes; ever since the beginning of the year 1798.

Q. Whom do you look upon as the discoverer thereof?

A. I consider certainly Dr. Jenner: for although since his publication it has appeared that it had been obscurely practised, the world would never have been acquainted with it but for Dr. Jenner.

Q. Have you introduced this practice into either of the hospitals of which you are physician?

A. Yes; into the Inoculation Hospital.

Q. Did you introduce this practice in consequence of Dr. Jenner's communications, or any other person's?

A. Certainly from the information of Dr. Jenner.

Q. Do you give the preference to the vaccine inoculation over the variolous?

A. Constantly.

Q. What are your motives for doing so?

A. Because, in the first place, I find it equally certain in securing the patient in future against the small-pox, as if the person were inoculated with small-pox itself: and in the next place I attain this without danger or risk to the life of the patient, as he is put to little or no inconvenience during the whole process of the inoculation.

Q. Is the cow-pox, like the small-pox, a contagious disorder?

A. Certainly not ...

Q. Is it necessary frequently to recur to the cow for original matter; or does the vaccine matter, after passing through a number of human bodies, retain its pristine mildness and efficacy?

A. I believe it retains its efficacy for any length of time while carried from one human subject to another; and I am now using matter which has passed through many hundred subjects, having been taken from the cow three years since.

Q. Have you ever inoculated with small-pox matter after the patient had taken the cow-pox, in order to try its efficacy—and what was the event?

A. The number that has been inoculated with the vaccine disease in the hospital, amounted on the first of January last to 7,500; about one half of which was since inoculated with small-pox matter, *in none of whom did the small-pox produce any effect.*

Q. Do you conceive Dr. Jenner to have made communications on this subject which have been the means of its being adopted in this kingdom and other parts of Europe; or was it any other person, or by any other means?

A. The whole entirely originated with Dr. Jenner.

Source: Jenner, George C. (1805). *Evidence at Large, as Laid before the Committee of the House of Commons, Respecting Dr. Jenner's Discovery of Vaccine Inoculation.* London: J. Murray.

ANALYSIS

Though textbooks and websites often speak of Edward Jenner's "discovery," the word is misleading. There are at least six other people who can plausibly claim to have inoculated patients with cowpox before him. We can better understand his innovation if we think of it as a solution to the social and scientific problems with smallpox inoculation developed in the last chapter. As we have seen, while inoculation could be shown to work, it was also controversial. While it might well save the lives of those inoculated, it might well also spread the disease to other vulnerable members of the community. It was really only an option for well-to-do households: most people lived in such crowded conditions that inoculating one child, or one family, could easily spread smallpox to the entire village or tenement.

What that meant was that every city, town, and village had a kind of reservoir of potential smallpox victims, one that renewed itself each time a child was born but not inoculated. In the second half of the 18th century, physicians and community leaders tried exhorting "the poor" to inoculate their children, assuring them the procedure was much safer than catching smallpox "the natural way," that is, during an outbreak. They found some success when inoculation was offered for free, either by the practitioner himself or—more usually—through medical institutions like public hospitals or dispensaries. The demand for inoculation went up dramatically whenever there was an outbreak. Yet, even then, practitioners complained that most residents neglected to get their free medical care. Or, having inoculated their children, they would not isolate themselves. Instead, recently inoculated children, still infectious, would sleep in the same room and the same bed as untreated children and go back out to work as soon as their strength returned.

By the 1790s, when Jenner began his investigation into the properties of cowpox, he was a well-established scientist and a member of Britain's prestigious Royal Society. His innovation consisted in his recognizing that if the folk belief were true, it would solve the problems posed by current inoculation methods. Cowpox was never fatal, and it was much less infectious: indeed, it could only be spread by direct, physical contact. If it could be introduced in the same way as the smallpox virus—two quick punctures with the lancet—physicians could simply substitute the new "matter" for the old. Doing so would completely eliminate the need for costly, ineffective public health measures like strict quarantine of smallpox hospitals.

Jenner tested this hypothesis by a series of careful experiments that culminated in his inoculating James Phipps (1788–1853), a healthy eight-year-old child, with cow-pox matter from the dairymaid Sarah Nelmes. Dairymaids typically developed cow-pox on their hands, that is, the part of their body that came in direct contact with the teats of cows. Jenner, though, inoculated Phipps with cowpox on the arm, as if he were following the standard procedure for smallpox. He was delighted to see that the pustules appeared in the same way as if he had used smallpox matter, but in a much milder form. He subsequently inoculated Phipps with live smallpox and found, again to his delight, that his patient experienced no sign of the disease whatever.

Jenner concluded that this new technology had worked, and his future experiments, and those of his contemporaries, supported that conclusion. This document indicates the extent of his contemporary support by medical practitioners and government officials. Vaccination, as inoculation with cowpox matter came to be called, spread rapidly throughout Great Britain, the European continent, and the United States. By 1810, Jenner noted in wonder, he was receiving thousands of letters from around the globe, including India and China.

FURTHER READING

Baxby, Derrick. (1981). *Jenner's Smallpox Vaccine. The Riddle of Vaccinia Virus and Its Origin.* London: Heinemann Educational Books.

Fisher, Richard. (1991). *Edward Jenner 1749–1823.* London: André Deutsch.

Fulford, Tim and Debbie Lee. (2000). "The Jenneration of Disease: Vaccination, Romanticism, and Revolution." *Studies in Romanticism* 39: 139–163.

Hammersten, J. F., W. Tattersall, and J. E. Hammersten. (1979). "Who Discovered Smallpox Vaccination? Edward Jenner or Benjamin Jesty?" *Transactions of the American Clinical and Climatological Association* 90: 44–55.

Simon, John. (1857). *Papers Relating to the History and Practice of Vaccination.* London: Her Majesty's Stationery Office.

"IT IS PASSING OVER A SAFE BRIDGE"

- **Document:** Philadelphia Dispensary, *A Comparative View of the Natural Small-Pox, Inoculated Small-Pox, and Vaccination in Their Effects on Individuals and Society*
- **Date:** 1803
- **Where:** Philadelphia, PA
- **Significance:** This broadsheet reproduces a table first produced by pro-vaccination advocates in London. Published by the Philadelphia Dispensary, which offered free vaccination, it was signed by the most prominent physicians in the city.

DOCUMENT

Natural Small-Pox	Inoculated Small-Pox	Vaccination
For twelve centuries this disorder has been known to continue its ravages, destroying every year an immense proportion of the population of the world. It is in some few instances mild, but for the most part violent, painful, loathsome, dangerous to life, and always CANTAGIOUS. One case in three dangerous, one in six DIES. At least half of mankind have it, consequently one in twelve of the human race perish by this disease.—In London 3000 die annually—40,000 in Great Britain and Ireland. The eruptions are numerous, painful, and disgusting. Confinement, loss of time and expence are certain, and more or less considerable.—Precautions are for the most part unavailing.—Medical treatment necessary, both during the disease, and afterwards. It occasions pitts, scars, seams, &c. disfiguring the skin, particularly the face. The subsequent diseases are scrophula in its worst forms; diseases of the skin, glands, joints, &c. and loss of sense, sight or hearing frequently follow.	For the most part mild, but sometimes violent, painful, loathsome and dangerous to life, always Contagious, and therefore gives rise to the Natural Small-pox, and has actually, by spreading the disease, increased general mortality 17 in every 1000. One in forty has a dangerous disease, one in three hundred dies.—And in London one in 100. Eruptions are sometimes very considerable—confinement loss of time and expence certain, and more or less considerable—preparation by diet, and medicine necessary—extremes of heat and cold dangerous—during ill health—teething and pregnancy to be avoided—medical treatment usually necessary. When the disease is severe deformity probable, and subsequent disorders as in the Natural Small-pox.	Is an infallible preventive of the Small Pox, always mild, free from pain or danger, NEVER FATAL, NOT CONTAGIOUS. No eruption but where VACCINATED.—No confinement loss of time or expence necessary. No precaution—no medicine required—no consequent deformity.—No SUBSEQUENT DISEASE.
It is attempting to cross a large and rapid stream by swimming, when one in six perish.	It is passing the river in a boat subject to accidents, where one in 300 perish, and one in 40 suffer partially.	It is passing over a safe bridge.

Source: Philadelphia Dispensary. (1803). *A Comparative View of the Natural Small-Pox, Inoculated Small-Pox, and Vaccination in Their Effects on Individuals and Society.* Philadelphia, PA: Jane Aikin.

ANALYSIS

The table in this document was published in a one-page newssheet and signed by 50 of Philadelphia's most illustrious medical practitioners. Based on a table first published in London, it set out what must have seemed to its authors completely unassailable logic. Smallpox was a deadly disease; inoculation with smallpox virus was less deadly but very unpleasant and highly contagious; vaccination was safe, pleasant, and effective. And they, the generous physicians of the city, were prepared to offer it for free at the Philadelphia Dispensary. The managers of the dispensary noted, "We do entirely accord with the sentiments of the Physicians, and earnestly recommend to the poor of the city, to embrace the means now offered to preserve themselves and families from a dangerous and loathsome disease by the newly discovered and happy mode of inoculation for the cow pock; which will be daily performed by the Physicians at the Dispensary."

And yet "the poor" did not instantly avail themselves of this offer or of similar offers from other city dispensaries. The reasons were to become clear during the next 100 years of public health measures aimed at the urban poor. The first was perhaps most obvious: urban residents in the lowest income groups often could not read. Instead, they would listen to broadsheets read to them, perhaps in church or in a tavern. This tabular form, so familiar to scientific readers, would have been completely lost on them.

Another problem was the terminology. Even wealthy, literate residents who had been previously familiar with smallpox inoculation found the new comparisons between "natural smallpox," "inoculated smallpox," "vaccination," and "inoculation for the cow pock" very confusing. The technique was simply a preventative for the smallpox. Poorer residents would have made the same assumption. If they had not wanted the old inoculation, we can imagine them asking, why should they want the new one, especially when they had to go out of their way to get it? "The Poor" to whom this broadsheet was addressed were the "working poor." That means they had to work every day to earn money to pay for food and rent. If they took time off from their work to go to the dispensary, they would not be paid.

There were other problems with the broadsheet, if its intent was to attract the majority of urban residents. Though signed by doctors, the sheet does not include any information from patients. Surely it would have been helpful to include some testimonials from members of "the poor" whose lives had been saved by the new methods. And why refer to them as "the poor" in any case? Most urban residents, no matter how little money they made, did not refer to themselves in that way. No one wanted to be labeled as a charity case: when patients did come to the dispensary, they were generally in such need of urgent medical care that labels no longer mattered.

In fact, it seems most likely that the intent of the broadsheet was not so much to attract poor patients as to advertise both the value of vaccination and the value of the dispensary as a public health institution to wealthy urban elites. Although vaccination did prove highly effective in reducing smallpox in Philadelphia, it was most successful when practitioners brought the vaccine to patients, rather than expecting the patients to make a special effort to get to practitioners. This lesson would be learned, unlearned, and relearned throughout the history of vaccination.

FURTHER READING

Finger, Simon. (2012). *The Contagious City. The Politics of Public Health in Early Philadelphia.* Ithaca, NY: Cornell University Press.

Klepp, Susan. (1991). "The Swift Progress of Population: A Documentary and Bibliographic Study of Philadelphia's Growth." Philadelphia, PA: American Philosophical Society.

Loetz, Francisca. (2010). "Why Change Habits? Early Modern Medical Innovation between Medicalisation and Medical Culture." *History and Philosophy of the Life Sciences* 32: 453–473.

Tunis, Barbara. (1982). "Public Vaccination in Lower Canada, 1815–1823: Controversy and a Dilemma." *Historical Reflections/ Réflexions Historique* 9: 264–278.

Unrau, William. (1989). "Fur Trader and Indian Office Obstruction to Smallpox Vaccination in the St. Louis Indian Superintendency, 1831–1834." *Plains Anthropologist* 34: 33–39.

SPREADING VACCINATION WORLDWIDE

- **Document:** Extracts, *Philadelphia Medical Museum*, John Redman Coxe, editor
- **Date:** 1805–1807
- **Where:** Philadelphia, PA
- **Significance:** Dr. John Redman Coxe of Philadelphia was one of the earliest adopters of Jenner's vaccination. He began vaccinating patients with cowpox matter sent to him by Thomas Jefferson, ultimately building up one of the largest practices in the city. As editor of the journal *Philadelphia Medical Museum*, he made a point of reporting the progress of vaccination around the world.

DOCUMENT

Dr. DeCarro, in a letter to the editors of the Bibliotheque Britannique, dated Vienna, March 27, 1804, giving an account of the success of vaccination in the East, states, "that it is now practiced every where from Cape Comorin to Delhi."

He adds, that he had succeeded in transmitting to Dr Milne, physician to the English factor at Bassora [Iraq], the vaccine infection on lint; the matter *still moist*, at the end of November, though the packet was dispatched from Vienna in the beginning of August."

Source: Philadelphia Medical Museum 1805, 1: 98.

The following valuable extract from a Paris paper ... will doubtless be read with the highest satisfaction by the friends of vaccination throughout America, as an ample proof, in addition to former testimonials, of the security obtained by that practice against the small-pox ...

"Six black children, the first who were vaccinated in the Isle de la Reunion [Réunion], and whose infection afterwards served for more than 5000 other individuals, were embarked in the vessel, the Young Caroline, (infected with the small-pox) and carried to one of the Isles des Seychelles, where the vessel was obliged to perform quarantine. These six children

DID YOU KNOW?

A Prayer for Inoculation

In Jenner's day, religious values could provide the strongest support for protection against smallpox. In urban centers, religious leaders promoted education and charitable institutions to encourage poor as well as rich to seek, first, inoculation and then vaccination. In the countryside, clergymen and wealthy elites gave their support to the new practice, often providing the necessary funds out of their own pocket.

In Scotland, in 1792, an influential local landowner, Lawrence Oliphant, decided to take especially decisive steps to promote the spread of inoculation. As his daughter later explained, he assembled "all the poor people in the neighborhood in his house who wished—or rather who would consent to have their children inoculated for the smallpox." He paid for a physician and several apprentices to stand by while he offered the following prayer:

O Lord from whom health only can come—look favorably on the endeavors used to soften the effects of a loathsome disease to the children of this parish and neighborhood & grant thy blessing on these endeavors, may the parents and all concerned by watchful in their care of the children, may they pass through this disease with ease and safety, and if agreeably in Thy sight may their recovery be a means of encouraging the neighboring country to follow the example, save distress to the children, make them thankful, give comfort to their parents, all be to the glory of the Father, through the merits of Jesus Christ our Lord, in whose name and words we further pray.

Then, the medical practitioners "gave the infection to about sixty children."

Oliphant's daughter was convinced that the prayers, as well as the medicine, were effective. "It pleased our Heavenly Father," she wrote, "so completely to hear the prayer of his servant (in which we all joined every day which any of them was in danger) that none of them had any alarming symptoms or even a mark remaining—excepting two —who recovered perfectly though they had not the disease so very easily, as all the others had."

Within 10 years, the inoculation Oliphant promoted had been replaced by Jenner's vaccination, but physicians and local elites continued to recognize the power of the clergy and prayer in spreading support for vaccination throughout their congregation.

Source: "Prayer by Lawrence Oliphant of Gask on Behalf of Inoculation against Small Pox, c. 1792." Edinburgh: National Archives of Scotland Mss. GD/155/1322.

remained three months on board, constantly placed in the focus of the infection; and pains were taken to make them live, eat, and sleep with the infected. They were also, during the quarantine, twice inoculated for the small-pox, each time with large incisions in both arms. It is stated by the register, daily kept, that these six children having slept under the bed-clothes of the persons having the small-pox, in contact with their pustules, eating and drinking out of the same utensils, having been twice inoculated from those, who afterwards fell victims to their disorder, were *preserved from all contagion, and continue at the present time in perfect health . . .*"

Source: Philadelphia Medical Museum 1805, 1: 353.

The society lately instituted at Lausanne, to exterminate the small-pox by vaccination, have publicly offered to pay 100 livres to any person who, after successfully undergoing vaccination under their care, shall take the small-pox.

Source: Philadelphia Medical Museum 1805, 1: 354.

Dr. Bremer, physician to the great Orphan Hospital at Berlin, observes, that in 100,000 cases of vaccination, that have more or less immediately come under his cognizance, not a single instance of subsequent small pox has occurred: he has himself vaccinated more than 4,000 subjects.

Source: Philadelphia Medical Museum 1805, 1: 453.

On Sunday the 7th of last September, Dr. Francis X. de Balmis, honorary surgeon of the Royal Chamber, had the honour of kissing the hand of his Majesty, on his return from a voyage round the world, undertaken with the sole view of carrying to all the Spanish dominions beyond sea, as well as to those of other nations, the inestimable blessing of vaccination. His Majesty deeply interested in the subject, informed himself of the principal events of the expedition, and was wonderfully gratified by finding that the happy results had far exceeded the expectations formed when it was planned.

The persons attached to the expedition were, several physicians, with assistants, and 22 children, who had not had the small-pox, and were destined to preserve the valuable fluid, by a successive vaccination from arm to arm, or one after another in the course of the voyage. They sailed from the port of Coruña, under the direction of Balmis on the 20th November, 1803. They first touched at the Canaries, then at Puerto Rico, and from thence proceeded to Caracas. On leaving the port of La Guaira in that province, they separated into two parties, the one sailing for South America under the care of the sub-director Dr. Francis Salvani; the other under Dr. Balmis for Havana, and from thence to Yucatan. In this province they again made a division. Dr. Francis Pastor proceeded from the port of Sisal to that of Villahermosa in the province of Tabasco, to propagate vaccination in the royal city of Chiapas, and as far as Guatemala, passing through a tedious and rough country for 400 leagues to Oaxaca; whilst the other party arriving safely at Vera Cruz, not only passed through the whole viceroy-ship of New Spain but the interior provinces, from whence they were to return to Mexico which was the point of reunion. Having profusely disseminated this preservative from the natural small-pox, through the northern parts of Spanish America, to the coasts of Sonora and Sinaloa, and even to the Pagans and new converts; having established in each capital a central *society*, composed of *the highest authorities* and most zealous medical characters, to preserve it as a sacred deposit, for which they were answerable to the king and posterity. The director determined, that this part of the expedition, which had been crowned with the most brilliant success, should carry to Asia this consolation of humanity; and having overcome some difficulties, they embarked at Acapulco for the Philippine islands, which was the ultimate point prescribed to them.

The great and pious designs of his Majesty being favoured by Providence, Dr. Balmis accomplished his passage in little more than two months, taking with him from New Spain 26 children to be successively vaccinated; and, as many of them were very small, they were placed under the care of a matron from the orphan house of Corunna; and in this, as in the former voyages, the greatest attention was paid to their cleanliness and comfort.

Source: Philadelphia Medical Museum 1807, 3:237–238.

ANALYSIS

In order to carry out vaccination, physicians had to solve two problems. The first was convincing patients to be vaccinated. This was not difficult in the case of many well-to-do families, especially in big seaport cities where inoculation had been practiced for years. Since patients were used to the technique of inoculation, it was easy for physicians to make the case for the milder cowpox. The "passing over a safe bridge" argument worked very well.

But not everyone found it easy to understand why being treated with one disease could prevent another. Preventing a deadly disease like smallpox with actual smallpox virus made sense in the way that many people, then and now, think about the disease. It could be thought of as "fighting fire with fire" or treating a hangover by taking a drink. But there was no folk-medicine analogy for using a mild disease to drive away a dangerous one. Some patients feared that there was no way to know if vaccination truly prevented smallpox until a dangerous epidemic came around. And surely then it would be too late.

Vaccination advocates had no more knowledge than their patients of exactly why cowpox worked. What they emphasized instead was all the practical demonstrations that it really did work. The six children kept on board a quarantine ship off the Seychelles, forced to eat, drink, and sleep with desperately sick sailors, makes for gruesome reading today. The point it conveyed to its readers was that vaccination was a kind of force field that kept the children safe, even directly in the path of contagion. Pro-vaccination writers carried out similar experiments with their own children, handing their recently vaccinated babies to smallpox patients to be held and kissed. As those children grew up, they became practical demonstrations of yet another value to vaccination: the force field did not wear off but instead lasted for the rest of their lives.

The very efficacy of cowpox brought about the second problem: how to propagate it so as to ensure enough of a supply. A key advantage of cowpox was that it was not contagious, but that became a disadvantage for any physician who wanted to be able to vaccinate on a regular basis. The physician had, in effect, to use people—generally children—as a kind of soil on which to grow cowpox matter, transplanting the material from one child to the next. Physicians soon found that it might be kept for several months if carefully preserved on a string or on a glass slide. But the most reliable way to ensure a supply was to have a large number of vaccine patients and to keep transplanting the matter from old patients to new ones.

Dr. Francis de Balmis's voyage to disseminate cowpox around the world provides an especially vivid depiction of the problem of supply. The 22 children who accompanied him from Spain to Mexico and the further 26 children—some of them babies—who traveled on to the Philippines were necessary to ensure that live, active cowpox reached the far side of the world. Since the children were not vaccinated all at once, the non-vaccinated ones would have been vulnerable to smallpox if they had encountered it on the voyage. But vaccinating them all at once would have eliminated the supply of cowpox matter after a mere 8–10 days at sea. We can only hope that they received some reward for their service to Spain beyond the "inestimable blessing" of vaccination.

FURTHER READING

Few, Martha. (2010). "Circulating Smallpox Knowledge: Guatemalan Doctors, Maya Indians and Designing Spain's Smallpox Vaccination Expedition, 1780–1803." *British Journal for the History of Science* 43: 519–537.

Huerkamp, Claudia. (1985). "The History of Smallpox Vaccination in Germany: A First Step in the Medicalization of the General Public." *Journal of Contemporary History* 20: 617–635.

Rigau-Perez, Jose. (1989). "The Introduction of Smallpox Vaccine in 1803 and the Adoption of Immunization as a Government Function in Puerto Rico." *The Hispanic-American Historical Review* 69: 393–423.

Thompson, Angela. (1993). "To Save the Children: Smallpox Inoculation, Vaccination, and Public Health in Guanajuato, Mexico, 1797–1840." *The Americas* 49: 431–455.

Walker, Brett. (1999). "The Early Modern Japanese State and Ainu Vaccinations: Redefining the Body Politic 1799–1868." *Past and Present* 163: 121–160.

"DISTRACTED WITH DOUBT, AND LABOURING UNDER GLOOMY APPREHENSIONS"

- **Document:** Benjamin Moseley, *A Treatise on Sugar with Miscellaneous Medical Observations*
- **Date:** 1800
- **Where:** London, United Kingdom
- **Significance:** Attacks on vaccination often came through appeals to the public. Documents 4 and 6, below, show the rhetorical strategies used by medical writers to discredit Jenner's methods in books, pamphlets, and newspaper articles, intended to win the hearts and minds of patients. Once published, critics could employ those same rhetorical strategies against the anti-vaccine writers, as we can see in Document 5.

DOCUMENT

The *Cow-Pox* has lately appeared in England. This is a new star in the Aesculapian system. It was first observed from the Provinces . . .

To preserve, as far as in my lies, the genesis of this desirable—this excelling distemper, to posterity,—I mention, that it is said to originate in what is called, the *greasy heel* distemper, in horses. These *greasy heels*, are said to infect the hands of people who dress and clean them. The hands of people thus infected, are said to infect the teats of cows in milking them. The teats of these infected cows in return, are said to infect the hands of others who milk them; and so the distemper, is said to be propagated among the country people.

The virtues of this charming distemper, are said to be an amulet against the small-pox; that it is mild and innocent; and communicated with safety by inoculation . . .

In this *Cowmania*, it is not enough for reason to concede, that the Cow-pox may *lessen, for a time*, the disposition in the habit to receive the infection of the *Small-pox* . . .

But no complaint to which people are repeatedly subject, as the Cow-pox, can perform all circumstances in the habit, equivalent to the Small-pox, which people never have but once . . . the Small-pox and the Cow-pox, then, are not analogous; but radically dissimilar.

The Small-pox is undoubtedly an evil; but we understand the extent of that ill; which we had better bear, "than fly to others that we know not of."

Inoculation has disarmed the Small-pox of its terrors, and reduced it to management.

I have inoculated in the West Indies, and in Europe, several thousands. I never lost a patient . . . I should not have mentioned this, but that it gives me an opportunity of saying many others, whom I know, have done the same, with the same success. Accidents, in the inoculated Small-pox, are uncommon; and we all know from experience, that disease, properly treated, leaves nothing after it injurious to the constitution. . . .

Can any person say what may be the consequences of introducing the *Lues Bovilla*, a *bestial* humour—into the human frame, after a long lapse of years?

Who knows, besides, what ideas may rise, in the course of time, from a *brutal* fever having excited its incongruous impressions on the brain?

Who knows, also, but that the human character may undergo strange mutations from *quadrupedan* sympathy . . .

Source: Moseley, Benjamin. (1800). "Cow-Pox." A *Treatise on Sugar with Miscellaneous Medical Observations*. London: John Nichols.

- **Document:** "Review of a Treatise on the Lues Bovilla, or Cow Pox," published in *The Critical Review*
- **Date:** 1805
- **Where:** London, United Kingdom

DOCUMENT

It were not very easy to characterize this serio-comic pamphlet. Waggery, ridicule, and sarcasm, transcripts of newspaper advertisements, of the addresses of committees and institutions, and of the evidence given before the House of Commons, and lastly, some cases, most uncircumstantially related, in which small pox is said to have occurred after cow pox, constitute the motley composition . . . It contains . . . some notable discoveries. In the first place . . . the cow pox is the parent of a host of diseases 'totally new' . . . In the next place, pustules have been seen, such as never appeared before; as large as cherries, and filled with matter, some green, some yellow, some blue! . . . Moreover, no disease has been found to be so singularly tormenting. 'I have seen *children* die of the cow pox,' says the author, 'without losing the sense of torment even in the article of death! I saw *one child*, in Chelsea, that died in the 16th day after inoculation; who shewed evident signs of severe anguish on being touched in the slightest manner, at the very moment she expired.' . . . But this is not all. 'Several children have died from diseases, brought on by the cow pox, when no ulcerations had appeared; and others have lost their nails, and end of their fingers, *several months* after inoculation.' . . . And besides . . . his 'accounts from the country are full of dismal histories of ulcerated arms, and mortifications, of which *one* person lately died.'

But we would be serious. All this may be admitted in an essay . . . in which vague allusion, appeals to prejudice, and ridicule may consistently enough supply the place of accuracy of detail, of philosophy, and of argument. But we have received our principles upon evidence alone, and are ready to abjure them only when that evidence is countervailed ... But the prejudice was unconquerable with Dr. Mosely. 'I thought then (in 1798,) as I do now, that *experience is not necessary*, to know that cow pox cannot be a preventive of the small pox.' ... This is giving the lie to Bacon and to Newton, and trampling inductive philosophy under foot. We believe indeed, that the investigation has not been complete and final; and fear that it has often been conducted carelessly ... But we cannot forget that, on a question of *fact*, analogy, ridicule, and general assertions, are but as a feather in the balance, when poised against the leaden weight of the results of experiment and induction.

Source: "Review of a Treatise on the Lues Bovilla, or Cow Pox." (1805). *The Critical Review* 5: 329–330.

- **Document:** John Birch, *An Appeal to the Public on the Hazard and Peril of Vaccination, Otherwise Cow Pox*
- **Date:** 1817
- **Where:** London, United Kingdom

DOCUMENT

THAT the enthusiasm with which Vaccination was at first adopted should subside, and that the Public should express regret that what ought to have been admitted as an experiment only, had been adopted as practice, are circumstances which it was easy to foresee, would sooner or later occur. In all investigations, and in all enquiries, Truth must ultimately prevail. In the present it would have long since prevailed, had not the patrons of Vaccination had recourse to such expedients to interest the passions, and mislead the judgment of the Public, as could hardly fail of obtaining for their system, a temporary kind of success. But the triumph of prejudice and novelty will always be transient. The empire of Truth alone is permanent. I entertain no doubt therefore but that we shall soon see what yet remains of popular opinion favourable to the cause of Vaccination, vanish into thin air; and that the speculatists in physic, like the speculatists in polities, will be brought back to the old standard of sober reason and experience.

Impressed with this conviction I should have patiently awaited the event, and contenting myself with having declared my opinion publicly, should have forborne taking any part in the controversy, had it not been for considerations of humanity, which supercede every other.

Wherever I go I find the minds of parents distracted with doubt, and labouring under gloomy apprehensions. They tell me that the fluctuations of medical opinion concerning the origin, and nature of the Vaccine disease fills them with alarm; and they say they are in the most fearful state of suspense, dreading lest what they were persuaded to do in the hopes of saving their children from one disease, may not prove the means of plunging them into another, at once novel and malignant.

Much as I lament their being in so distressing a state of suspense, I cannot wonder at it. For while on the one hand they hear of repeated instances of the failure of Vaccination, on the other they find, that reports from the Jennerian Committee, subscribed by names, some of the highest respectability, are widely circulated, full of seeming arguments and assertions in favour of the experiment; assertions which they have not the means of contradicting; and arguments just plausible enough to excite doubt, but not sufficiently strong to operate conviction.

Source: Birch, John. (1817). *An Appeal to the Public on the Peril and Hazard of Vaccination, Otherwise Cow Pox.* London: J. Harris.

ANALYSIS

Vaccination had its medical critics in the early 19th century, like inoculation before it. The most outspoken opponents of the new practice were those who had established their professional reputations through inoculation of live smallpox virus. Benjamin Moseley (1742–1819) was a successful medical practitioner in Jamaica. He published treatises on dysentery, coffee, and sugar, all subjects of interest to the British families in the Caribbean, and was appointed surgeon-general. His books make painful reading today for their racism, intolerance, and inaccuracy, but they sold well and helped promote his business investments in Caribbean plantations. On returning to London, he established a successful practice among the London elite.

Moseley seems to have taken the success of vaccination and Parliament's patronage of Jenner as personal attacks. He responded by publishing a series of pamphlets on the dangers of what he called the "Lues Bovilla" or cattle (bovine) plague. This would have been clear to his contemporaries as a reference to *Lues Venerea*, the medical Latin name for syphilis. Moseley invented a whole new set of diseases that, he claimed, affected children who had been vaccinated: Facies Bovilla, or Cow Pox Face, Scabies Bovilla, Cow Pox Itch or Mange, Tinea Bovilla, or Cow Pox Scaldhead, and Elephantiasis Bovilla, or Cow Pox Farcy. He made up case histories, such as Sarah Burley, "whose face was distorted, and began to resemble that of an Ox," "Edward Gee who was covered with sores, and afterwards with patches of Cow's Hair," and little William Ince, "vaccinated when four months old," who broke out in all manner of sores and eruptions all over his body. They eventually dried up but then there "appeared on his back and loins, patches of hair; not resembling his own hair, for that was of light colour, but brown; and of the same length, and quality, as that of a Cow." The message was clear: vaccinate your child, and he will turn into a cow. And not even a healthy cow: as Moseley concluded, the child "remained in a miserable state, under various changes, until he was three years and a half old, when he languished and died."

The reviewer in the literary journal *The Critical Review* could afford to treat such case histories as jokes, but pro-vaccination physicians found they had to take them seriously. The excerpt from John Birch (1745–1815), another London practitioner who had built a lucrative inoculation practice, shows why: families were puzzled by a new technique that seemed to divide the medical profession. Birch did his best to spread doubt among them. He pointed to the fact that Jenner himself had described his early vaccination efforts as "experiments" and that none of the pro-vaccination physicians could say why, precisely, cowpox worked. He asked, did parents want to be part of an experimental trial? Did they want to inject this foreign, animal substance into their children?

Both Moseley and Birch contributed to the medical journal *Medical Observer*, started ostensibly to enlighten the public about quack medicines, but which in fact was the mouthpiece of anti-vaccination writers. As late as 1808, the journal continued to describe smallpox inoculation as "that mild, safe, and certain process," which "this country and the world enjoyed without interruption, until the springing up of that empirical and unphilosophical idea of attempting to prevent the Small-pox, by introducing a bestial humour into the human frame" (*Medical Observer* 3: 258).

By that time, anti-vaccination combatants were fighting a rearguard action: cowpox vaccination had become mainstream medical practice among elite practitioners and their patients, and new public health measures were underway that made it standard practice in many countries. But writers like Moseley and Birch highlighted a major weakness in the way many medical professionals approached vaccination advocacy. Medical writers for the next 200 years assumed that if they could marshal scientific evidence in favor of vaccines, they would be able to convince their patients. What they found, however, is that patients expected more from their practitioners than just scientific evidence: they also wanted certainty and trust: certainty, to ensure that the prescribed treatment actually worked as specified, and that it did no harm; trust, to ensure that their doctors always told them the truth, and the whole truth. Promoting uncertainty and fomenting distrust remained tactics of anti-vaccination rhetoric to the present day.

FURTHER READING

Brunton, Deborah. (2004). "Birch, John." "Moseley, Benjamin." *Oxford Dictionary of National Biography*. http://www.oxforddnb.com/.

Lee, Debbie. (2002). *Slavery and the Romantic Imagination*. Philadelphia, PA: University of Pennsylvania Press.

Richardson, Alan. (1993). "Romantic Voodoo: Obeah and British Culture, 1997–1807." *Studies in Romanticism* 32: 3–28.

Rosner, Lisa. (2012). "What's in a Name? Or, Will Vaccination Turn Your Children into Cows?" *History of Vaccines*. http://www.historyofvaccines.org/content/blog/what's -name-or-will-vaccination-turn-your-children-cows.

Schiebinger, Londa. (2004). *Plants and Empire: Colonial Bioprospecting in the Atlantic World*. Cambridge, MA: Harvard University Press.

WHO SHOULD BE AUTHORIZED TO VACCINATE?

- **Document:** Report from the Academy of Medicine
- **Date:** 1837
- **Where:** Paris, France
- **Significance:** These two documents illustrate a key component of vaccination as a public health initiative: the requirement that safe, effective vaccines be distributed by health-care professionals who are both well trained and trusted by prospective patients and their families. This is as necessary today as it was in the 19th century.

DOCUMENT

After the discussion on statistics at the Academy of Medicine, a discourse was made on one of the discoveries most important to society, which incontestably is vaccination; its happy influence has so powerfully contributed to the prolongation of human life, and has preserved us from the infirmities which so often followed the fatal action of variola [smallpox].

Notwithstanding its undoubted utility, it has long been the subject of unfounded and undeserved criticism. Soon after the discovery of vaccination, Government understood its importance, and placed it under its protection; yet its triumph was difficult, and unforeseen, and unexpected obstacles were daily encountered.

Vaccination has this year again proved a certain preservative against variola. M. Barrey de Besancon, who has vaccinated for two-and-thirty years, wrote to the Academy, to state that he had never seen a single case of variola in any person who had been vaccinated: he observes, that in many places, children are vaccinated by ignorant apothecaries, or midwives, unable to distinguish good vaccination from bad, and who only desire to perform the operation frequently, but are wholly indifferent as to its results; should the small-pox be afterwards caught, they attribute it to vaccination, and not to their own carelessness.

Source: "Varieties. Paris and London." (1837). *Continental and British Medical Review* 1: 422.

- **Document:** Antoine Barthelemy Clot, "On the Medical Institutions of Cairo"
- **Date:** 1838
- **Where:** Cairo, Egypt

DOCUMENT

The hospital and school of medicine formerly existing at Abou-zabel have lately been removed to Cairo. Here also are formed an establishment for pharmacy, a new botanical garden, a museum of natural history, a civil hospital, and a "matern-ité" [maternity hospital] ... It was required to find in Cairo a building sufficiently large to contain from one thousand to fifteen hundred patients, accommodation for three hundred students, and rooms appropriate for their instruction ... The building is surrounded by fine walks. Its form is square: it has two stories above the ground-floor. All the wings consist of a double row of wards, separated by a corridor. Each wing is divided into four wards, each ward containing fifty beds. The first floor consists of vaulted chambers, which are used as stores. In the center of the building is a large court, planted with trees. Connected with the south wing are four large buildings, separated one from the other. The first is employed for amphitheatres, chemical laboratories, cabinets of physics and natural history; the second for dormitories and refectories; the third for pharmacy; the fourth for kitchens, baths, and waiting places ...

The necessity of a *maternité* has been strongly felt. The negresses and Abyssinian women have hitherto learned the art of midwifery in a school at Abou-zabel. Thirteen of them have already learned to write Arabic very correctly: they have studied the art of midwifery in a treatise translated into that language, together with demonstrations on an anatomical figure conducted by an European female teacher; and a professor to whom the teaching of the art is entrusted. A small hospital for females annexed to their school has afforded them an opportunity of superintending some deliveries; together with the practice of bleeding, vaccination, and surgical dressing. They have been instructed in some simple medical subjects, and in the preparation of some medicines. A distinguished student from the Maternité of Paris (Madame Gault) has been attached to the establishment as [chief midwife]. She has found the female students very much advanced, and very capable of advancement ...

The females of the capital and of the provinces will be admitted, instructed, fed, and clothed, at the expense of the government. They will receive rewards in the same manner as the students of the school of medicine. Orphans, and the daughters of soldiers who have died or who are in active service, will be chiefly selected as students. The capital will furnish twenty students, and each province will supply four; making upwards of a hundred. A body of educated midwives will thus be formed ...

Source: Clot, Antoine Barthelemy [Clot Bey]. (1838). "On the Medical Institutions of Cairo." *British and Foreign Medical Review* 11: 592–594.

ANALYSIS

As techniques for vaccination spread, the question arose, who should be authorized to offer it to patients? As with many other aspects of the history of vaccines, the answer was contested.

In many cities in Europe and in the United States, university-trained physicians competed with many other types of practitioners to attract paying patients. To do so, they emphasized their main assets: extensive education and scientific credentials. Vaccination became a new scientific technique that they could use to attract patients. Though not especially lucrative in itself, a vaccination practice was a way of advertising to patients that a physician was up-to-date, efficient, modern—that is, that he or she could provide the best of care.

The difficulty was that the largest group of potential patients were young children, and in the early 19th century, medical care of young children was generally in the hands of another group of medical practitioners, midwives. In fact, midwives continued to dominate obstetric practice even in industrialized countries until the early 1900s. The actual technique of vaccination was very simple to master. It did not require a university education—after all, Edward Jenner himself did not have a university degree. What it did require was initial access to "cow-pox matter." Wherever possible, physicians made a point of limiting access to cowpox to their own professional circle, thus keeping the technique in their own hands. They justified this by saying that only properly trained physicians could perform the technique properly and by blaming all accounts of infection or mistakes on "ignorant apothecaries and midwives," as in the Academy of Medicine's excerpt above.

This was, quite simply, self-serving propaganda. Since the majority of vaccinations were performed by physicians, the majority of mistakes can be traced directly to their doors. John Redman Coxe even published a list in the *Philadelphia Medical Museum* of 12 things that could go wrong in vaccination. It seems likely, though, that many midwives would have recognized that incorporating the new technique into their practice could involve them in controversy. Rather than fighting with physicians, they found a better professional strategy in forming alliances, by referring their young patients—and their parents—to physicians who had a ready supply of the cowpox matter.

That may have solved the problem to the satisfaction of physicians, but national governments were not as well satisfied. As the 19th century progressed, government officials increasingly promoted public health practices, including vaccination. They confronted the problem that limiting vaccination practice to university-trained physicians meant limiting it to major cities. What could they do about the countryside, where there were not enough paying patients to support a university-trained physician? Surely there were other people who could be trained to offer vaccination.

France confronted this problem in two areas: obstetric practice and education for girls. The solution was to offer scholarships for smart young women from the provinces to study in Paris, with the understanding that they would then go back and teach or practice in their own villages. In Paris, young women received obstetric training in the famous maternity hospital La Maternité, where vaccination was incorporated into the curriculum. That education was subsequently transplanted to Egypt, as described in the excerpt from Antoine Clot (1793–1868). Clot Bey, as he was known, was the chief medical advisor to the Viceroy of Egypt and founder of the Cairo hospital and medical school. His belief in his educated midwives was sincere, but his efforts to promote vaccination met with considerable resistance in many Egyptian villages, where families believed that vaccination would be the first step toward conscripting their sons for military service. Like many top-down approaches to vaccination, this one did little to promote support at the local level.

The Swedish government's approach was more effective. In 1802, vaccination was officially sanctioned by the Board of Health, and, in 1816, the Swedish Parliament made it compulsory. The Board of Health also made the commonsense decision that the best way to disseminate vaccination was to bring it to families, rather than expecting families to come to the vaccine. Any local official could be authorized to perform vaccination, with church assistants being most common in the first half of the century and midwives taking over in the second half. As a result of these measures, childhood mortality from smallpox decreased to insignificance in Sweden.

FURTHER READING

Fahmy, Khaled. (1997). *All the Pasha's Men. Mehmed Ali, His Army, and the Making of Modern Egypt.* Cairo: American University in Cairo Press.

Margadent, Jo Burr. (1990). *Madame Le Professeur: Women Educators in the Third Republic.* Princeton, NJ: Princeton University Press.

Nguyen, Thuy Linh. (2010). "French-Educated Midwives and the Medicalization of Childbirth in Colonial Vietnam." *Journal of Vietnamese Studies* 5: 133–182.

Skold, Peter. (1996). "From Inoculation to Vaccination: Smallpox in Sweden in the Eighteenth and Nineteenth Centuries." *Population Studies* 50: 247–262.

Weiner, Doris and Michael Sauter. (2003). "The City of Paris and the Rise of Clinical Medicine." *Osiris* 18: 23–42.

4

EPIDEMICS IN THE INDUSTRIAL AGE (1840s–1860s)

MAKING THE CASE FOR EXPERIMENTAL MEDICINE

- **Document:** Claude Bernard, *An Introduction to the Study of Experimental Medicine*
- **Date:** 1865
- **Where:** Paris, France
- **Significance:** To mid-19th-century European and American observers, the triumphs of science were everywhere. Progress in physics and chemistry had led directly to inventions that were rapidly transforming everyday life, such as the steam engine, the electromagnet, and the aniline dye industry. This progress was based upon careful, controlled experiment. Physicians, too, looked for progress in medicine. The question is, how could it be achieved? In this passage, Claude Bernard, a prominent physiologist, calls for the same experimental standards in physiological research as scientists adhered to in other sciences. That would lead, he believed, a truly scientific medicine.

DID YOU KNOW?

The Coffin Ships

The rise of industrialization led to unprecedented movements of people, which unfortunately could lead to unprecedented public health tragedies. From 1845 to 1852, the potato crop in Ireland was decimated by potato blight, and the resulting Great Famine led to an estimated 1 million deaths from starvation and another million Irish immigrants to the United States and Canada.

In 1847, a quarantine station in Grosse Isle, Quebec, Canada, became the site of a terrible epidemic of typhus that killed more than 20,000 men, women, and children on their way from Ireland to what they expected would be their new homes. In the middle of May, the first ship arrived from Great Britain with over 400 fever victims. Another 36 ships arrived by the end of the month, each with hundreds of patients suffering from dysentery, typhus, and other fevers. The hospital facilities at Grosse Point were not built to accommodate such numbers and soon were filled to bursting. Every bed was taken, and health authorities had to put patients in tents and hastily constructed fever sheds, without clean water or sewage

DOCUMENT

To Conserve and to Cure Disease: Medicine is still pursuing a scientific solution of this problem, which has confronted it from the first. The present state of medical practice suggests that a solution is still far to seek. During its advance through the centuries, however, medicine has always been driven into action and from numberless ventures in the realm of empiricism has gained useful information. Though furrowed and overturned by all manner of systems so evanescent that, one by one, they have disappeared, it has none the less carried on research, acquired ideas and piled up precious materials which in due time will find their place and meaning in scientific medicine. Today, thanks to the great development and powerful support of the physico-chemical sciences, study of the phenomena of life, both normal and pathological, has made progress which continues with surprising rapidity.

It is therefore clear to all unprejudiced minds that medicine is turning toward its permanent scientific path. By the very nature of its evolutionary advance, it is little by little abandoning the region of systems, to assume a more and more analytic form, and thus gradually to join in the method of investigation common to the experimental sciences.

In order to embrace the medical problem as a whole, experimental medicine must include three basic parts: physiology, pathology and therapeutics. Knowledge of causes of the phenomena of life in the normal state, i.e., physiology, will teach us to maintain normal conditions of life and to conserve health. Knowledge of diseases and of their determining causes, i.e., pathology, will lead us, on the one hand, to prevent the development of morbid conditions, and, on the other, to fight their results with medical agents, i.e., to cure the diseases.

In the empirical period of medicine, which must doubtless still be greatly prolonged, physiology and therapeutics could advance separately; for as neither of them was well established, they were not called upon mutually to support each other in medical practice. But this cannot be so when medicine becomes scientific: it must then be founded on physiology. Since science can be established only by the comparative method, knowledge of pathological or abnormal conditions cannot be gained without previous knowledge of normal states, just as the therapeutic action of abnormal agents, or medicines, on the organism cannot be scientifically understood without first studying the physiological action of the normal agents which maintain the phenomena of life.

facilities. As the numbers grew, desperately ill patients were kept on ships, unable to land, because there were no facilities for them. In an effort to make room for new arrivals, many patients were transferred to quarantine quarters in Montreal. There, too, hospital facilities could not contain the disease, and the typhus epidemic spread to surrounding areas.

The ships carrying the immigrants became known as "coffin ships," and a contemporary author, writing under the name Robert Whyte, gave a firsthand account of the voyage. "Poor creatures," he wrote, of the farming families who agreed to leave Ireland, "they thought that any change would be for the better. They had nothing to risk, everything to gain. 'Ah! Sir,' said a fellow passenger to me after bewailing the folly that tempted him to plunge his family into aggravated misfortune, 'we thought we couldn't be worse off than we war but now to our sorrow we know the differ for sure supposin' we were dyin' of starvation or if sickness overtuk us, we had a chance of a doctor and if he could do no good for our bodies sure the priest could for our souls and then we'd be buried along wid our own people, in the ould churchyard, with the green sod over us, instead of dying like rotten sheep thrown into a pit, and the minit the breath is out of our bodies flung into the sea to be eaten up by them horrid sharks'"(Whyte, 1848, 94).

In 1997, 150 years after the epidemic, the National Famine Monument in Murrisk, Ireland, commissioned artist John Behan (b. 1938) to create a memorial sculpture depicting a coffin ship filled with skeleton bodies.

Sources:
Ireland's Great Hunger Museum. http://ighm.org.
Whyte, Robert. (1848). *The Journey of an Irish Coffin Ship.* http://xroads.virginia.edu/~hyper/sadlier/irish/rwhyte.htm.

But scientific medicine, like the other sciences, can be established only by experimental means, i.e., by direct and rigorous application of reasoning to the facts furnished us by observation and experiment. Considered in itself, the experimental method is nothing but reasoning by whose help we methodically submit our ideas to experience,—the experience of facts . . .

To be worthy of the name, an experimenter must be at once theorist and practitioner. While he must completely master the art of establishing experimental facts, which are the materials of science, he must also clearly understand the scientific principles which guide his reasoning through the varied experimental study of natural phenomena. We cannot separate these two things: head and hand. An able hand, without a head to direct it, is a blind tool; the head is powerless without its executive hand . . .

The ideas which we shall here set forth are certainly by no means new; the experimental method and experimentation were long ago introduced into the physico-chemical sciences, which owe them all their brilliancy . . . Our single aim is, and has always been, to help make the well-known principles of the experimental method pervade medical science.

Source: Bernard, Claude. (1927). *An Introduction to the Study of Experimental Medicine*, trans. Henry Copley Greene. New York: Henry Schuman, Inc.

ANALYSIS

It may seem self-evident that medicine should be scientific, and if by *scientific* we mean the word *rational*, then there would be little room for debate. But if by *scientific* we mean "following the scientific method of hypthothesis and controlled experiment," then we might find numerous obstacles. The first has to do with the setting in which medical treatment takes place. Traditionally, that setting is initiated when a patient falls sick or is injured. He or she calls a healer, whose charge is to treat that particular patient to the best of his or her ability. In every culture that has a healing profession—there are very few that do not—an individual healer has the ethical charge of treating an individual patient according to the best established methods. The healer is emphatically not supposed to try uncertain or experimental methods. Patients throughout history and across cultures have always wanted the best possible care. They do not, in fact, want to be made a part of an experiment.

The second obstacle has to do with the complexity of the human body. It is extremely difficult to carry out experiments that isolate one particular organ or one particular physiological system, without affecting the others.

And the third has to do with the complexity of disease. Until the second half of the 19th century, as we will see, disease was generally considered to be an organic part of the human body, not a separate biological entity. Different diseases might even create the same set of symptoms. How could anyone create experiments to study disease? The more obvious approach was to classify them, as one might classify plants or animal species.

Claude Bernard (1813–1878) called for a new, scientific medicine that would overcome those obstacles. A prominent physiologist and professor at the Museum of Natural History in Paris, his *An Introduction to the Study of Experimental Medicine* provided the key statement of purpose for researchers in physiology and pathology. His own research established the role of the pancreatic gland in digestion, the function of the liver, and the existence of vasomotor nerves. He was especially interested in the way in which the human body maintained an internal equilibrium, such as temperature and blood pressure, in response to changes in the external environment.

Bernard and like-minded scientists did not do experiments on people. Instead, they expected that their physiological discoveries would yield insights that would ultimately help physicians treat their patients. Instead, they carried out experiments using animals, a process called vivisection. Many of his contemporaries were horrified by what they saw as cruelty to animals, and as the use of animal experimentation in physiological experiments increased, so did the membership of antivivisection societies. Bernard's wife, Marie Françoise, née Martin, (1819–1901), was very distressed by his experiments. They separated, and she became antivivisection advocate.

Whatever his personal sorrows, Bernard's experimental methods transformed physiological research and laid the basis of modern scientific medicine. As he wrote, "The science of life is a superb and dazzlingly lighted hall which may be reached only by passing through a long and ghastly kitchen."

FURTHER READING

Debru, Claude. (1997). "On the Usefulness of the History of Science for Scientific Education." *Notes and Records of the Royal Society of London* 51: 291–307.

Holmes, Frederic. (1974). *Claude Bernard and Animal Chemistry*. Cambridge, MA: Harvard University Press.

Rudacille, Deborah. (2000). *The Scalpel and the Butterfly. The Conflict between Animal Research and Animal Protection*. Berkeley, CA: University of California Press.

Sinding, Christiane. (1999). "Claude Bernard and Louis Pasteur: Contrasting Images through Public Commemorations." *Osiris* 14: 61–85.

Weinger, Dora and Michael Sauter. (2003). "The City of Paris and the Rise of Clinical Medicine." *Osiris* 18: 23–42.

EXPERIMENT AND OBSERVATION IN ACTION: DIFFERENTIAL DIAGNOSIS OF DIPHTHERIA

* **Document:** Pierre Bretonneau, *Memoirs on Diphtheria*
* **Date:** 1826
* **Where:** Academy of Medicine, Paris
* **Significance:** One of the key features of scientific medicine was research to detect specific changes in the body caused by specific disease. The difficulty was that many diseases seemed to produce the same symptoms. In the excerpt below, Pierre Bretonneau, describing an epidemic in his district in France, gives the first clear clinical description of diphtheria, supported by postmortem dissection.

DOCUMENT

The Memoir which I have the honour to submit to the judgment of the Academy, is extracted from a collection of observations on the special phlegmasia [inflammation] of the mucous membranes. The result of my labours tends to prove, that many inflammatory lesions of the mucous tissue have been confounded together, while the gradations of the same affection have often been mistaken for so many different diseases.

The inflammations of the mucous membranes exhibit, perhaps, some characters no less varied than those of the cutaneous phlegmasia, the classification of which has exercised so fully the talent of nosographers. The exudation which accompanies them, presents, in itself, remarkable varieties; sometimes it is a diffluent serosity, sometimes it is mucus variously altered; sometimes it is a coating, which has the whiteness and consistence of cheesy matter; at other times it is an intimately adherent membranous substance, or simply an adherent membraniform pellicle. The degree of thickness, or of induration, the force of cohesion, the colour, the amount of elevation of the affected tissue, and the more or less limited nature of the inflammation, furnish a multitude of other varieties, which I shall not undertake even to indicate. I shall only add, that some very frequent combinations of these different alterations co-exist too constantly with the symptoms of certain diseases, to prevent us from seeing in them the relations of cause and effect.

So far from entering into these distinctions, and insisting upon the difference of the inflammatory conditions of the mucous tissue, I undertake at present to prove, by the testimony of facts, that the Scorbutic Gangrene of the gums, Croup, and Malignant Angina, are only one and the same form of phlegmasia. These facts, which are supported by numerous researches in pathological anatomy, have been noticed and collected together, during the course of an epidemic which prevailed at Tours, from 1818 till 1820; and they have been obtained either in the town, the population of which amounts (1826) to upwards of twenty thousand souls, or in the Hospital, where the number of patients varies from one hundred and twenty to four hundred. They are similar in their nature to those facts which have been seen in our own time, or have been observed from the most remote antiquity, and by bringing together the notions of modern times, and those which have been transmitted to us by the ancients, their anomaly and discordance are explained …

But the truth has only to exhibit itself, in order to surmount these obstacles. From the moment when chance presented it to me, I thought that before publishing my conclusions, it was my duty to direct my attention again to the observation of facts, to review them, to examine them a second time, and to consider them under all their aspects.

Sixty bodies were opened during the course of the epidemic. Although the examination of certain viscera, which had not presented any sign of morbid alteration during life, was sometimes neglected, the state of the digestive canal and of the air-passages was always studied with the most minute exactness.

I endeavoured to prosecute my researches on the bodies of those, who had more particularly presented, either the characteristic symptoms of Croup, or those of Malignant Angina, whether the progress of the disease had been left to take its course without any treatment, or had been fruitlessly opposed by the most energetic and most opposite remedies.

In a great number of subjects, I was able to follow the decreasing modifications of the disease up to its perfect cure, which was obtained under the influence of special, general, or local treatment.

A hundred and thirty soldiers, and twenty individuals of all ages, presented the different gradations, acute or chronic, of scorbutic gangrene, confined to the mouth, or extending to the pharynx …

Source: Semple, Robert, ed. (1859). *Memoirs on Diphtheria from the Writings of Bretonneau, Guersant, Trousseau, Bouchut, Empis, and Daviot.* London: The New Sydenham Society.

ANALYSIS

When we get sick, what does that do to our body? At one level, we certainly know the answer. We speak of getting headaches, feeling chills, getting sick to our stomachs. But what, exactly, is going on inside of us?

In the days before X-rays and other modern technology, the answer was hard to come by. The body was a kind of black box: physicians could see what went into it and what came out but only rarely could they detect what was going on inside. If patients recovered from what ailed them, their physicians might never know what had gone wrong. But if they died, there was a chance to find out. Physicians, who had studied their symptoms while they were alive, could carry out dissections after their death. That process would allow them to relate the symptoms to the part of the body affected.

Though the technical language of this excerpt may be hard to follow, Bretonneau is actually describing a very clear, well-researched set of medical observations. He set out to investigate a long-standing problem in medicine: why some forms of sore throat simply get better, while others have fatal consequences. He took advantage of a particularly virulent epidemic in his district to show that a nasty sore throat, known by a variety of names, was really the same disease. Though the coating on the throat might take different forms, it was always present; the disease was always highly contagious; though it could result in a "perfect cure," it was more likely to have fatal consequences. In Paris, it was the primary cause of epidemic mortality for children under the age of seven, with 1,800–2,000 deaths per year.

In advanced cases of diphtheria, the mucous covering the trachea could be so thick that patients died of suffocation. Bretonneau pioneered a form of surgery that involved cutting a whole in the trachea and inserting a tube to allow air to reach the lungs. This was always a last resort, attempted only when there was no other hope of saving the patient. By 1835, there had been 18 cures out of a total of 60 operations. It says much for the seriousness of the disease that a treatment which saved just over 25% of the patients was considered a success.

FURTHER READING

Day, Alison. (2013). " 'The Magical Formula': Reactions and Responses to Diphtheria Immunisation in New Zealand 1920–1960." *Health and History* 15: 53–71.

Hooker, Claire. (2000). "Diphtheria, Immunisation and the Bundaberg Tragedy: A Study of Public Health in Australia." *Health and History* 2: 52–78.

Lewis, Jane. (1986). "The Prevention of Diphtheria in Canada and Britain 1914–1945." *Journal of Social History* 20: 163–176.

Singh, J., A. K. Harit, D. C. Jain, R. C. Panda, K. N. Tewari, R. Bhatia, and J. Sokhey. (1999). "Diphtheria Is Declining but Continues to Kill Many Children: Analysis of Data from a Sentinel Centre in Delhi, 1997." *Epidemiology and Infection* 123: 209–215.

Smith, F. B. (1999). "Comprehending Diphtheria." *Health and History* 1: 139–161.

CAN WE EXPERIMENT ON DISEASE?

- **Document:** Abraham Jacobi, "Rudolf Virchow"
- **Date:** 1881
- **Where:** New York
- **Significance:** Rudolf Virchow's lectures and textbook did for pathology what Bernard had done for physiology: they established scientific experimental methods. His textbook, *Cellular Pathology*, was published in 1858 and immediately recognized as a medical classic. In the extract below, Abraham Jacobi, professor of pathology at Columbia University, used Virchow's ideas to explain to his students how pathology became a scientific discipline in its own right.

DOCUMENT

The emancipation of pathology, its rise into the number of independent sciences, with, in its turn, its fertilization of anatomy and physiology, dates from April, 1847, when [Rudolf] Virchow wrote on the standpoints in scientific medicine ... At that time he wrote as follows:

"We ought not to deceive ourselves or each other in regard to the present condition of medical science. Unmistakably, medical men are sick of the large number of new hypothetical systems which are thrown aside as rubbish only to be replaced by similar ones. We shall soon perceive that observation and experiments only have a permanent value. Then, not as the outgrowth of personal enthusiasm, but as the result of the labors of many close investigators, pathological physiology will find its sphere. It will prove the fortress of scientific medicine, the outworks of which are pathological anatomy and clinical research."

Five years afterward he could say: "The scientific method of medical research is firmly established. It is not my merit to have discovered it. Without me it would have been found, and the new trail would have been followed. But I trust that the battle against the existing mixture of arbitrary rationalism and gross empiricism ... in which I aided by the introduction of genetic investigation, must have contributed much in procuring new aims for pathology."

You remember that, but little more than forty years ago, Schleiden discovered the cell to be the elementary basis of the vegetable tissue. Schwann recognized the same element as the foundation of the structure of all animal tissues. A long series of observations and experiments convinced Virchow of the continuous propagation and proliferation of cells within the individual. After five years of hesitation he published the first preparation for, or introduction to, his cellular pathology ...

He proved, and all our experience proves, that life requires a special formation to manifest itself, and certain conglomerates of substance. These conglomerates are the cells and their compounds. Like the individual in its totality, the cell in its turn is the physical body with which the action of mechanical substance is connected, and within which the latter can retain its functions which alone justify the name of "life." In the normal state of this conglomerate it is a mechanical substance which acts, and acts only, on chemical and physical principles.

The pathological process within the elements, according to cellular pathology, is as follows: a living cell is acted upon by something outside. The latter works a mechanical or chemical change in the cell. This mechanical or chemical change is disorder or disease . . .

Source: Jacobi, Abraham. (1881). "Rudolf Virchow. An Address, Introductory to the Course of Lectures of the Term, 1881–2." Reprinted from *The Medical Record*. New York: Trow's Printing, 11–12.

ANALYSIS

The emphasis on scientific medicine transformed the medical curriculum. In the 18th century, anatomy and physiology had been taught in the same course: anatomy, which described the parts of the body, took up most of the academic year, while physiology, covered in the last couple of months, explained the functioning of major organs, like heart and lungs. Diseases were taught in a course called Medical Practice, which took students through the major diseases, their treatment, and cure. In the early 19th century, this began to change. Physiology became a research-based discipline in its own right, increasingly viewing the body as a series of systems working together to maintain homeostasis (the technical term for Bernard's inner equilibrium). Pathology, too, became an independent science, focusing on tissues (histology), rather than entire organs. The discoveries of Matthias Schleiden (1804–1881) and Theodor Schwann (1810–1882) established the cell as the unit of structure and function in organisms, and biological research labs turned their attention to cellular processes. Most of the cellular structures known to modern science had been identified by the end of the 19th century.

Rudolf Virchow (1821–1902) took the theory of the cell one step further: if it was the unit of structure and function in a healthy person, he reasoned, it must also be the unit of structure and function in disease. His contemporaries established that all the metabolic processes necessary to life—respiration, assimilation, reproduction—take place at the cellular level. Disruption to those metabolic processes—that is, disease—must also take place at the cellular level. In other words, when people got sick, the disease was not working on whole organs like the heart or lungs. It was, instead, working on the cells. Without this insight and the accumulating research to support it, the germ theory would not have been possible.

By the 1870s, Virchow was the most famous name in pathology. He was a prolific writer and was the founding editor of several prestigious journals. That might have been reason enough for Abraham Jacobi (1830–1919) to make him the focus of his introductory lecture. Certainly there would seem to be few points of connection between the eminent Berlin professor who was also an elected member of Germany's national government and the German-Jewish immigrant who corresponded with Karl Marx and Friedrich Engels. Yet, the two men had many things in common. Both came from poor backgrounds, and their families had worked hard to allow them to study medicine. Both were committed to public health initiatives. Both were involved in the Revolutions of 1848 in Germany, which sought— unsuccessfully—to promote political reform. Virchow's involvement led to his being dismissed from his hospital position, though he was later reinstated. Jacobi was imprisoned for several years and after his release, traveled first to Great Britain and then to the United States. He became a leader of the newly emerging field of pediatrics and one of the founding contributors to the *American Journal of Obstetrics and Diseases of Women and Children*.

And finally, both Virchow and Jacobi were staunch advocates of vaccination.

FURTHER READING

Ackerknecht, Erwin. (1953). *Rudolf Virchow. Doctor, Statesman, Anthropologist*. Madison, WI: University of Wisconsin Press.

McNeely, Ian. (2002). *"Medicine on a Grand Scale": Rudolf Virchow, Liberalism, and the Public Health*. London: Wellcome Trust.

Truax, Rhoda. (1952). *The Doctors Jacobi*. Boston, MA: Little, Brown, and Co.

Viner, Russell. (1998). "Abraham Jacobi and German Medical Radicalism in Antebellum New York." *Bulletin of the History of Medicine* 72: 434–463.

Warner, John Harley. (1991). "Ideals of Science and Their Discontents in Late Nineteenth-Century American Medicine." *Isis* 82: 454–478.

YELLOW FEVER SPREADS THROUGH
THE ATLANTIC WORLD

- **Document:** James Ormiston McWilliam, "Some Account of the Yellow Fever Epidemy by Which Brazil Was Invaded in the Latter Part of the Year 1849"
- **Date:** 1851
- **Where:** Bahia, Brazil
- **Significance:** Disease has always followed human transportation networks. In the 19th century, as steamships replaced sail, the speed of human transportation accelerated the spread of human epidemics. The same occurred on land as canals and train travel improved communication across continents. In this document, Dr. James McWilliam, naval surgeon turned medical officer for the London custom office, is not just documenting the spread of a disease. He is also arguing for a new field of medicine, epidemiology, the study of epidemic disease.

DOCUMENT

Notwithstanding the geographical position of Brazil, its great variety of climate, and its abounding in those elements which theoretically are supposed to induce the more aggravated forms of tropical disease, endemic disease, except in a mild form, is little known; from sweeping epidemic disease, of any kind, with the exception of small-pox— introduced by slavers—the country has, until lately, been generally considered as wholly exempt.

It was, therefore, with astonishment not unmixed with doubt, that information of the existence of yellow fever in the city of Bahia, in the month of November, 1849, was received in the other parts of the empire; and it was not until the disease had extended to Pernambuco and Rio de Janeiro, that the people in general could be led to believe that so formidable an invader had arrived among them.

I shall now endeavour to trace the origin and progress of the yellow fever epidemy of Brazil, commencing with Bahia, and then taking up the other ports of the empire in the order, so far as my information enables me, according to which they were respectively invaded by the disease . . .

On the 17th day of December, 1849, the French bark Alcyon arrived at Pernambuco from Bahia, having lost two men on the passage from yellow fever. Notwithstanding this she was admitted to pratique [allowed to land], and anchored among the other vessels in the harbour. Some fresh cases of fever occurring on board, they were sent to the French hospital (situated in San Antonio;) but one of them having terminated fatally on the 19th, the authorities ordered the rest to be re-embarked, and interdicted all communication with the Alcyon. The Consul, writing on the 21st December, says, "No cases have as yet to my knowledge occurred within the city. The authorities have ordered all vessels from Bahia to be placed under quarantine for eleven days." In a postscript to the same letter, he adds, "Two cases have since been reported on shore." On the 25th December, Dr. Paton, an English medical man, young, healthy, and robust, and but a short time in the country, was attacked with fever in the British Hospital at Boa Vista, and died on the 27th. The immediate cause of death was at first supposed to have been epilepsy. He laboured for some days under low fever, and was found upon the floor of the room, and almost instantly died, the body turning bright yellow. On the day of Dr. Paton's death, another gentleman, the house apothecary, Mr. Pitt, also residing at the British Hospital, was seized with fever, and died on the fourth day with suppression of urine and black vomit. At this time there were only three other patients in the hospital—one with phthisis, one with ulcer, and the other with paronychia. On the evening of the day on which Mr. Pitt was attacked, the seaman with paronychia, was seized with similar symptoms. Next morning his countenance was anxious, and his extremities were cold, and he died on the following day with black vomit. Dr. May and his housekeeper, who attended Mr. Pitt, were next attacked. Both recovered, but the housekeeper's escape was a narrow one. During Dr. May's illness, the seaman with ulcer was taken ill, and, although sedulously attended by a friend, he also died. After this, all Dr. May's black servants in the house were attacked, but none of them died. The man with phthisis escaped . . .

Dr. May and Dr. Arckbuckle, the two chief practitioners of the place, both declared that Mr. Pitt died of yellow fever; but it was resolved, at a consultation held by the chief men in the profession, with the view of preventing alarm, to conceal the existence of the disease in the city.

The Consul, writing at this time, says, "It is hoped that the general purity and breadth of the streets, intersected as they are in all directions by the rivers, the perpetual sea breeze, and the clearness of the atmosphere, will at once check the disease, although for the present the city may be looked upon as threatened by invasion from without, and by pestilence within."

The disease, however, radiated in all directions from the Boa Vista Hospital, so that, by the 14th of January, most of the inhabitants in that part of the city had been attacked; and its course, say the best authorities, could be traced step by step, from one district to another, all over the city, and even throughout the province.

So early as the 6th of January, the disease had spread to the shipping anchored in the harbour near the Alcyon, proving extremely fatal to those newly arrived in the country.

On board a Prussian vessel lying in the same tier with the Alcyon, a man was attacked shortly after the Alcyon's arrival with excruciating pains in the loins and legs, and died on the third day with black vomit. Although the Prussian vessel was quite new and remarkably clean, the captain had her fumigated, and used chloride of lime daily. Still in a day or two after another man was attacked, and he also died in a few days with black vomit. Others followed in rapid succession, until this vessel had lost eight men out of a crew of twelve.

The next vessel in which the fever broke out was an English barque, called the Esther Anne, a perfect model of cleanliness. She was also in the same tier with the Alcyon, and she lost her mate and four or five of her crew all from yellow fever. During the whole of this time, not a single case occurred in any other ship in the port, except among those in the same tier with the Alcyon.

The fever gradually extended from ship to ship, until all, with very few exceptions, were infected.

One English ship, the Columbus, anchored very high up the harbour, far from every other vessel, escaped entirely.

Another vessel, laden with guano, escaped for a long time, and the captain attributed his good fortune to the nature of his cargo. A day or two, however, before this vessel left Pernambuco, one of her sailors went on a visit to an infected ship. He was soon seized with fever and died, as did also the mate who attended him. Hundreds of similar instances might be narrated.

By the 20th of February, not less than 30,000 persons had been attacked on shore by the fever, and it had also extended to English, Portuguese, and Imperial men-of-war in the harbour. On board the Imperial corvette there were twenty cases of fever. At this time the business of many of the public departments could scarcely be carried on, from the number of employees affected.

The weather was at this time very hot. "On the 27th," says the Consul, "the sun will be vertical, and it is to be hoped that shortly afterwards we may have a change for the better."

These hopes were not, however, realised, for early in March the fever had increased in intensity, no longer confining itself to persons newly arrived in the country, but proving fatal to natives as well as foreigners. By this time eleven of the British community, and probably two thousand residents, had perished. The Consul had already established an hospital on one of the islands in the bay, to which, during the month of February, seventy seamen, American, Hamburghian, and Swedish, were admitted, of whom forty-one died. Of forty-one British seamen, twenty-seven died.

This increased mortality of the disease was considered the more remarkable, as the Consul at this period observes, "the arrangements are all improved, the weather latterly uncommonly cool for the season; the medical men have increased experience, and the people invariably adopt habits of precaution; but nevertheless the plague increases both on board and on shore."

Nothing could be better than the judicious arrangements suggested by Mr. Cowper, the English Consul, for the accommodation of the sick. Finding that the hospital was crowded, he, with the permission of the President of the Province, caused tents to be erected on Cocoa Nut Island, and afterwards had the sick treated on board their own ships, lying on deck, under awnings, exposed to a free circulation of air.

Mr. Cowper, to whom I am indebted for so much valuable information regarding this epidemy, thus classifies those that were attacked by fever at Pernambuco:— "1. New comers; 2. Seamen; 3. Residents of less than two years, not perfectly acclimated; 4. Natives of the first class from the southern provinces and from the interior, including North and South Americans, and even Brazilians. Of the second class, during the first month, the deaths were 1 in 3; during the second month, 1 in 2; during the third month, 2 in 3; during the fourth month, 4 in 5; and the mortality increased in proportion as the number attacked decreased. Of the third class very few escaped attack, and certainly not more than half death. Of the fourth class scarcely one escaped attack, but the disease was in a mild form; whilst nearly 100 per cent, of the two first classes, and 50 per cent, of the third, fell victims, not more than 3 per cent, of this class died."

Without reference to race, 16 per cent, of all foreigners attacked died, and 3 per cent, only of the natives.

The Sardinians, from some unknown cause, suffered more severely, both afloat and on shore, than other foreigners. According to Dr. May, the mortality afloat was 60 per cent, of those attacked.

Source: McWilliam, James Ormiston. (1851). "Some Account of the Yellow Fever Epidemy by Which Brazil was Invaded in the Latter Part of the Year 1849." *Medical Times* 23: 424–426.

ANALYSIS

In the 19th century, the world population is estimated to have grown from 900 million to 1,600 million. And this was a population on the move: 33.6 million people emigrated from Europe to the United States; 2.3 million immigrated to Canada, and another 2 million to Australia and New Zealand; 3.6 million immigrated to South America, a substantial proportion of whom were slaves; French emigrants went to Algeria and Morocco, and Russians moved into Siberia; Chinese immigrants moved to Siam, Java, the Malay Peninsula, California, British Columbia, and New South Wales; and Indian emigrants moved to East Africa and to the Caribbean. In industrial countries, the percentage of the population who lived in urban centers increased dramatically; cities overflowed their traditional boundaries in an effort to accommodate their millions of new residents.

This meant that epidemics were now global phenomena. Yellow fever had long been endemic on the West Coast of Africa. Now, the frequency with which ships, both slave ships and British Naval vessels assigned to stop the slave trade, stopped at West African ports before heading across the Atlantic ensured that yellow fever was a frequent fellow traveler. The increased use of steam ships meant that a ship anchored at Sierra Leone could be in the Azores within a few days. If the ship continued to follow the warm weather to Brazil, the mosquitoes that carried the virus could continue to breed, disembarking with the humans they fed on. Contemporaries noted that a ship infected with yellow fever could stop the spread of disease by immediately heading for a colder climate. The cold, fresh air was believed to be more healthful than heat and humidity; we now think that it worked by killing the mosquitoes. Not until the early 20th century was the connection between mosquitoes and yellow fever clinically proven. According to modern estimates, up to 50% of those severely afflicted with yellow fever may die.

James Ormiston McWilliam (1808–1862) was a founding member and secretary of the Epidemiological Society of London, founded in 1850 to promote the scientific study of epidemics. Part of his job was to plot epidemics as they appeared throughout the world so as to promote scientific research into their causes and treatments. The society also tried to influence government policy with respect to prevention of infectious diseases.

McWilliam's article may appear to be a simple report, but it is, in fact, part of an ongoing argument in favor of stricter measures to prevent the spread of disease from ships to the ports at which they land. McWilliam makes the point that Brazil, though it may have appeared to be tropical, had previously been free from serious epidemic diseases. He notes that neither the climate nor the location of the port near water could account for the development of the epidemic. Yellow fever spread from specific ships to specific populations on shore, with nearly 30,000 sick after three months; local authorities, McWilliam says, traced the disease, "step by step, from one district to another, all over the city, and even throughout the province." Ships that escaped the disease were those, like the Columbus, that stayed far away from any reported illness.

McWilliam points out the failures of public health policy. The problem was exacerbated, he notes, by officials who refused to believe that the ports were vulnerable to yellow fever and who therefore allowed ships to land. Medical officers made matters worse by concealing information about the disease in order not to alarm the population. As a result, yellow fever spread not only through Pernambuco but also Rio de Janeiro and Sao Paulo. It became endemic in Brazil and remains a risk factor for travelers to remote parts of the country to the present day.

FURTHER READING

Crosby, Alfred. (2004). *Ecological Imperialism. The Biological Expansion of Europe 900–1900*. New York: Cambridge University Press.

Curtin, Philip. (1973). *The Image of Africa. British Ideas and Action, 1780–1850*. 2 vols. Madison, WI: University of Wisconsin Press.

McNeill, J. R. (1999). "Ecology, Epidemics and Empires: Environmental Change and the Geopolitics of Tropical America, 1600–1825." *Environment and History* 5: 175–184.

Ngalamulume, Kalala. (2004). "Keeping the City Totally Clean: Yellow Fever and the Politics of Prevention in Colonial Saint-Louis-du-Sénégal, 1850–1914." *The Journal of African History* 45: 183–202.

Watts, Sheldon. (1999). *Epidemics and History. Disease, Power, and Imperialism*. New Haven CT: Yale University Press.

CHOLERA SPREAD THROUGH TRADE

- **Document:** Duane Simmons, *Cholera Epidemics in Japan*
- **Date:** 1880
- **Where:** Japan
- **Significance:** Cholera was another unwelcome fellow traveler. Thousands died in Great Britain and America in three epidemics— 1832, 1849, and 1866. Those three epidemics were part of five pandemics (worldwide epidemics) that are estimated to have killed 15 million people in India and 2 million in Russia.

  Until the 1850s, Japan had successfully limited foreign access to its ports. Commercial treaties imposed by the United States and European powers ended those restrictions and opened the door to disease as well as trade. An estimated 100,000–200,000 people died in Tokyo during the 1859–1860 cholera outbreak.

DOCUMENT

As for 1861 and 1862, the disease was then raging, as already stated, in many parts of China. This country was at that time open to foreign trade; and communication was constant, both by steam and sail, with continental Asia. No measures, as indeed is still the case, were taken to prevent the importation of the disease, and the result, as I have every reason to remember, from weeks of day and night work, was a terrible epidemic, attended with great loss of life. An epidemic of measles, brought into the country for the first time in 27 years (it was introduced by a foreigner, no less a personage than the English Chargé d'Affaires), had immediately preceded that of cholera. The consequence was that many persons were attacked by the latter before they had fully recovered from the former malady. For this cause, according to impressions formed at the time, I consider that a much higher mortality rate was reached than is usual from cholera alone. The subject of establishing a quarantine, or taking some means for preventing the importation of contagious diseases into the country by means of ships, was discussed at this period; and I then met, at the United States legation in Tokio, by request of the Japanese government, a delegation of medical men appointed by the Tycoon for the purpose of drafting some regulations on the subject. As, however, the epidemic had by that time nearly exhausted itself, and the moment of immediate necessity for enforcement of stringent preventive measures had passed away, nothing came of this conclave's deliberations.

From 1862 until 1877, or during a period of 15 years, no case of cholera is known to have occurred here, notwithstanding that the disease did not entirely cease its ravages in China until 1867—five years later than its temporary disappearance from Japan.

I subjoin extracts from a translation, which recently appeared in the *Hiogo News*, of a native "brief history of cholera" in this empire.

In the summer of the 6th year of Shotoku (2376, era of Jimmu) (A.D. 1718) ... fever prevailed, and the mortality in the city of Great Yedo exceeded 80,000 per month. Owing to the rapid spread of the disease and the number of deaths, the carpenters were unable to keep pace with the demand for coffins, and empty salt casks had therefore to be employed for the purpose. The graveyards were at length all filled up, no space remained for more burials, and the priests of the various sects refused to permit the interment of the remains, insisting that the bodies should be burned, and only the ashes be buried.

At the various cremation grounds, therefore, coffins in countless numbers were seen piled on top of each other, the burning of bodies being done in regular succession, according to the order of their arrival. Numbers of corpses, mostly of poor persons, had to be left unburnt for upwards of half a month, and the head-man of the ward was at his wit's end what to do in the matter. The government was therefore asked for instructions, and an order was issued that the bodies should be wrapped in coarse mats, and that (after the performance over them of a brief religious ceremony) they should be conveyed in boats to the Bay of Yedo, and sunk in the sea.

This we read in the *Shokio Kanki*, and we may judge from the virulence of the disease that it was quite different from ordinary fever. We are inclined to think that it was what we now call cholera, and that this was the first appearance of the pest in our Toyoashihara ["fertile sweet flag plain"—Japan]. We, however, invite an expression of opinion from antiquarians.

Again, in the 5th year of Ansei ... [A. D. 1850], an epidemic prevailed in Yedo [Edo], as many persons will recollect. This disease first manifested itself in the neighbourhood of Akasaka, in the beginning of the 7th month of that year; according to some, it was brought from the Tokai-do. Reiganjima became infected, and soon it spread in all directions. During the first half of the 8th month the epidemic raged most furiously. At the gates of every temple there were hills of coffins; the men who worked at the cremation furnaces in the evening were themselves changed into smoke the next morning, and the tombstone-cutter of one day found his own name carved on a stone on the morrow. The panic amongst the populace beggared description. The epidemic was regarded with even far greater dread, by both high and low, than is the prevailing one in this 12th year of Meiji, for medical knowledge was in such a crude state that no one was able to ascertain the cause of the disease, and the people could do nothing but sit down in dread suspense and await the approach of death.

The disease was generally attributed to diabolical agency ... It was also believed that all water and all fish were poisoned, so that people dared not draw water even from the pure stream of the upper Tamagawa, nor eat any fresh fish, even when it was brought to their doors alive. Each one adorned his gate with branches of pine and bamboo, and straw ropes, and prayed that so dreadful a year might pass away as quickly as possible; some praying to the *kami*, and some td Buddha The whole city was filled with horror and dismay, and a state of things existed to which that in Osaka at the present time bears but a faint resemblance.

If we may believe the ... *Record of the Ravages of Dysentery*, which was published in the 9th month of the 5th year of Ansei, there were then in Yedo 1,775,215 houses, and a population of 7,101,318. The disease was most virulent between the 1st and the 30th of the 8th month, during which space of time the number of deaths was 12,492, as appears from the statistics of death reported to the Government daily. Besides these, 18,737 persons, whose names had not been properly registered at the ward offices, died. For the first three or four days in the beginning of the 9th month there were 50 or 60 deaths daily; after that the number gradually decreased, and at length the disease entirely disappeared, and tranquility was once more restored.

Source: Simmons, Duane. (1880). *Cholera Epidemics in Japan.* Shanghai, China: Statistical Department of the Inspectorate General of Customs, 4–10.

ANALYSIS

Cholera had been an endemic disease in human society for millennia. It is caused by a bacteria that propagates in the human digestive tract, leading to vomiting and diarrhea and, if left untreated, death by dehydration. If contaminated feces from its victims get into the water supply, it can spread throughout the community. For much of the world's history, it was a seasonal disease, because all human communities understand the importance of depositing human excrement far away from drinking water. In hot weather, though, the water table might drop, leading to sewage seeping into the water supply. In the Northern Hemisphere, cholera tended to appear in late summer and then disappear when the autumn rains arrived.

The industrial revolution and the massive growth of population that accompanied it completely overwhelmed traditional sewage facilities in cities around the globe. With no knowledge of bacteria, observers could not understand where cholera came from or how it spread. It was clear that it did not spread person-to-person, like smallpox, because doctors who worked among their poor patients did not get sick. Yet, entire households could become sick and die within 36 hours of the first appearance of the disease.

John Snow (1813–1858), a London physician, demonstrated the connection between cholera and the water supply in his groundbreaking work, *On the Mode of Communication of Cholera* (1849). By analyzing what became known as the "Broad Street Pump" incident, in which a cluster of deaths were linked to a single contaminated pump, he argued that cholera was spread when sewage containing human excrement seeped into the water supply. He also posited that the cause might be a living agent propagating itself first in the water and second, most dangerously, in people. John Snow documented his findings by mapping the incidence of cholera in London; detailed mapping became one of the most valuable tools in the new science of epidemiology.

Modern laboratory techniques for identifying disease agents had not yet been invented in Snow's time, and he relied above all on careful observation. It is possible that the Japanese families in Edo, during the 1850 outbreak of cholera, did the same. For although the narrator says that "the disease was generally attributed to diabolical agency," he also records the belief that "all water and all fish were poisoned, so that people dared not draw water even from the pure stream of the upper Tamagawa, nor eat any fresh fish, even when it was brought to their doors alive." It may well be that local people made the same observation that John Snow did in London: that water may look "pure" while still carrying some kind of "poison," or as we might say now, an infectious agent.

By the end of the 19th century, improved sanitation had all but eliminated cholera in industrialized nations, but it remains a serious threat anywhere sanitation facilities break down, whether 19th-century Japan or, after Hurricane Katrina, 21th-century New Orleans.

FURTHER READING

Echenberg, Myron. (2011). *Africa in the Time of Cholera. A History of Pandemics from 1817 to the Present*. New York: Cambridge University Press.

Fuess, Harald. (2014). "Informal Imperialism and the 1879 'Hesperia' Incident: Containing Cholera and Challenging Extraterritoriality in Japan." *Japan Review* 27: 103–140.

Hamlin, Christopher. (2009). *Cholera: The Biography*. New York: Oxford University Press.

Johnson, Steven. (2006). *The Ghost Map: The Story of London's Most Terrifying Epidemic—and How It Changed Science, Cities, and the Modern World*. New York: Riverhead Books.

Rosenberg, Charles. (1987). *The Cholera Years: The United States in 1832, 1849, and 1866*. Chicago, IL: University of Chicago Press.

SLAVERY AND THE SPREAD
OF INFECTIOUS DISEASE

- **Document:** Solomon Northup, *Twelve Years a Slave*
- **Date:** 1855
- **Where:** New York
- **Significance:** The slave trade carried diseases as well as human victims. It is clear from Solomon Northup's account that he and his enslaved friends received medical treatment to protect their owner's investment, rather than from humanitarian motives.

DOCUMENT

We were all prepared, and impatiently waiting an opportunity of putting our designs [for escape from the slave ship Orleans] into execution, when they were frustrated by a sad and unforeseen event. Robert was taken ill. It was soon announced that he had the small-pox. He continued to grow worse, and four days previous to our arrival in New Orleans he died. One of the sailors sewed him in his blanket, with a large stone from the ballast at his feet, and then laying him on a hatchway, and elevating it with tackles above the railing, the inanimate body of poor Robert was consigned to the white waters of the gulf.

We were all panic-stricken by the appearance of the small-pox. The captain ordered lime to be scattered through the hold, and other prudent precautions to be taken. The death of Robert, however, and the presence of the malady, oppressed me sadly, and I gazed out over the great waste of waters with a spirit that was indeed disconsolate . . .

That night, nearly all who came in on the brig Orleans, were taken ill. They complained of violent pain in the head and back. Little Emily—a thing unusual with her—cried constantly. In the morning a physician was called in, but was unable to determine the nature of our complaint. While examining me, and asking questions touching my symptoms, I gave it as my opinion that it was an attack of smallpox—mentioned the fact of Robert's death as the reason of my belief. It might be so indeed, he thought, and he would send for the head physician of the hospital. Shortly, the head physician came—a small, light-haired man, whom they called Dr. Carr. He pronounced it small-pox, whereupon there was much alarm throughout the yard. Soon after Dr. Carr left, Eliza, Emmy, Harry and myself were put into a hack and driven to the hospital—a large white marble building, standing on the outskirts of the city. Harry and I were placed in a room in one of the upper stories. I became very sick. For three days I was entirely blind. While lying in this state one day, Bob came in, saying to Dr. Carr that Freeman [the slave auctioneer] had sent him over to inquire how we were getting on. Tell him, said the doctor, that [he] is very bad, but that if he survives until nine o'clock, he may recover.

I expected to die. Though there was little in the prospect before me worth living for, the near approach of death appalled me. I thought I could have been resigned to yield up my life in the bosom of my family, but to expire in the midst of strangers, under such circumstances, was a bitter reflection.

There were a great number in the hospital, of both sexes, and of all ages. In the rear of the building coffins were manufactured. When one died, the bell tolled—a signal to the undertaker to come and bear away the body to the potter's field. Many times, each day and night, the tolling bell sent forth its melancholy voice, announcing another death. But my time had not yet come. The crisis having passed, I began to revive, and at the end of two weeks and two days, returned with Harry to the pen, bearing upon my face the effects of the malady, which to this day continues to disfigure it. Eliza and Emily were also brought back next day in a hack, and again were we paraded in the sales-room, for the inspection and examination of purchasers.

Source: Northup, Solomon. (1855). *Twelve Years A Slave.* New York: Miller, Orton, and Mulligan, 72–85.

ANALYSIS

Solomon Northup (1808–1863?) was a free African American from New York who was kidnapped in Washington, DC, and sold into slavery. He was eventually rescued, and the book he wrote about his experiences, *Twelve Years a Slave*, fueled the abolitionist cause. Steve McQueen directed the 2013 movie version, which won three Academy Awards, including Best Picture, thus bringing Northup's story to a wider 21st-century audience.

The African slave trade was so effective at spreading infectious diseases that it might have been invented for that purpose. The process began when men, women, and children were captured from widely dispersed communities and brought to population centers on the West African coast. This allowed infectious diseases to attack susceptible victims. Then, victims of slavery were transported under unspeakable conditions rapidly across the Atlantic, where ships typically put in at a succession of ports. This ensured that the diseases would be spread from the ships to the ports and thus to the local residents.

From 1808 onward, the British Navy spearheaded the task of ending the African slave trade. The West African Squadron patrolled the coast, sending boats into the shallow, mosquito-infested inlets in order to seize slave ships and free the Africans on board. It is estimated that they were able to disrupt the trade considerably, seizing approximately one-third of the slave ships and freeing 150,000 enslaved people. But the West African Squadron was notoriously unhealthy, and it seems clear that sailors who rejoined their ships after several months patrolling the coast brought yellow fever and dysentery with them.

Some slave owners promoted smallpox inoculation or vaccination, even employing a slave as the vaccinator. As in Northup's account, this was not done for humanitarian reasons but in order to protect the health of their property.

FURTHER READING

Alden, Dauril and Joseph Miller. (1987). "Out of Africa: The Slave Trade and the Transmission of Smallpox to Brazil, 1560–1831." *The Journal of Interdisciplinary History* 18: 195–224.

Gates, Henry Louis Jr. "'12 Years a Slave': Trek from Slave to Screen." *The African Americans: Many Rivers to Cross.* http://www.pbs.org/wnet/african-americans-many -rivers-to-cross/history/12-years-a-slave-trek-from-slave-to-screen/.

Lloyd, Christopher. (1968). *The Navy and the Slave Trade. The Suppression of the African Slave Trade in the Nineteenth Century.* London: Frank Cass & Co. Ltd.

Mustakeem, Sowande'. (2008). "'I Never Have Such a Sickly Ship Before': Diet, Disease, and Mortality in 18th-Century Atlantic Slaving Voyages." *The Journal of African American History* 93: 474–496.

Smith, Benjamin Allen Concannon. (2013). "Impatient and Pestilent: Public Health and the Reopening of the Slave Trade in Early National Charleston." *The South Carolina Historical Magazine* 114: 29–58.

QUARANTINE CONTROVERSIES

- **Document:** Gavin Milroy, *The Cholera Not to be Arrested by Quarantine*
- **Date:** 1847
- **Where:** London, United Kingdom
- **Significance:** By the 1840s, anyone with a map could trace the movements of ships and of diseases around the globe. The question was, were those two movements connected? The answer was complicated by the fact that microorganisms had not yet been identified as the cause of disease and also by the fact that worldwide movement of ships, men, and goods had become a key component of politics, diplomacy, and commerce. The two documents below show how both sides of the argument could marshal convincing medical evidence.

DOCUMENT

"There is [a] circumstance . . . which is utterly incompatible with the idea of infection playing the chief part in the diffusion of the Cholera; and that is the sudden seizure of hundreds of persons in a place on one and the same day. How can any one seek to reconcile such an occurrence with the notion of the disease being communicated from one person to another, and of its proceeding, as it were, step by step, until it has overspread a space of several miles in circumference within 24 or 36 hours? . . .

When . . . it is remembered that nine-tenths, I might rather say 99 out of every 100, of the medical men in India entirely reject the idea of the disease being propagated by infection,—that it has over and over again broken out in places remote from, and having no direct communication with, those where it chiefly prevailed,—that the attendants upon the sick are not a whit more liable to be attacked than others, a fact quite as true in Europe and America as in the East Indies,—that the pestilence every now and then unexpectedly bursts out in some district previously healthy with amazing fury, sweeps off its thousands, and then, in the course of a week or so, ceases altogether, sometimes after a thunder-storm, at other times without any appreciable cause,—that in its migratory course it has frequently appeared in numerous points of a large and scattered city at the very same time, while in other instances, the distance of a few hundred yards has made all the difference between a region of almost inevitable death and one of complete exemption and even of health . . . —that the Russian Government, in 1831, having found their utter inefficacy, speedily abandoned all [quarantine] attempts,—that the Austrian Emperor formally declared that, "he had committed an error in adopting the vexatious and worse than useless quarantine and cordon regulations against cholera," freely admitting that he did so before the nature of the disease was properly understood,—that Prussia, too, having in vain had recourse to the same expedients, was forced to give them up,—that, in our own country, the Government intimated, in the Speech delivered from the Throne, if not their positive disbelief, at least their emphatic incredulity as to the importation of the disease from the continent by shipping or otherwise;—that one of the latest acts of the Central Board of Health in London was to announce that cholera patients should be as freely admitted into our public hospitals as any other sick,—that the Board of Health in Ireland candidly admitted that "they were not able to trace the disease to any communication by which it might have been introduced into the neighbourhood of Dublin,"—that the leading physicians and surgeons in Paris drew up a formal memorial, declaring their disbelief in its infectiousness, and that the French Academy of Medicine adopted and confirmed this opinion,—that the Government of the United States, too, at first tried the effects of quarantine protection, but quickly abandoned it, the chief medical men in New York, Philadelphia, and other leading cities of the Union having pronounced against it ... —can any one, after impartially thinking upon all these things, reasonably entertain a doubt as to the utter inadequacy of personal infection to account for the career of Cholera, or hold to the folly and wickedness of ever again attempting to arrest its march by measures which have been proved to be wholly valueless?

Source: Milroy, Gavin. (1847). *The Cholera Not to be Arrested by Quarantine.* London: J. Churchill.

- **Document:** Thomas Spencer Wells, "On the Practical Results of Quarantine"
- **Date:** 1854
- **Where:** London, United Kingdom

DOCUMENT

Those who think a rational system of quarantine necessary for the public safety and tranquility are among the most earnest advocates of those measures which are calculated to remove preventable causes of disease ...

For instance, [in a recent report, the author states that] "during the plague in Alexandria, in 1834, the squadron of 16,000 persons remained perfectly well, and this not on account of removal from the seat of infection, because other ships in the same situation, which had communication with the shore, lost many persons. The arsenal, with 6,000 labourers, was situated close to the infected quarters, but kept in strict quarantine. During six to seven months, five or six cases of sudden death occurred, but no decided case of plague ... The land hospital was very favourably situated, but the physician was a non-contagionist, did not adopt precautionary measures, and the disease "carried off many victims, and subjected the government to great sacrifice." ... During the plague, the college with its hospital, the populous harem of the viceroy, other inferior establishments, and numerous private families who *shut up*, escaped entirely; while of the Turks, who took no such precautions, it is said, "when the malady declined, more than a hundred keys were found at the police office, of houses where the inhabitants had all perished" ...

I say, therefore, now, as I wrote in 1849: "Experience has most fully established the great efficacy and real security to be derived from quarantine regulations when properly practised. Until the last twelve years, plague was so regularly a yearly visitor in the Levant, that it was believed to be indigenous in the whole Ottoman dominions. Russia occupied some of the Turkish provinces, the sanitary condition of which, as regards the local origin of disease, has not been much ameliorated by the change of dynasty; but quarantine was established, importation of plague was prevented, and these districts have since been as free from plague as the rest of Europe. Since the new kingdom of Greece has been separated from Turkey, and plague has been kept from its seaports by quarantine, no plagues has been known in the kingdom, although those best acquainted with the country know that no other sanitary improvements of importance have been effected. In the Barbary States, since quarantine has been established, no plague has existed ..." I claim, therefore, for these regulations an enormous saving of human life, infinitely overbalancing any pecuniary mischief caused by impediments to commerce, or any personal inconvenience to which travelers have been subjected ...

I cannot conclude without protesting against the absurdity of those who talk of the *substitution* of quarantine by sanitary measures, as if quarantine when rationally practised was not a sanitary measure of the very first importance. I contend that those who most firmly believe in the good that quarantine can do and has done, but at the same time are anxious to remove its inconsistencies and to reduce it to a system based on science and experience, those, I say, are the men who are the most earnest and practical supporters of other sanitary measures. They fully recognise the importance of drainage, ventilation, and cleanliness; the necessity for improving the dwellings of the poor, and labouring hard to raise the social condition of the people; but they say at the same time, do not neglect another great means of preserving health; do not, in case of contagious epidemics, hesitate to separate the sick from the healthy; not by crowding the sick together, but by separating them from each other in well ventilated institutions, and thus prevent them from communicating the disease under which they labour to the rest of the community.

Source: Wells, Thomas Spencer. (1854). "On the Practical Results of Quarantine." *Association Medical Journal* 2: 831–834.

ANALYSIS

Controversies over quarantine are as old as the practice itself, which goes back to the ancient world. Quarantine is designed to prevent ships, people, and goods that might carry disease from coming into contact with the local population. It imposed a period—originally 40 days, but by the 19th century, ranging from several weeks to as much as six months—during which the incoming ship or person had to wait outside a port before being admitted. Some cities had special quarantine hospitals for people suspected of carrying an illness. Others required the affected persons to wait on board ship.

From the point of view of the residents or officials on land, quarantine was necessary to protect them from infectious diseases. But from the point of view of persons on board ship, it was at best a nuisance, and at worst, a death sentence. Local officials had full authority to decide whether they were, or were not, carrying disease. Even if they did not have a single sick person on board ship, they could still be refused permission to land if they had previously stopped at a port where a contagious disease was present. And if they did have sick persons on board, keeping them on board might well make their illness worse. Refusing permission for their—for the moment—healthy colleagues to land might lead to more people contracting the illness. For those reasons, medical opinions on whether a disease was, or was not, contagious were literally a matter of life or death.

As maritime traffic increased throughout the 19th century, hundreds of ships might converge on a single port, each carrying its complement of sailors, soldiers, civilian passengers, and, of course, diseases. The world leader in this traffic was the British Navy, and British naval authorities therefore had considerable incentive to argue that diseases like cholera and yellow fever were not contagious. Gavin Milroy (1805–1886), one of the foremost authorities on public health with close ties to the navy, was also one of the chief proponents of this position. Cholera, he said, came from improper sanitation; yellow fever, from local environmental conditions of heat, humidity, and stagnant water. His arguments were based on medical observations that showed that neither disease is propagated from person to person like smallpox. He concluded that neither could be transported by ships, their human occupants, or their cargo. The proper preventative was sanitary measures, both at sea and on land.

Thomas Spencer Wells (1818–1897) spent the early part of his career as a naval surgeon. But a long tour of duty in the Mediterranean, with its many ports and strict quarantine requirements, convinced him of the importance of quarantine in protecting residents on land from the ever-expanding maritime traffic. In arguing for quarantine, he, too, used careful medical observations, but he emphasized a disease that served his purpose: bubonic plague, the most terrifying epidemic disease then known to medical science.

Milroy and Wells were not always on opposite sides of medicine. Both served in the Crimean War and saw firsthand the serious sanitary problems created by the modern warfare.

Neither writer addressed one of the most persistent problems with quarantine: passengers, residents, or officials on land and at sea, who actively hid or did not report cases of suspected illness. Even the most well-regulated ship might have a surgeon who decided that a medical case was not serious enough to support; even the most well-guarded quarantine hospital had smugglers who, for a fee, would help a resident over a wall or across a channel. As the next hundred years would show, the most effective way to allow free trade while preventing the spread of disease was not quarantine but vaccination.

FURTHER READING

Booker, John. (2008). *Maritime Quarantine. The British Experience 1650–1900.* Farnham, England: Ashgate Publishing.

Harrison, Mark. (2012). *Contagion: How Commerce Has Spread Disease.* New Haven, CT: Yale University Press.

Morman, Edward. (1984). "Guarding against Alien Impurities: The Philadelphia Lazaretto 1854–1893." *The Pennsylvania Magazine of History and Biography* 108: 131–151.

Wald, Priscilla. (2008). *Contagious: Cultures, Carriers, and the Outbreak Narrative.* Durham, NC: Duke University Press.

Williamson, James. (1828–1835). "Packet Surgeon's Journals." *National Maritime Museum of Cornwall.* http://maritimeviews.nmmc.co.uk/index.php?/packet_surgeons_journals/.

SOLDIERS' HEALTH AND INFECTIOUS DISEASE IN THE CIVIL WAR

- **Document:** Henry Bellows, Notes of a Preliminary Sanitary Survey of the Forces of the United States, Washington, 1861
- **Date:** 1861
- **Where:** Washington, DC
- **Significance:** The U.S. Sanitary Commission was set up in early 1861 with two main purposes: advising the government on matters relating to the health of the armed forces and raising money and volunteers to support military hospitals. The two documents below show the scope of the Sanitary Commission's work.

In Great Britain, the importance of well-run army hospitals had been learned the hard way in the Crimean War (1853–1855), in which thousands of British soldiers died due to poor sanitation and, even worse, medical administration. The Parliament appointed a series of sanitary commissions to monitor conditions and propose reforms. Florence Nightingale (1820–1910) is the best known of the sanitary reformers associated with the war. In 1861, the U.S. government hoped to avoid the British army's mistakes by instituting reforms before troops died from preventable infectious diseases.

DOCUMENT

JUNE 28, 1861. Camp Dennison, Ohio,

Is situated on the line of the Cincinnati and Columbus railroad, about fifteen miles north of Cincinnati. It is a wide and open common, well adapted as a whole to the purpose. The drainage is imperfect. The general police of the camp is only tolerable—the sinks not being carefully situated, and, in parts, the odor from them both disagreeable and dangerous, as the prevailing winds have not been considered in their position. Little attention had been given among the medical men to sanitary considerations, up to the time of our visit. They generally complained of inability to procure supplies, of unacquaintance with the forms of officials through whom they were to be obtained, and of the carelessness and inefficiency of the State authorities, both in the original outfit of the soldiers and in the attention paid to their wants

DID YOU KNOW?

Quinine and the Civil War

During the Civil War (1861–1865), both Union and Confederate medical officers worked hard to safeguard their supply of quinine, the only medication known to be effective against malaria. Many of the major battles took place in low-lying, swampy areas, the breeding grounds for mosquitoes that carry the debilitating and often-fatal disease. Though the precise connection between mosquitoes and malaria was not established until the end of the 19th century, everyone knew that quinine, derived from the cinchona plant, was essential to protect the health of armies and civilians alike.

In the production and distribution of quinine, the Union army had the clear advantage. Union Surgeon General William Hammond (1828–1900) established the U.S. Army Laboratory and hired German-educated chemist John Michael Maisch (1831–1893) to oversee the production of quinine. Maisch had the tremendous industrial resources of the northern states at his command, including well-equipped pharmaceutical companies and extensive railroad networks. He was therefore able to implement a large-scale process to obtain cinchona bark, process it to obtain the active ingredients for quinine, package the medication in standard doses, and distribute it to army medical staff and base hospitals.

The Confederate Surgeon General, Samuel P. Moore (1813–1889), had a much harder time. The southern states had no pharmaceutical companies with the manufacturing expertise to produce quinine, and the Union blockade made it very difficult to import in sufficient quantities. "I write now to beg you to send in your next letter a quarter of an ounce of quinine," wrote one South Carolina resident. "You know, in this climate, life depends upon quinine—and though large quantities come in every ship, it is taken up so immediately for the army that it is exceedingly difficult for private individuals to procure it even at a very high price."

Moore believed that the key to keeping his armies healthy lay in finding a native southern plant that could serve as a substitute for quinine. He commissioned surgeon Francis Peyre Porcher (1825–1895) to create a compendium of southern plants and their medicinal properties. Porcher had only one year to complete the work, and he pressed his wife, mother, and scientific friends into service to find and test medicinal properties of local flora. The result was *Resources of the Southern Fields and Forests, Medical, Economical, and Agricultural,* published in 1863. It is still cited today as a guide to native plants in the southern United States. But no native plant could replace quinine in the treatment of malaria.

Both northern and southern armies suffered from the Confederate's quinine shortage. Confederate army surgeons were no more able to treat their injured or captured Union patients than they were to treat their own soldiers. The impact of this, and other deadly conflicts, led to the founding of the Red Cross in Switzerland in 1864, to help ensure that humanitarian aid, including medications, might be made available to all combatants.

Source: Hicks, Robert. (2013). " 'The Popular Dose with Doctors': Quinine and the American Civil War." *Chemical Heritage Magazine* 31. https://www.chemheritage.org/distillations/article/%E2%80%9C-popular-dose-doctors%E2%80%9D-quinine-and-american-civil-war.

since. A general burst of dissatisfaction was directed towards Governor Dennison, who was pronounced good-natured and well meaning, but wretchedly inefficient, and easily managed by designing speculators. A contract which he had made for feeding the troops at sixty cents apiece a day (more expensive than hotel fare in all but the best hotels for regular boarders in that region) had been broken up by public indignation.

The cooking of the camp seemed conducted in a very uneconomical and shiftless manner, and the general appearance of the men, and their manners and ways, in my cursory visit of three hours, (which can boast no accuracy of observation,) did not strike me as favorably as in the other camps I have visited. General Bates, in command, appeared a dignified and commanding soldier, and is no doubt doing the best for his men, who are officered in the semi-political and semi-accidental fashion of most volunteer regiments. They complained of the difficulty of keeping the men from passing the lines; and I saw one man, a little under the influence of strong drink, a soldier, brutally knocked down, and his scalp cut open to the depth of a finger, by a sentry whom he was wrangling with about passing out. An officer was brought into the hospital who, twenty minutes before, had been thrown from his horse, and who appeared paralyzed on one side, and was probably fatally injured. A good deal of drinking was complained of in this camp.

The hospitals (regimental) were comfortable, and decently furnished, although there seemed to be a scarcity of attendance, particularly in the general hospital, which was roomy and already quite full of patients. Diarrhea, pneumonia, measles, and typhoid fever had been the common complaints. It was obvious that the recruiting had been careless, and the men who were sick were mainly those who should never have been permitted to enter the service ...

The United States Marine Hospital [in Cincinnati] —a fine edifice, built three or four years ago at an expense, it is said, (land and all,) of $200,000 ... had laid entirely idle since its erection, being in charge of a steward at $600 a year, who presided over the empty building. Meanwhile the real and proper claimants on its privileges, the boatmen, sick and disabled on the rivers, were farmed out to the Commercial Hospital in Cincinnati at $5 per week. I visited them there, and found about fifty in the uncomfortable ward of that miserable, not to say disgraceful, building—an old tumbledown edifice, behind-hand in all respects—with men eating at table in the same ward in which they slept, and with poor evidence in any department of the cleanliness and order now demanded by humanity in such institutions. The steward, a highly intelligent man, seemed doing his best, and grieved over the lack of a proper building in which to lay out his pains. A very excellent and distinguished surgeon attends it ...

The abuses of the United States Marine Hospitals are worthy of the attention of a special committee, directed to visit every one of them, and report minutely their separate history, cost, age, use, and present condition. It is feared that they would turn out to be a systematic fraud on the public treasury, made with the connivance or inadvertence of successive administrations, under the alleged necessities of party spoils. They afford opportunities for the sale of costly pieces of ground, and the erection under profitable contracts of expensive edifices, and then the appointment to lazy offices of resident stewards, and the salarying of attendant physicians. Being under the control of the Treasury Department, they fall into the hands of the collectors of the ports where they are situated, and by them are, I suspect, generally administered, as at St. Louis, in a perfectly careless manner. Their combined cost, and the money expended in maintaining them, often in a ruinous state, would, considering the small amount of usefulness reaped from them, present them, taken altogether, as one of the most unjustifiable abuses of the public funds; and if they are sustained, as is affirmed, out of the money paid by the marines themselves, it makes the misconduct of their trustees, the United States Government, only additionally reprehensible.

JULY 1, 1861. Cairo

This highly important strategical point, at the confluence of the Ohio and Mississippi rivers, now holds, within two miles of its apex, about five thousand men. Two regiments are at Bird's Point, just opposite, on the Missouri shore, and a few companies are stationed a few miles up on the west bank of the Ohio. The ground, which is very low, is defended, by a lofty and now quite solid levee or dyke on three sides, from overflow from the occasional sudden and excessive freshets of the two rivers. It is deemed already quite secure against any future flood, as much has been done since 1858, when it suffered seriously, to strengthen these embankments. A feud exists between the three companies representing the business of the place—the original Cairo City Company, the Illinois Central, and the Wharf Company—who are at loggerheads with each other and with the citizens, who are opposed to them all. The land company, by holding its lots at excessive prices, stands in the way of the city's growth, and in its own light. The Illinois Central, it is complained, has not fulfilled its own contracts with this company; and the wharf monopoly discourages the citizens. The consequence of all this is a discouraged and paralyzed community, where nature and circumstances have provided for a prosperous and growing city. Neither the exposure nor the climate warrants the bad reputation and slow growth of Cairo. It is perfectly defensible from the waters at a moderate expense, and is capable of being thoroughly drained, and, indeed, of being raised throughout its whole area to the height of its levees, which ought to be the level of the future city. An enlightened policy would effect this in a very few years after war has ceased, provided the companies that now smother the place would enter with zeal and alacrity into it. The back country on both sides of Cairo is undeveloped, and, perhaps, is not promising; but the Illinois Central, running through that immensely fertile State, and terminating here, is a back country in itself, capable of building up a great city. The immense commerce concentrating at this point of perpetual open navigation, low enough down to escape all serious influence from ice, and at a point where water never fails for large boats, would itself, properly utilized, create a fine city here. The necessity of erecting a United States fortress at this point is now very apparent, and probably the problems of the health of the point and its commercial importance will be so tested by the necessary presence of thousands of troops through the war, as to do for the reputation and making of the place more than peace itself could have done in many years.

Cairo, though low, is now neither damp, muddy, nor unhealthy. The water which stands in the plain a few inches deep, after a heavy rain, very soon, owing to the sandy character of the soil, disappears. Engines are at work, also, to drain the surplus surface water off into the river. The army has cleared away some thousands of stumps from the central plain of Cairo, and created a very fine parade of two or three miles long, and a mile or so broad. Col. Paine's regiment was chiefly active in this good work, which will prove of lasting service to Cairo. The general health of the place is testified to by an intelligent resident physician (a Virginian) as being better than at most points on the Ohio and Mississippi. Fever and ague does not abound, and there seemed to be a general testimony among the army surgeons there that the health of the troops was as good as at any other point where so many men were collected. The sick list showed us about 250 on their hacks in a force of 6,000, which, at the close of June and 1st July, is not an excessive number. The open, airy character of Cairo, situated between two rivers, which act by their unequal currents as perpetual ventilators, saves it from the influence of the malarious airs which seem to blow over it, and produce their mischievous effects in the high lands beyond, on bluffs crowned with wood, at Villa Ridge, clothed with a forest obstructing the free passage of winds, and occasioning, perhaps, by a cooler atmosphere, a precipitation of the poison at a particular level. Cairo proves more healthful than would be supposed from its apparently exposed position.

The Mississippi water has a general reputation for wholesomeness. The Missouri mud, with which it is charged, in settling, carries down whatever vegetable or animal substance may exist in the water, and leaves it, though still colored, comparatively pure. The Ohio water, being more conveniently reached, is, however, chiefly used by the troops. They had all suffered diarrhea from the use of this water, or from change. It took about a fortnight to accustom them to it. The surgeons were doubting the expediency of going into the use of the Mississippi water, from fear that another change might produce another access of the same complaint. But it was promised that careful experiments should be made in the relative effects of the two kinds of water. A filtering system was proposed. Fortunately, large ice-houses already existed in Cairo, well filled, which have been a great comfort to the troops.

The camp police of Cairo was not good; the men being shockingly remiss in the use of the sinks, which are badly situated and poorly constructed. Cleanliness was not observed; the camp showed a great deal of garbage and waste water lying about. The officers complained bitterly of the carelessness of the men in all these respects.

The medical force was very excellent in quality and service; the hospitals usually good and cleanly; always too much crowded, and even when this was not necessary. There was the same difficulty about procuring stores. The regiments had fortunately come from Chicago chiefly well provided in these respects with medicines, &c.; but all their fresh wants they did not know how to provide for. Some of the physicians were absent at the examination at Springfield and Washington. The arrival of the medical director, Dr. Simmons, U. S. A., an intelligent and earnest gentleman, seemed to promise relief, as he at once undertook to instruct them in the means of procuring what they needed from the regular sources. There were no ambulances in the place, and few surgical instruments. The same kind of complaints—measles, diarrhea, pneumonia, rheumatism, and typhoid fever—prevailed; but the types of disease were commonly mild.

JULY 2, 1861. St. Louis, MO

I have just visited the 13th Illinois regiment, Col. J. D. Wyman, and the 22d regiment from the same State, volunteers, at Caseyville, Camp McClellan.

Col. Wyman, of the 13th regiment, is in command of both regiments. The camp of the 13th is very much crowded, and needs nearly double the number of tents it has to make the men comfortable. Col. Wyman complains of the inattention of the quartermaster general at Springfield, and is very much perplexed, because he has conflicting orders from General McClellan and from General Lyon, both of whom claim his obedience. Of course his men must suffer many evils until the question is finally determined. The colonel has been paying out his own money to make his men comfortable. Owing to the goodness of his position, on an open and dry plain, and to the convenience of good well water, there is no sickness of any importance in his camp, eight being the total number in the hospital. He is likely to move either to the St. Louis arsenal or to Cairo at any moment.

The 22d regiment, Col. Dougherty, is in a wretched condition. It is encamped only half a mile to the east of the 13th. But it is in a valley, beneath very shady trees, and under the lee of some hills, all which combine to make the miasmatic atmosphere stagnate at the spot, as the winds have no circulation. They have been there only 13 days, but have at least 250 men out of about 900 more or less sick with camp dysentery. This is due in part to the situation, but in part also to the water, which is positively black and disgusting. It is taken from some pits sunk in a kind of half stagnant gutter, in the other end of which the pigs are rooting. All the water they have is from this wretched source, and they have not enough even of this. Of course they mix worse rum with this bad water, and the men are poisoned.

The hospital is in a room hired for the occasion, which is a perfect pig-sty for nastiness. The accommodations are only for, say five and twenty, and the sick are 250. The steward (for both surgeon and assistant were absent) had made fifty prescriptions to-day, and was not through yet. This camp has no hospital tents or stores, except what it borrows from the 13th. The surgeon of that regiment is also absent. There is evidently a gross neglect in these easy absences, granted at a time when no excuse should suffice to absent the doctor, who is so sadly wanted. The 22d should be moved immediately.

The camp police is very imperfect. Rotten bones and other nuisances lay about the camp. Col. Wyman appeared to be very solicitous to do his duty, but was puzzled how to get what he needed for his men.

There had been five men carelessly wounded by bayonets in his regiment, and one valuable officer shot dead in consequence of the inexperience of a sentry.

Source: Bellows, Henry. (1866). Sanitary Commission No. 26. Notes of a Preliminary Sanitary Survey of the Forces of the United States, in the Ohio and Mississippi Valleys, near Midsummer, 1861. Reprinted in Documents of the U.S. Sanitary Commission. New York.

- **Document:** A Report to the Secretary of War on the Operations of the Sanitary Commission, and upon the Sanitary Condition of the Volunteer Army
- **Date:** 1861
- **Where:** Washington, DC

DOCUMENT

The following statement exhibits a classification of the cases of disease in the volunteer army during a portion of the campaign, showing, also, the per centage of casualties of all kinds (wounds, accidents, etc.) for the same period, compared with like returns from the army of the Crimea, from April 10, 1854, to June 30, 1856:

	Army of the Potomac	Army of the West	Army of the Crimea, Ap. 10, '53 to June 30, 1856
Zymotic [acute infectious] disease, (per cent.)	61.1	76.3	69.8
Constitutional	1.2	.6	.5
Local	30.7	17.8	15.6
Developmental	3.4	3.5	.1
Violence	3.6	2.2	14.0
All cases	100.0	100.0	100.0

Two most important facts appear on the face of this table: first, the immense disproportion between cases of disease and of violence, fully justifying all that has been asserted as to the loss an army in the field must expect to sustain from these causes respectively; and, secondly, the great excess of zymotic [acute infectious] diseases, nearly all of which are, in a greater or less degree, preventable by proper precautions. For instance, typhus can be almost certainly averted by systematic attention to cleanliness and ventilation, smallpox by vaccination, and malarious diseases (intermittent fever, etc.) by quinine. It seems apparent, therefore, that it is within the power of Government, either by the action of the War Department or by legislation, to enforce rules that will most materially diminish the waste of efficiency by disease, and the consequent cost of the present war.

Source: Sanitary Commission No. 40. (1866). A Report to the Secretary of War on the Operations of the Sanitary Commission, and upon the Sanitary Condition of the Volunteer Army, Its Medical Staff, Hospitals, and Hospital Supplies. Washington, DC: McGill and Witmerow, Printers, 1861. Reprinted in Documents of the U.S. Sanitary Commission. New York.

ANALYSIS

By the mid-19th century, military leaders throughout the world were facing health-care crises brought on by a number of factors: the increasing size of armies and navies, improved transportation networks that brought soldiers together from all parts of the country and sent them quickly throughout the globe, and improvements in military technology that created ever more deadly wounds. Training camps, if improperly managed, could become incubators of smallpox, cholera, and typhus. Army and navy hospitals became death traps as infectious diseases spread after every battle. Even improvements in military surgery could pose logistical challenges: since more soldiers recovered even from amputation and other severe injuries, military hospitals had to care for more convalescing patients.

The U.S. Sanitary Commission sent out inspectors to over 400 regimental camps in the summer of 1861. As the document indicates, preventative medicine had not been very high on the list of priorities for recruiters or for regimental officers. Epidemic diseases—"diarrhea, pneumonia, measles, and typhoid fever"—abounded: as Henry Bellows (1814–1882), the president of the U.S. Sanitary Commission noted, "It was obvious that the recruiting had been careless, and the men who were sick were mainly those who should never have been permitted to enter the service." Officers were not paying enough attention to clean water or hospital sanitation. A hospital that was a "perfect pigsty" before a battle even started would surely prove a death trap when filled with the sick and the wounded. Bellows also paid attention to camp "police," that is, military order, cleanliness, and discipline. Lack of good order led to obvious health hazards, such as "rotten bones and other nuisances." In Bellows's view and that of his contemporaries, it could also interfere with soldiers' health: lack of discipline, they thought, led to demoralized troops, which would, in turn, lead them to be more susceptible to illness.

The Report to the Secretary of War shows how much the medical disasters of the Crimean War influenced the U.S. Sanitary Commission. It also shows the sanitary commissioners' strategies for influencing the war effort. Since, as an advisory body, they had no power to compel military officers to listen to them, they turned their efforts to the Secretary of War. The key points were first, that infectious diseases killed many more soldiers than battle wounds, and second, that those diseases could be held in check with proper sanitary measures. Preventing "typhus . . . by systematic attention to cleanliness and ventilation, smallpox by vaccination, and malarious diseases . . . by quinine" would ensure that the army could be kept in full strength through prevention and at a fraction of the cost of treatment.

As the Sanitary Commission had feared, the new Army of the Potomac suffered attacks again and again from diseases in the first year of the war. Fortunately, in June 1862, Jonathan Letterman (1824–1872) was appointed medical director of the army, with the explicit charge from General George McClellan (1826–1885) to take any measures he thought necessary. The result was a sweeping reorganization of army medical administration that became the basis of modern military practices. Among other reforms, he instituted efficient use of ambulance corps to transport the wounded quickly from the battlefield and railroads to send them to base hospitals. In doing so, Letterman turned the transportation technology that spread disease into means for preventing and alleviating it. He was buried at Arlington National Cemetery and honored at the National Museum for Civil War Medicine.

FURTHER READING

Devine, Shauna. (2014). *Learning from the Wounded: The Civil War and the Rise of American Medical Science*. Chapel Hill: The University of North Carolina Press.

Humphreys, Margaret. (2013). *Marrow of Tragedy: The Health Crisis of the American Civil War*. Baltimore, MD: Johns Hopkins Press.

Letterman, Jonathan. (1866). *Medical Recollections of the Army of the Potomac*. New York: Appleton and Company.

McGaugh, Scott. (2015). *Surgeon in Blue: Jonathan Letterman, the Civil War Doctor Who Pioneered Battlefield Care*. New York: Arcade Publishing.

Rutkow, Ira. (2005). *Bleeding Blue and Gray: Civil War Surgery and the Evolution of American Medicine*. New York: Random House.

Schroeder-Lein, Glenna R. (2008). *Encyclopedia of Civil War Medicine*. New York: ME Sharpe.

CIVIL WAR NURSING

- **Document:** Cornelia Hancock, Letter from the Army of the Potomac
- **Date:** 1864
- **Where:** Washington, DC
- **Significance:** Civil War medical professionals, men and women, were as passionate about their cause as the soldiers they cared for. The war was a turning point for the American nursing profession, as a generation of young women learned firsthand about the realities of battlefield medicine.

DOCUMENT

Where are the people who have been professing such strong abolition proclivity for the last thirty years?—certainly not in Washington laboring with these people whom they have been clamoring to have freed. They are freed now or at least many of them, and herded together in filthy huts, half clothed. And, what is worse than all, guarded over by persons who have not a proper sympathy for them. I have been in the Washington Contraband Hospital for the past two months—it is in close proximity to the Camp of Reception—and I have had ample opportunity to see these people, the persons in charge of them, and the whole mode of proceeding with them. Their wants are great and appeal in every way for aid from the North . . .

The situation of the Camp is revolting to a degree, 12 or 14 persons occupy a room not 15 ft. square, do all their cooking, eating, etc. therein. The Camp has but one well of water and that out of order most of the time. All the water used by nearly 1,000 persons is carted from Washington so one can judge of the cleanliness of the Camp. In "the hall," consisting of nothing conducive to comfort, neither light nor beds, probably some fifty sleep and the consequence is in a few days several of these people are seized with some aggravated disease and have to be carried to the hospital on stretchers and lay there to be supported by this same government that the authorities here say refuses to give them better accommodations when they first arrive.

Now, I maintain an ounce of preventative would be worth a pound of cure, if the object is to save the government expense. The Hospital here is under the care of colored surgeons. It was built under the supervision of Dr. Breed of Washington, and is supplied just as other hospitals are. It is the most humane establishment for the accommodation of contrabands that there is in Washington. We have here all sick and wounded black soldiers, all sick servants serving officers in the army, and the sick in general around Washington. Smallpox has raged here to a great extent but a separate hospital has been established for that now. The order now is to remove all contrabands south of the Potomac. It may be better there than here, but we remain under the same authority and let me state emphatically that nothing for the permanent advancement of these people can be effected until the whole matter is removed from the military authority and vested in a separate bureau whose sole object is the protection and elevation of these people. Now this whole contraband business is under military regulation and under officers that think to spend government money for contrabands all waste. Now I can see the abuses here plainly but to remedy them is the trouble. Many wise and good people visit here and exclaim "this must not be," go away fully convinced they will do all in their power to rectify matters; go to some military functionary, who probably cares as little and less for a contraband than his riding horse. He informs them all is done for contrabands that the government allows; so you might go to numerous military men and receive the same answer. I say all is not done for contrabands that government allows. The designs of the government are not carried out by subordinate authorities.

And the only way to ever get justice done to these people is to separate the whole matter from the military authority, make a separate bureau, have men at the head of this bureau with living souls in them large enough to realize that a contraband is a breathing human being capable of being developed, if not so now. Let them have the power to appoint officers to have charge of these camps, good energetic, anti-slavery persons who will take an interest in the improvement of those under their charge. I feel this to be the duty of every individual to urge upon every senator and congressman that this step be taken, but meanwhile as we stand at present, our needs are very pressing and any contributions of any land of clothing, old or new, shoes and stockings especially, both men's and women's, will prevent much immediate suffering. There is much charity being extended to our poor soldiers and I would not that any one should withhold one mite from them, but I maintain that persons living in their comfortable homes in the North should give liberally to those so sadly situated as these forlorn contrabands, as well as to the soldiers. A national Sanitary Commission for the Relief of Colored Persons of this class would save lives and a great deal of suffering. The slaves generally get free when our army advances; they come into our lines several hundred at a time, follow the army for a while, then come into Washington, some probably having walked 50 miles. One woman carried one child in her arms and dragged two by her side. Judge of the condition of that woman when she arrives. Should not some comfortable quarters await her weary body?

Source: Hancock, Cornelia. (1937). *South after Gettysburg: Letters of Cornelia Hancock from the Army of the Potomac, 1863–1865.* Philadelphia, PA: University of Pennsylvania Press, 40–43.

ANALYSIS

Having carefully studied the British experience in the Crimea, members of the U.S. Sanitary Commission wholeheartedly recommended recruiting female nurses to staff military hospitals. The exact number of nurses cannot be known, because records were kept very sporadically, but historians estimate between 3,000 and

8,000 women contributed their services. Dorothea Dix (1802–1887), already noted for her work to improve care of the insane, was appointed superintendent of nurses for the army. Clara Barton (1821–1912) worked as a hospital administrator on the front lines of the Union army; she later went on to found the American branch of the International Red Cross. The writer Louisa May Alcott (1832–1888), best known as the author of *Little Women*, served as a nurse in Washington, DC, hospitals. Her account of her experiences, *Hospital Sketches*, sold very well to a civilian audience eager for news of the war. Alcott earned five cents in royalties for every book sold, and the publisher donated five cents per book to a charity for children orphaned by the war.

Hospital nurses were typically well educated, resourceful, independent-minded women with a strong sense of social justice. It is no wonder they frequently clashed with the military authorities that were ultimately responsible for their patients and for overall hospital management. Cornelia Hancock (1840–1927), a Quaker from New Jersey, made it clear in her letters to her family that she was exasperated by the indifference of the military to her patients. She was only 22 when she joined the Union army—so young, in fact, that Dorothea Dix turned down her application. Not to be deterred, Hancock simply arrived after the battle of Gettysburg and went to work. She stayed with the Army of the Potomac until the end of the war, moving south with them to Washington and then through Virginia to Richmond.

Hancock was appalled by the way her own army handled the group dismissively known as "contraband" but whom we might better characterize as refugees: former slaves who sought protection from the Union troops moving through Confederate states. The attitude she encountered, that "contrabands" were not worth spending money on, was completely misguided from a medical standpoint. As she notes, "An ounce of preventative would be worth a pound of cure," for so many people, coming from so many separate parts of the country, under such hardship conditions, were bringing a host of diseases within range of both troops and civilians. The conditions were such as to almost guarantee not only smallpox outbreaks but also typhus and cholera—and all within close proximity to the nation's capital and a vulnerable civilian and military population.

Hancock's account illustrates one of the key lessons to emerge from the medical reforms of the Civil War: if sanitary and medical measures are to be effective in protecting everyone, everywhere, then they must be available to everyone, everywhere. As a later generation would phrase it, that is what puts the "public" in "public health."

FURTHER READING

Alcott, Louisa May. (1863). *Hospital Sketches*. Boston, MA: James Redpath.

Dammann, Gordon and Alfred Jay Bollet. (2008). *Images of Civil War Medicine*. New York: Demos.

Pryor, Elizabeth. (1987). *Clara Barton: Professional Angel.* Philadelphia, PA: University of Pennsylvania Press.

Ropes, Hannah Anderson. (1980). *Civil War Nurse: the Diary and Letters of Hannah Ropes,* edited by John Brumgardt. Knoxville, TN: University of Tennessee Press.

Schultz, Jane. (1992). "The Inhospitable Hospital: Gender and Professionalism in Civil War Medicine." *Signs* 17: 363–392.

5

THE GERM THEORY AND VACCINATION (1870–1900)

THE GERM THEORY AND THE SCIENCE OF IMMUNOLOGY

- **Document:** Louis Pasteur, "Prevention of Rabies"
- **Date:** 1885, 1886
- **Where:** Paris, France
- **Significance:** Louis Pasteur, together with Robert Koch (see next section), was one of the founders of the germ theory, the theory that a specific microorganism causes a specific disease. He made bacteriology, the study of microorganisms, his life's work. His research showed that an attenuated, or weakened, version of certain microorganisms could produce immunity to the disease in animals and inaugurated a worldwide effort to produce vaccines. In the section below, Pasteur explained the circumstances that led him to switch his efforts from producing immunity to rabies from dogs to people, specifically a nine-year-old boy, Joseph Meister (1876–1940).

DOCUMENT

Of twenty dogs treated, I could not render more than fifteen or sixteen refractory to rabies. Further, it was desirable, at the end of the treatment, to inoculate with a very virulent virus—a control virus—in order to confirm and reinforce the refractory condition. More than this, prudence demanded that the dogs should be kept under observation during a period longer than the period of incubation of the disease produced by the direct inoculation of this last virus. Therefore, in order to be quite sure that the refractory state had been produced, it was sometimes necessary to wait three or four months. The application of the method would have been very much limited by these troublesome conditions . . .

After making almost innumerable experiments, I have discovered a prophylactic method which is practical and prompt, and which has already in dogs afforded me results sufficiently numerous, certain, and successful, to warrant my having confidence in its general applicability to all animals, and even to man himself.

This method depends essentially on the following facts:

The inoculation of the infective spinal cord of a dog suffering from ordinary rabies under the dura

---

DID YOU KNOW?

Timeline of Human Vaccine Development, 1798–1900

Disease	Year
Smallpox	1798
Rabies	1885
Typhoid	1896
Cholera	1896
Bubonic plague	1897

Source: Plotkin, Stanley, Walter Orenstein, and Paul Offit, eds. (2013). *Vaccines.* Philadelphia, PA: Elsevier Saunders.

mater of a rabbit, always produces rabies after a period of incubation having a mean duration of about fifteen days.

If, by the above method of inoculation, the virus of the first rabbit is passed into a second, and that of the second into a third, and so on, in series, a more and more striking tendency is soon manifested towards a diminution of the duration of the incubation period of rabies in the rabbits successively inoculated.

After passing twenty or twenty-five times from rabbit to rabbit, inoculation periods of eight days are met with, and continue for another interval, during which the virus is passed twenty or twenty-five times from rabbit to rabbit. Then an incubation period of seven days is reached, which is encountered with striking regularity throughout a new series extending as far as the ninetieth animal . . .

The virus of rabies at a constant degree of virulence is contained in the spinal cords of these rabbits throughout their whole extent.

If portions, a few centimeters long, are removed from these spinal cords with every possible precaution to preserve their purity, and are then suspended in dry air, the virulence slowly disappears, until at last it entirely vanishes. The time within which this extinction of virulence is brought about varies a little with the thickness of the morsels of spinal cord, but chiefly with the external temperature. The lower the temperature, the longer is the virulence preserved. These results form the central scientific point in the method.

These facts being established, a dog may be rendered refractory to rabies in a relatively short time . . .

[Pasteur then explains his method, which involves giving the dog a series of inoculations, starting with the weakest form of the virus and ending with the most virulent.]

The dog has now been rendered refractory to rabies . . .

Never having once failed when using this method, I had in my possession fifty dogs, of all ages and of every race, refractory to rabies, when three individuals from Alsace unexpectedly presented themselves at my laboratory . . .

Théodore Vone, grocer, of Meissengott, near Schlestadt, bitten in the arm, July 4th, by his own dog, which had gone mad.

Joseph Meister, aged 9 years, also bitten on July 4th, at eight o'clock in the morning, by the same dog. This child had been knocked over by the dog and presented numerous bites, on the hands, legs, and thighs, some of them so deep as to render walking difficult. The principal bites had been cauterized at eight o'clock in the evening of July 4th, only twelve hours after the accident, with phenic acid . . .

The third person, who had not been bitten, was the mother of little Joseph Meister.

At the examination of the dog, after its death by the hand of its master, the stomach was found full of hay, straw, and scraps of wood. The dog was certainly rabid. Joseph Meister had been pulled out from under him covered with foam and blood.

M. Vone had some severe contusions on the arm, but he assured me that his shirt had not been pierced by the dog's fangs. As he had nothing to fear, I told him that he could return to Alsace the same day, which he did. But I kept young Meister and his mother with me . . .

[Pasteur, who was not a physician, consulted with two professors from the medical school in Paris. They examined Joseph Meister and noted that he had 14 wounds.]

The opinion of our learned colleague ... was that, owing to the severity and the number of the bites, Joseph Meister was almost certain to take rabies. I then communicated to [them] the new results which I had obtained from the study of rabies ...

The death of this child appearing to be inevitable, I decided, not without lively and sore anxiety, as may well be believed, to try upon Joseph Meister the method which I had found constantly successful with dogs ...

Consequently, on July 6th, at 8 o'clock in the evening, sixty hours after the bites on July 4th, and in the presence of [two doctors], young Meister was inoculated ...

In the following days fresh inoculations were made. I thus made thirteen inoculations, and prolonged the treatment to ten days. I shall say later on that a smaller number of inoculations would have been sufficient. But it will be understood how, in the first attempt, I would act with a very special circumspection ...

On the last days, therefore, I had inoculated Joseph Meister with the most virulent virus of rabies, that, namely, of the dog, reinforced by passing a great number of times from rabbit to rabbit, a virus which produces rabies after seven days incubation in these animals, after eight or ten days in dogs ...

Joseph Meister, therefore, has escaped, not only the rabies which would have been caused by the bites he received, but also the rabies with which I have inoculated him in order to test the immunity produced by the treatment, a rabies more virulent than ordinary canine rabies.

The final inoculation with very virulent virus has this further advantage, that it puts a period to the apprehensions which arise as to the consequences of the bites. If rabies could occur it would declare itself more quickly after a more virulent virus than after the virus of the bites. Since the middle of August I have looked forward with confidence to the future good health of Joseph Meister. At the present time, three months and three weeks have elapsed since the accident, his state of health leaves nothing to be desired.

Source: Pasteur, Louis. (1885). "A Method by Which the Development of Rabies after a Bite May Be Prevented." In *Recent Essays by Various Authors on Bacteria in Relation to Disease*, edited by W. Watson Cheyne. (1886). London: New Sydenham Society, 635–640.

ANALYSIS

Rabies is one of the most fearsome diseases known to humankind. It is primarily a disease of mammals, attacking dogs and their wild cousins, wolves, foxes, coyotes, and jackals; it also appears in bats and skunks. In dogs, the virus travels from the original source of infection—generally a bite from a wild animal—to the brain, leading to wild, aggressive behavior. People contract rabies primarily from being attacked by rabid dogs, and the process repeats itself: the virus begins to travel from the site of the bite to the brain, leading to fever, muscle pain, hallucinations, and increasingly erratic behavior. Left untreated, it is 100% fatal. But from an early period in human history, there was one treatment that, if applied early enough, sometimes arrested the disease: cauterizing the bite by applying a red-hot iron. The more bites there were, though, the more painful this treatment, and the less chance of cure.

We now know that cauterization would have worked by killing the virus before it could reach the nervous system. The reason we know it is the tremendous research achievement of scientists like John Snow (1813–1858), Louis Pasteur (1822–1895), Robert Koch (1843–1910), and many others, known as the germ theory of disease. It provided both an explanation of previously existing treatments like Jenner's cowpox vaccination and a way forward for developing new treatments for infectious diseases. The premise was simple: when a patient contracted and survived certain kinds of diseases—like smallpox, for example—the microorganism responsible for the disease created a biological response in the patient. That biological response created immunity to that disease so that the microorganism had no further impact on that patient. The problem was that only smallpox seemed to come with its own, naturally occurring preventative microorganism. Scientists would have to come up with ways of creating the others in the laboratory.

Pasteur claimed that his first attempt at creating a vaccine, for cholera in chickens, came about because of an accident, when he used a weakened form of the microorganism without realizing it. Scholars who have examined his notebooks have found a very careful, thorough pattern of research into all aspects of bacteriology, including the laboratory production of vaccines for a range of diseases affecting agricultural production, including both chicken cholera and anthrax, a disease of cattle. Pasteur was well aware of both the public and professional importance of his research. He was one of the earliest scientists to make use of national and international patents to protect the vaccination processes he devised, and he sometimes took public credit for work actually carried out by his assistants. The name "Pasteur" became a kind of national brand, with his patent for "pasteurization"—the process by which organic products, like wine and milk, were heated to sterilize them and prevent the propagation of microorganisms—and the founding of the Pasteur Institute in Paris. To contemporary accusations that he spent too much time seeking public recognition, he insisted that it was for his work, not for himself: it was essential that the public recognize the existence of germs, those tiny killers, invisible to the naked eye, and the awful consequences of neglecting their impact. One of his ardent admirers was Joseph Lister (1827–1912), who introduced sterile practices into surgery, credited with saving countless lives.

We can recognize Pasteur's careful research methods in this document, as he painstakingly developed the procedures for creating a vaccine, as he intended, that would protect dogs from rabies. If dogs could be rendered immune from the disease, that would shut down the main vector transmitting the disease to humans. Despite—or perhaps because of—his reputation as a showman, therefore, we can believe that trying the method on a dangerously ill small boy, even under the supervision of two physicians, aroused "lively and sore anxiety." By this time, anything Pasteur did would have made the headlines, and if Joseph Meister had died, both his own reputation and that of the fledgling science of bacteriology could have suffered. Fortunately, his research was sound, and Joseph survived both the disease and the treatment. He worked as a caretaker at the Pasteur Institute for much of his adult life.

Pasteur, in acknowledgment of Jenner's pioneering efforts, proposed that the term *vaccine* be expanded from smallpox and applied to the process of induced immunity for all diseases.

FURTHER READING

Dubos, René. (1960). *Pasteur and Modern Science*. Garden City, NY: Anchor Books.

Geison, Gerald. (1978). "Pasteur's Work on Rabies: Reexamining the Ethical Issues." *The Hastings Center Report* 8: 26–33.

Geison, Gerald. (1995). *The Private Science of Louis Pasteur*. Princeton, NJ: Princeton University Press.

Latour, Bruno. (1988). *The Pasteurization of France*. Cambridge, MA: Harvard University Press.

Vallery-Rodot, René. (1919). *The Life of Pasteur*. New York: Doubleday.

GROWING CHOLERA IN THE LABORATORY

- **Document:** George Lewis, "The Methods to be Employed in the Cultivation and Detection of the Comma Bacillus of Asiatic Cholera"
- **Date:** 1885
- **Where:** Berlin, Germany
- **Significance:** Though Robert Koch and Louis Pasteur are inextricably linked in the history of vaccines, they were fierce rivals during their own lifetime. This was in part because of the animosity between their countries, France and Germany. That animosity was responsible for bitter warfare during the 19th and 20th centuries, but it had one small silver lining: as the reputation of Pasteur's laboratory achieved international stature, the German government responded by founding its own laboratory, which, as described below, invited scientific delegations from all over the world to learn the new bacteriological techniques.

DOCUMENT

On October 1, 1884, the German government completed arrangements with Dr. Robert Koch by which he was to establish, in the city of Berlin, a laboratory well equipped with apparatus and assistants for the purpose of acquainting the German physicians with his theory of the cause of cholera, and the mode of cultivation of the so-called "comma-bacillus." The time specified for the duration of this course was to extend from October 1, 1884, to the end of January, 1885, and the four months were to be divided into periods of ten days each, that time being sufficient for a thorough understanding, not merely of the theory, but also of the practical work necessary in the cultivation and detection of the cholera bacillus. Delegations from the principal cities and towns were to be received in groups of from four to six at a time, and all their work was to be under the direct supervision of Dr. Koch, aided by a competent corps of assistants, most of whom have accompanied him during his investigations in Egypt, Italy and France. At the expiration of the ten days allotted to a single group, another was to take its place and receive a similar course.

Some two weeks ago I had the good fortune to receive one of the two appointments granted to Americans, and should like to give the reader some idea of the thoroughness and practicability of such instruction. Before doing this, however, a few words with regard to the present understanding of the disease may not be entirely out of place. Perhaps no visitation of the epidemic has afforded a better opportunity for studying its characteristics and tendencies than the recent outbreak in Italy and France, and for this reason most of our knowledge comes from these sources. The idea that cholera is of spontaneous origin is now no longer entertained by those who have given particular attention to the subject. Dr. Koch, who is undoubtedly the oldest investigator in this direction, is of opinion that its home is in the Delta of the Ganges, and his reasons for thus closely confining its limits seem at least plausible. The conditions that favor the spread of cholera in India are of a very peculiar nature. It was formerly maintained that the disease was indigenous in Ceylon, Madras and Bombay, but later research indicates that the almost constant existence of the infection in these places is due to the active traffic between them and certain parts of the Delta. The only region, however, in India where the cholera prevails continuously and without apparently any fluctuation, is the Delta of the Ganges. This entire tract is the unceasing home of the epidemic. It even extends up the banks of the Ganges as far as Benares. The upper part of the Delta is densely inhabited, while the lower part or base of the triangle is unapproachable to man on account of the inundations and pernicious fevers which invariably attack any one who passes its borders. In this uninhabited district may be found a luxuriant vegetation and an abundant variety of animal life, and one can easily imagine what quantities of animal and vegetable matter are here exposed to putrefaction. As Dr. Koch maintains, there is perhaps no better place in the world for the development of micro-organisms, and especially micro-organisms of an infectious character. In this respect the boundary between the inhabited and uninhabited parts of the Delta would seem to be exceptionally favorable, where the refuse from an extremely thickly populated country is floated down by the small streams, and mixes with the brackish water below, which flows backwards and forwards and is already saturated with putrefied matter.

The theory that the comma-bacillus belongs to a special fauna and flora of micro-organisms whose growth and development are adapted to these surroundings, is very probable, for everything points to the fact that cholera derives its origin from this frontier territory. This statement may appear more valuable when we consider that all the greater epidemics have been accompanied by a corresponding increase of the disease in the south of Bengal. We now know that the comma-bacillus finds, in the districts adjoining the supposed habitat, the most favorable conditions for obtaining a footing and transferring itself from man to man. The entire stretch of country known as Lower Bengal is only slightly raised above the sea-level, and during the rainy season almost the whole extent is submerged. For this reason the inhabitants are compelled to build their huts upon raised ground. This is effected by taking the earth near where the hut is built in order to raise the ground on which the house stands. The result of thus displacing the earth is to leave a large tank adjoining each but in which soiled water and putrefied matter from the household rapidly collect. Strange as it may seem this very water is used for drinking and other household purposes, and in turn receives much of the refuse matter which is necessarily thrown out. Under these circumstances can it be wondered at that the deadly cholera germ should take its origin and be transferred from one to another until it reaches all Europe and America? . . .

Through the discovery of the cholera bacillus, which has received the very characteristic name of "comma" bacillus, a speedy diagnosis is rendered possible. In spite of all opposing assertions, this characteristic biological and microscopical bacillus is found in no other infection save cholera, and by means of Dr. Koch's simple yet comprehensive method of "pure culture," every physician would be able to detect the existence of the organism with perfect certainty. The possibility of thus being able to speedily diagnose a case of cholera will undoubtedly, in time, render a most valuable aid in checking its spread, and by taking the proper precautions after recognizing its presence, the danger of an epidemic will be greatly lessened. From a medical point of view, however, its utility at the present time is very slight, but it must be remembered that rational therapeutics for the majority of diseases, and especially for those of an infectious character, cannot be obtained until we have ascertained their precise causes. It is certainly to be hoped that the presence of the comma-bacillus may be of service in diagnosing Asiatic cholera, and more especially so, in the early cases of its visitation. For the diagnosis, however, cultivation experiments are indispensable, and few have either the knowledge or the conveniences to enable them to carry this out. It is with a view of relieving the former of these wants that I have written this paper. No doubt, if Dr. Koch's theory is confirmed, some steps will be taken, in places threatened with an epidemic, to have means at hand for the satisfactory and rapid determination of the disease in suspicious cases. At present, if the discharges from suspicious cases were forwarded for examination to those who are interested in this work, much useful knowledge might be acquired, and an early intimation of its existence gained.

The method in itself is so easily understood that a physician possessing an ordinary knowledge of microscopical research would have little difficulty in cultivating, in the pure state, any bacillus with which he may be especially interested, and in a comparatively short time. The method is essentially the same as that employed in the cultivation of many of the different classes of bacilli known to us at the present time. Among these may be mentioned the typhus bacillus and tuberculosis bacillus, both of which are of recent discovery. A single week, perhaps, would be sufficient for developing and studying the peculiarities of any one species, but in order to appreciate minute differences, several species should be cultivated at the same time. In the course under Dr. Koch are cultivated, side by side . . . the comma-bacillus, the typhus bacillus, besides several forms of micrococci, all to render stronger the contrast between them . . . Nor is the same nourishing medium employed in all cases. Gelatine, bouillon, agar-agar, blood-serum and potatoes are all used as nourishing substances, and the various methods of preparing them will be explained further on.

The one precaution to be observed in bacteria cultivation is to thoroughly sterilize all vessels and instruments used in the promotion of the culture. This is effected either by a dry heat of 160° Centigrade, or a vapor heat of 100° Centigrade. The former is on all accounts the more satisfactory, although somewhat destructive to the fine tempering of steel instruments. The substance known as "food-gelatine" is most commonly employed as a breeding medium by the students in Dr. Koch's laboratory and its mode of preparation is as follows: Take 250 grams of fresh beef as free from fat as possible, and, after cutting it up into fine particles, add 500 grams of distilled water. Allow this to stand over night in an ice-chest or cellar and then strain it through a towel of ordinarily fine texture. The resulting mass will amount about to 400 com. Place the jar containing this substance in a metal vessel partly filled with water, and over a gasjet allow it to reach the body-heat. Now add 40 grams of stick gelatine, 4 grams of peptone and 1 gram of salt. It requires one-half hour for the gelatine to become thoroughly dissolved although this time may be somewhat less-ened by occasionally stirring the mass with a sterilized glass-rod. The addition of a little carbonic acid will enable one to prove the reaction. For this purpose small pieces of red and blue litmus paper are used. Enough of the carbonic acid should be added to prevent the blue paper from changing color when a drop of the nourish-ing substance has been poured upon it. As a further test a single drop should cause the red paper to become blue in color. When this result is obtained, the whole mass is to be thoroughly cooked until it has the appearance of the white of an egg. In order to insure the utility of the entire mass, a little should now be strained into a sterilized re-agent glass and the reaction again be taken as above mentioned. If this proves satisfactory, the whole solution is to be strained through a double thickness of filter-paper arranged in the form of a funnel. Of course this process is an exceedingly slow one, and, if possible, it is best to have several funnels at work at the same time. . . . After filling the requisite number of glasses and carefully replacing the cot-ton corks, they are to be placed together in a metal pot and boiled for the period of one hour. At the end of twenty-four, forty-eight and seventy-two hours respectively, they are to be again boiled for the period of three-quarters of an hour. We now have the medium in which all future cultivations can be carried on in the most satisfac-tory manner, and although certain characteristics may, perhaps, be better observed in some of the substances to be described further on, this food-gelatine is the one to which the greatest preference is given . . .

To give the dimensions of comma-bacillus would, indeed, be useless, because only a very poor idea could be derived from the extremely small numbers which would be necessary to represent its length, breadth and thickness. To compare it, however, with some other well-known bacillus, such as the "tubercle," will enable the reader to form at least some notion of its size, and at the same time admit of a comparison as to form and general appearance. The comma-bacillus is about three-fifths as long as the "tubercle," but much thicker and more bulky. A very evident curve, similar to that of a "comma," is noticed midway between the two extremities, hence its name. Occasionally the curve is so marked that it resembles a semi-circle. Then, again, two bacilli may cling together, but in opposite directions, thus presenting the appear-ance of the letter "S" . . .

Source: Lewis, George W. (1885). *Ten Days in the Laboratory with Dr. Robert Koch.* Buffalo, NY: Times Print.

ANALYSIS

Robert Koch (1843–1910) was in many ways the opposite of Pasteur: his careful, thorough research was reported in scientific periodicals, not in national and international newspapers. He began his professional career as a country physician, and one day, bored by his practice, decided to investigate the outbreak of anthrax among cattle in his district. He took a drop of blood from an animal that was sick with anthrax and put it on a slide. Then, following standard laboratory procedure, he took a drop of blood from an animal that was not sick with anthrax and put it on a slide as well. When he compared the two slides, he found something odd: a set of rod-shaped microorganisms in the blood of the sick cow. Could they be responsible for anthrax?

At that point, Koch had done no more than what many other scientists were doing, as knowledge of bacteriology spread among researchers: put substances on a slide and look for distinctive features. It is what he did next that would lead him to be regarded as one of the founders of the germ theory. Instead of assuming that the rod-like organisms were the cause of anthrax, he realized that there were other explanations: they might be a by-product of the disease or else a breakdown of existing cellular structures. To prove they caused the disease, he had to first prove they were really organisms—that is, they were really independent, living creatures. Then, he had to prove that they could cause the disease, not merely appear when it was present.

Koch did manage those two things: he worked out a technique for growing the anthrax bacilli, as it came to be called, on a medium outside the original animal. After growing it for numbers of generations—so that no trace of the original set remained—he injected it into a new, healthy animal. The animal developed anthrax. Koch did that many times, until he was confident that he had proof that the bacilli he had isolated were the cause of anthrax. In 1890, he codified his methods in what has become known as Koch's Postulates:

1. The microbe is present in every case of the disease.
2. The microbe can be taken from the infected host and grown independently.
3. The disease can be produced by introducing a pure culture of the microbe into a healthy host.
4. The microbe can be isolated and identified from the host in Step 3 (http://www.historyofvaccines.org/content/koch's-postulates).

Koch's work on anthrax led to a research position in Berlin, and in the early 1880s, he traveled to Egypt and India to investigate the cause of cholera. He was successful in isolating the microorganism, *vibrio cholerae*, also known as the "comma bacillus" because of its distinctive shape. In 1885, when George Lewis went to Berlin, he noted that the "medical utility at the present time is very slight"; Koch's process was expected to be useful in the area of public health, to help identify whether a water supply was infected. Within another two years, however, cholera vaccines had been developed by Jaime Ferran (1852–1929) in Spain and Waldemar Mordechai Haffkine (1860–1930) in Russia. This was a medical breakthrough, which both marked the end of a single deadly disease—cholera—and heralded the application of a scientific research method that would end still more diseases worldwide.

FURTHER READING

Brock, Thomas. (1988). *Robert Koch, a Life in Medicine and Bacteriology*. Berlin: Springer-Verlag.

Coleman, William. (1987). "Koch's Comma Bacillus: The First Year." *Bulletin of the History of Medicine* 61: 315–342.

Gradmann, Christophe. (2009). *Laboratory Disease : Robert Koch's Medical Bacteriology.* Baltimore, MD: Johns Hopkins University Press.

"Koch's Postulates." *History of Vaccines.* http://www.historyofvaccines.org/content/koch's-postulates.

Schlicht, Thomas. (2000). "Linking Cause and Disease in the Laboratory: Robert Koch's Method of Superimposing Visual and 'Functional' Representations of Bacteria." *History and Philosophy of the Life Sciences* 22: 43–58.

YELLOW FEVER AND MOSQUITOES

- **Document:** Walter Reed, "The Prevention of Yellow Fever"
- **Date:** 1901
- **Where:** American Public Health Association, 29th Annual Meeting, Buffalo, NY
- **Significance:** Though Walter Reed never developed a vaccine for yellow fever, his research on its most common vector, the *Aedes aegypti* mosquito, was the basis of successful prevention efforts.

DOCUMENT

The prevention of yellow fever since its first importation into the United States in 1693, and especially during the latter half of the past century, has commanded, perhaps, more attention on the part of those who were concerned with matters pertaining to the public health than the prevention of any of the other acute infections. This has not been occasioned by the fact that its total sickness and mortality have exceeded that of other acute infectious diseases, such as typhoid fever or croupous pneumonia, but because rather of the proximity of its source to our shores; the lack of knowledge of its specific agent; the consequent mystery surrounding its origin and propagation; the alarmingly rapid spread and course of this disease, when once it had obtained a foothold, and the high mortality with which its epidemics have generally been attended. Although the duration of its presence in our seaports was plainly limited by certain seasonal conditions, yet during its brief reign—July to October—its ravages were such as to completely paralyze both the social and commercial interests of a given city, and even of an entire section of our country.

The interval between 1793 and 1888 is almost 100 years, but upon the appearance of yellow fever we observe no difference of behavior on the part of the inhabitants of Jackson, Miss., in 1888, from that shown by the citizens of Philadelphia in 1793, except that the terror of the former was greater and their flight from their homes more precipitate than in the case of the latter.

The recurrence of succeeding epidemics has, therefore, served to increase rather than to lessen the public alarm.

It would be difficult to determine with accuracy the loss of life occasioned by the 95 invasions of our territory by yellow fever during the past 208 years. We have endeavored to collect from the most available sources the mortality caused by this disease, but have been unable to obtain any reliable data for the earlier epidemics. If we confine ourselves to the epidemics which have occurred since 1793, we find that there have not been less than 100,000 deaths from this cause. The greatest sufferer has been the city of New Orleans, with 41,348 deaths, followed by the city of Philadelphia, with 10,038 deaths. The epidemics of 1855, 1873, 1878, and 1879 claimed 7,759 victims in the city of Memphis, Tenn. From 1800 to 1876, Charleston lost 4,565 of its citizens by attacks of yellow fever. New York, during the earlier and later invasions of this disease, has had 3,454 deaths, while the epidemic of 1855 in Norfolk, Va., caused over 2,000 deaths. During our brief occupation of the island of Cuba (July, 1898–December, 1900), with every precaution brought into exercise to ward off the disease, there have occurred among the officers and men of our Army 1,575 cases of yellow fever, with 231 deaths.

If we reckon the average mortality at 20 per cent, there have not been less than 500,000 cases of yellow fever in the United States during the period from 1793 to 1900.

Turning for a moment to other countries, we find that the great epidemic of 1800, in the province of Andalusia, Spain, caused 60,000 deaths, and that 20,000 more deaths attended the invasion of the city of Barcelona by this disease in 1821. From 1851 to 1883, the deaths from this cause in the city of Rio de Janeiro were 23,338, while in the city of Habana, between the years 1853 and 1900, 35,952 deaths have been recorded from yellow fever.

We have no means of computing the damage done to the commercial interests of the United States by epidemics of yellow fever. At the sixth annual meeting of this association, held in Richmond, Va., in 1878, Dr. Samuel Choppin, president of the State board of health of Louisiana, estimated the actual cost of the epidemic of that year to the material resources of the city of New Orleans as $10,752,500. Dr. Benjamin Lee, the present distinguished occupant of the presidential chair, at the seventeenth annual meeting of this association, held in Brooklyn, N. Y., in 1889, contributed a paper having the title, "Do the Sanitary Interests of the United States Demand the Annexation of Cuba?" From this we quote the following sentence: "A single widespread epidemic of yellow fever would cost the United States more in money, to say nothing of the grief and misery which it would entail, than the purchase money of Cuba." That this was no exaggeration, witness the language of the petition which the chairman of the committee on the etiology of yellow fever, in conjunction with other prominent members of this association, presented to the President of the United States on November 15, 1897, and again, on November 21, 1898, in accordance with a resolution adopted at the meeting of this association, held at Ottawa, Canada, in 1897. In addressing President McKinley, Dr. Horlbeck said: "It is hardly necessary to call your attention to the serious results of the recent epidemic of yellow fever in the States of Louisiana, Mississippi, and Alabama, but we may be permitted to mention the fact that the great epidemic of 1878 resulted in the loss of nearly 16,000 lives, and that it has been estimated that the total loss to the country resulting from this epidemic was not less than $100,000,000."

The importance of the study of the causative factors entering into the propagation of a disease so capable of quickly destroying the lives of the citizens and wrecking the commercial interests of the cities of the United States could hardly be overestimated ...

Notwithstanding the importance of the work and the efforts put forth by students in this and other countries, we believe that we are safe in saying that no results had been obtained which would enable us to combat successfully this disease when once imported into our larger centers of population, and no means found to keep it out of our ports except such as would place very heavy burdens upon commerce. This inability to control the disease grew not only out of our ignorance as to the way or ways in which yellow fever was propagated, but also out of certain false opinions which we had formed as to the mode of its spread. The doctrine of the spread of yellow fever by fomites and by filth had taken such hold on the professional mind as completely to overshadow all other views, and to direct into false channels the work of those who were engaged in the investigation of this disease. The efforts to isolate or to discover the specific agent of yellow fever, if successful, would possibly have greatly simplified the problem; in the absence of such discovery, the first step in our knowledge of how to prevent this disease could only be found, we think, along another line, viz., that of its propagation from the sick to the well. This step we endeavored to take in connection with our colleagues, Dr. Agramonte and the late Dr. J. W. Lazear of the United States Army, during our recent investigations into the causation and spread of yellow fever at Quemados, Cuba.

The results of our earlier work relative to the etiology and propagation of this disease we had the pleasure of presenting to this association at its last meeting, held in Indianapolis, IN. You will recall that one of the conclusions which we then submitted was as follows: "The mosquito serves as the intermediate host for the parasite of yellow fever" . . .

Continuing our studies, especially as regards the means by which yellow fever is spread from individual to individual, and as to the manner in which houses become infected, we were able, under strict rules of isolation and quarantine, to bring about an attack of yellow fever in 10 nonimmune individuals (and always within the period of incubation of this disease) out of a total of 13 (76.84 per cent) whom we attempted to infect by means of the bites of mosquitoes—*Stegomyia fasciata*—that had previously been fed with the blood of yellow-fever patients during the first, second, and third days of their attacks. These results were reported in part to the Pan-American Congress held in Habana during February of this year, and in part to the Association of American Physicians at its last meeting, held in the city of Washington.

It will be seen that we were able to establish in the most conclusive manner that the mosquito does serve as the intermediate host for the parasite of yellow fever. At this same experimental sanitary station we were also able to demonstrate that an attack of yellow fever can not be induced by the most intimate and prolonged contact with the clothing and bedding of yellow-fever patients, even though these articles had been previously thoroughly and purposely soiled with the excreta of such patients. In other words, we were able to prove that the garments worn, and the bedding used, by yellow-fever patients were no more concerned in propagating this disease than the clothing and bedding of patients suffering from malarial fever are concerned in the spread of the latter malady. The doctrine of the spread of yellow fever by fomites having, at the first touch of actual experiment on human beings, burst like a bubble, we may hereafter cast it aside, with other exploded beliefs, to the very great simplification of the problem how to prevent yellow fever. Indeed, in our opinion, the time has now arrived when the latter problem may be reduced to measures which shall prevent the propagation of this disease by mosquitoes. Although this specific agent of yellow fever has not, as yet, been discovered, this must remain largely a matter of scientific interest, and does not in the least lessen the efforts which we, as sanitarians, are now able for the first time to bring into action for the prevention of the spread of this disease, since in dealing with the mosquito we are dealing with the intermediate host which carries the specific agent from the sick to the well . . .

Since the mosquito, especially that species of stegomyia which has recently been designated . . . as *Stegomyia fasciata* . . . has become so prominent a factor in the spread of yellow fever, it becomes necessary to consider this insect from the point of view of its identification; its habitat; its breeding places; the length of its generation; its hours of feeding; the influence of temperature upon both its propagation and stinging; the interval after contamination before the insect becomes capable of propagating the disease; the length of time during which it remains dangerous; the measures that should be used not only to protect the sick against the bites of these insects, but also to prevent the latter from infecting the healthy individual; and, finally, a consideration of the several agents which may be successfully employed both to prevent the breeding of mosquitoes as well as directed toward their destruction in the adult stage.

Aside from the standpoint of scientific interest, it is certainly a matter of hygienic importance, in taking up the question of how to prevent the spread of yellow fever, when imported into the United States, that the health authorities of our several coast cities, and, indeed, of some of our inland towns, should be able to determine whether the only species of mosquito, which, up to the present time, has been shown capable of conveying yellow fever, is or is not present in these cities. If it should hereafter be proven that only species of the genus *stegomyia* are capable of acting as intermediate hosts for the specific agent of yellow fever, as appears to have been demonstrated for the genus *anopheles* in the spread of malaria, the presence or absence of the former genus will definitely determine whether yellow fever will or will not spread in a given locality. The presence or absence of mosquitoes that can propagate the disease is the only intelligible explanation of what has heretofore been considered an inexplicable problem, viz., the capability of this disease to propagate itself in certain localities, while in other places it could be introduced with perfect impunity to the public health. In other words, our present knowledge of this question solves, at last, the problem of the portability or nonportability of yellow fever.

Source: Reed, Walter. (1911). "The Prevention of Yellow Fever." In *Yellow Fever, A Compilation of Various Publications*, James Carroll, William Crawford Gorgas, Robert Latham Owen, and Walter Drew McCaw. Washington, DC: Government Printing Office, 131–148.

ANALYSIS

The study of bacteriology grew to encompass all aspects of microorganisms, including their vectors, that is, the mechanisms by which they moved from host to host. A combination of vaccination and sanitary measures, including animal and insect control, led to enormous decline in once-terrifying epidemics. Laws regulating clean water supplies in cities eradicated cholera as a threat to health in industrialized countries. Housing codes and pest control reduced the rat population and the threat of bubonic plague. Animal control and a safe, effective method for vaccinating dogs led, as Pasteur had hoped, to eliminating the terror inspired by rabies.

Though the microbe that produced yellow fever was not isolated until 1927, the Cuban scientist Carlos Finlay (1833–1915) had determined by 1881 that it was spread by mosquitoes. Walter Reed (1851–1902) followed up on Finlay's research, using it as the basis for his own investigation in 1901. He and the rest of the U.S. Army Yellow Fever Commission laid to rest many of the historic controversies over the spread of yellow fever: that it was spread by dust fomites or by dirt; that it was not contagious or only contagious for certain social groups; that it could not be transported from ship to port. Even more important, as he noted in his address to the American Public Health Association, "We, as sanitarians, are now able for the first time to bring into action for the prevention of the spread of this disease, since in dealing with the mosquito we are dealing with the intermediate host which carries the specific agent from the sick to the well." The next stage of research could focus on the mosquito itself, its life cycle and mechanisms to prevent its propagation.

Reed focused on the potential loss to American commerce if yellow fever should break out so as to underline the value of the public health measures he proposed to institute. Mosquito eradication was costly, as he well knew; his point, however, was that a yellow fever outbreak would be more costly still. It would also be detrimental to the national interest. The U.S. Army had first taken an interest in yellow fever during the Spanish-American War in 1898, when over 5,000 American soldiers were stricken with the disease. The problem was exacerbated when Cuba became a U.S. protectorate at the end of the war; the army faced the problem of a permanent military presence, without any effective protection against yellow fever. The success of the Yellow Fever Commission made it possible for the United States to take on the task of completing the Panama Canal in 1904.

Sadly, Walter Reed died of appendicitis, a condition which the germ theory had made eminently treatable.

FURTHER READING

The Great Fever. The American Experience. PBS.org. http://www.pbs.org/wgbh/amex/fever/index.html.

Historical Collections at the Claude Moore Health Sciences Library, University of Virginia. *The U.S. Army Yellow Fever Commission.* http://exhibits.hsl.virginia.edu/yellowfever/.

Kelly, Howard. (1923). *Walter Reed and Yellow Fever.* Baltimore, MD: Norman Remington Co.

Pierce, John and Jim Writer. (2005). *Yellow Jack.* Hoboken, NJ: John Wiley and Sons.

Stepan, Nancy. (1978). "The Interplay between Socio-Economic Factors and Medical Science: Yellow Fever Research, Cuba and the United States." *Social Studies of Science* 8: 397–423.

MEDICAL SCIENTIST AS INTERNATIONAL HERO

- **Document:** "A Thirtieth Anniversary—Pasteur and Rabies"
- **Date:** 1915
- **Where:** Chicago, IL
- **Significance:** By the early 1900s, the germ theory had become integral to the understanding of medical theory and practice. The medical practices of the period before the 1860s—that is, before vaccines for anthrax, rabies, and cholera, before antiseptic practices in surgery, before modern sanitation and pest control—appeared in hindsight to be barbaric, scarcely better than medieval amputation and bloodletting. Edward Jenner's great discovery of the efficacy of cowpox shone all the brighter for having been surrounded by so much darkness. His work appeared as a torch, passed down to his successors, the medical heroes of the late 19th and early 20th centuries. The three documents that follow celebrate those heroes while holding the torch aloft for future generations of medical scientists.

DID YOU KNOW?

Vaccinating Animals

Louis Pasteur is most famous for his development of human vaccination, which allowed him to save Joseph Meister's life. But most of his initial work was in animal vaccination. In an agricultural country like France, epidemics that attacked sheep and cows could mean economic disaster. Pasteur's first public triumph, in 1881, came from a public exhibition to test his newly developed anthrax vaccine, organized by a regional agricultural society in the small town of Pouilley-le-Fort. Sixty sheep were divided into three groups. Twenty-five were vaccinated with Pasteur's vaccine, while 25 were left unvaccinated. All 50 were then injected with a quadruple dose of live anthrax, certain to produce the disease. The remaining 10 sheep were given neither preventative treatment nor disease, to act as controls. Within a month, all the unvaccinated sheep were dead of anthrax, while those vaccinated showed no signs of the disease at all. The popular press spread the news, and agricultural societies and researchers worldwide took note of the value of vaccination for their own livestock.

DOCUMENT

July 4, 1885, Joseph Meister, an Alsatian boy 9 years of age, was severely bitten by a rabid dog. This was the first human patient on whom, July 6, 1885, Louis Pasteur used the protective treatment for rabies which he had proved on animals. In a delightful little volume entitled "Pasteur and After Pasteur," Stephen Paget has well said that there ought to be a calendar of the healing art to remind us of all such days. In these turbulent times when men and nations are gaining everlasting reputations in the death-dealing art, when the names of great generals and brave admirals are on the lips of old and young alike, it is fitting that we should recall the glory of those who have succeeded in the beneficent work of rescue and in preserving rather than destroying life.

The story of Pasteur's great accomplishment in effecting the cure of rabies is fascinating in its details. By September, 1884, he had attained the last step of his method: he had proved that he could prevent the disease in dogs already bitten. Then came the crucial test on man, which event took place thirty years ago next Tuesday.

Pasteur's original method is still observed in essence if not in details in many parts of the world. Pasteur institutes devoted to the treatment of rabies are found in every civilized country. There are more than sixty of these antirabic clinics now in operation, the original Pasteur Institute of Paris having been opened in 1888.

What they have meant to humanity is best appreciated by comparing the prognosis of the past with the accomplishments of Pasteur treatment. When the infected wounds are promptly cauterized, the protection may be great. Usually this help is of little or no avail when the bites are multiple and lacerated; and when they are about the face and head, thorough cauterization is difficult or impossible. The statistics of Proust show that in a series of 117 cases which were not cauterized, there were ninety-six deaths; whereas there were only eighty-nine deaths among 249 cases in which cauterization was practiced. Let us contrast with these statistics of two generations ago the outlook as influenced by Pasteur's work. From 1886 to 1914 the world's record of death from rabies after antirabic treatment has been kept down to less than 1 per cent. Hogyes has collected statistics for 54,620 persons treated at twenty-four institutes with a mortality of only 0.77 per cent. Bernstein's figures include 104,347 patients with a mortality of 0.54 per cent.

Surely these figures tell a victory against death in a way that puts the inhuman warfare of civilized nations in a sad light in comparison with this record, the fruits of one man's genius as a human benefactor. At this eventful anniversary we may recall the words of the chairman of the French Academy of Sciences when he arose to speak at the gathering before which Pasteur had described his first success in the treatment of rabies in man. "The date of the present meeting," he said, "will remain for ever memorable in the history of medicine and glorious for French science; for it is that of one of the greatest steps ever accomplished in the medical order of things—a progress realized by the discovery of an efficacious means of preventive treatment for a disease the incurable nature of which was a legacy handed down by one century to another. From this day, humanity is armed with a means of fighting the fatal disease of hydrophobia and of preventing its onset. It is to M. Pasteur that we owe this, and we could not feel too much admiration or too much gratitude for the efforts on his part which have led to such a magnificent result." Thirty years later these achievements have lost nothing of their original splendor.

Source: "A Thirtieth Anniversary—Pasteur and Rabies." (1915). Journal of the American Medical Association 65: 30.

Similar anthrax vaccination trials were carried out in many parts of Europe over the next few years. While most were successful, vaccinated animals sometimes died, for reasons no one could predict or explain. One of the Pasteur Institute scientists in charge of animal trials wrote to his colleague in Paris, "Hidden in the depths of your laboratory, you have no worries, whereas I, when a poor animal seems to lower its head a little, see all eyes going from the head of the animal to mine and back again. I can assure you that this situation is not amusing. And it is all the worse when I must lead the mourning for vaccinated animals that have died by my hand, and must make a speech at the grave" (cited in Bazin, 2011, 204).

The way in which Pasteur's vaccine spread around the world reflected the increasing speed of global medical communications. In 1888, another scientist from the Pasteur Institute carried out an anthrax vaccination experiment in Australia on 39 sheep and six cows. It succeeded, and he was invited to set up a vaccine production center on a small island near Sydney. By 1887, laboratories in India, then under British rule, were producing anthrax vaccine, and by 1892, Indian veterinarians successfully applied it to elephants.

Many additional livestock vaccines were developed over the next 30 years, and vaccine research and development are currently an essential part of global agricultural policy and practice.

Source: Bazin, Hervé. (2011). Vaccination: A History from Lady Montagu to Genetic Engineering. Esher, England: John Libbey Eurotext.

- **Document:** William Ford, "The Life and Work of Robert Koch"
- **Date:** 1911
- **Where:** Baltimore, MD

DOCUMENT

Paul Ehrlich, possibly the greatest mind in modern medical Germany, certainly the most prolific investigator in those fields of Medical Science in which his path has lain, said when Koch died that our entire knowledge of the infectious diseases and the various related branches of learning rests upon the foundations which he established; that he devised the methods which gave science the possibility of solving the problems in immunity on an exact experimental basis, the problems of immunity which Pasteur for the first time freed from the confusion of pure empiricism: and that even in the realm of experimental therapy Koch holds the first place, since he taught the world how to transmit the infectious diseases artificially from animal to animal, thus enabling us to apply therapeutic measures experimentally.

This praise by Ehrlich seems at first an extravagant tribute of admiration for a devoted friend and an honored colleague; but when we remember that every well-trained physician and surgeon of the present generation uses in his daily work the knowledge which came from the investigations of Koch; that every properly organized medical school and hospital has a laboratory founded on the methods which Koch devised and the apparatus which he invented; that every municipality in the fight against the great pestilences of the world, cholera, tuberculosis, typhoid fever, diphtheria, and in the efforts to provide for its citizens milk, water, and food which cannot serve as the vehicle of infection, depends for its preventive measures upon the doctrines which Koch proved; when we reflect that all modern bacteriology has been made possible by the discoveries of Robert Koch, then we are minded to regard Ehrlich's tribute as expressing even less than the truth . . .

Let us inquire into the circumstances of Koch's life and study for a moment his early publications to try and determine why he occupies such a pre-eminent place in medical science . . .

. . . on April 30, 1876, Koch, began a three-day demonstration before [Professor Ferdinand] Cohn in the Botanical Institute [in Breslau]. He brought with him many of his preparations and carried out a number of fundamental experiments. He showed Cohn how he could cultivate the anthrax bacillus in sterile blood serum or in the aqueous humor of a bullock's eyes, and how it went through a definite phase of development. During the course of this development the short rods originally present in the blood of animals dead of [anthrax] grew out into long threads or chains of bacilli in each of which a spore appeared. These spores became free from the organisms which disintegrated and disappeared, and under proper conditions of temperature and moisture underwent certain peculiar changes. As a result of these changes, projecting from each spore there appeared the short rod, characteristic of the bacillus of anthrax as observed in the blood of infected animals. Thus the complete life cycle of the anthrax bacillus was established, the first complete life cycle to be described for any of the bacteria. Koch further showed Cohn how the inoculation of animals always resulted in artificial anthrax when the material employed contained the bacillus or its spores, and only under these conditions, actually inoculating frogs, mice, and rabbits with infectious material in Cohn's presence. He finally proved to Cohn that the nature and the distribution of the disease could be amply explained by the facts which he had brought to light in regard to the life history of the anthrax bacillus. This demonstration took place in the presence of a number of professors in the University of Breslau besides Cohn, notably the physiologist Leopold Auerbach, the pathologist Julius Cohnheim and his assistant Karl Weigert . . .

It is said that Cohnheim was so astonished and delighted by Koch and his work that he rushed back to the Pathological Institute, called his assistants together and told them to stop their work and hasten to the Botanical Laboratory where they could see the demonstration for themselves. He said Koch had made a startling discovery which in the simplicity and exactness of the methods employed was the more to be wondered at since he was shut off in his life from all scientific intercourse, and yet everything he had done was absolutely original and absolutely complete. "It leaves nothing more to be proved," said Cohnheim. "I regard it as the greatest discovery that has ever been made with bacteria, and I believe that this is not the first time that this young Robert Koch will surprise and shame us by the brilliancy of his investigations."

Source: Ford, William. (1911). "The Life and Work of Robert Koch." *Bulletin of the Johns Hopkins Hospital* 22: 415–425.

- **Document:** William Gorgas, Report, Office of Chief Sanitary Officer, Havana
- **Date:** 1902
- **Where:** Havana, Cuba

DOCUMENT

General: I herewith forward the report of the sanitary department, bringing the account of the work up to May 20 of the present year.

This being the final report of the sanitary department of the city of Habana under the military government, it might be useful to review, in a general way, the work of the department since its inception in 1899.

The great object of sanitation for Cuba, and particularly for Habana, as far as the United States was concerned, was the eradication of yellow fever. For over 200 years this disease had, at short intervals, devastated the Atlantic and Gulf coasts of the United States, causing great loss of life, and still greater financial loss, due to the entire cessation of commerce which occurred during the epidemic. It is estimated that the money loss caused directly by the epidemic of 1878, which affected particularly the lower Mississippi Valley, amounted to $100,000,000, and in years when there was no epidemic quarantines had to be kept up against the infected regions around the Gulf of Mexico, which stopped almost all travel and greatly interfered with commerce. The United States had come to look upon Habana as the particular point from which infection was spread. Yellow fever has been continuously present in this city since 1762. Every month in every year during that time there have been some cases. In all other localities of North America where yellow fever occurred, it occurred epidemically; that is, the locality was free from the disease for a longer or shorter time. In places above the frost line winter always puts an end to the disease, and in localities in the Tropics it always terminates after a greater or lesser period of years from the exhaustion of the non-immune material. It was therefore hoped by the military authorities that if yellow fever could be controlled in Habana the United States would be free from danger of epidemic invasion.

One of the most prominent objects, then, that the military government had before it during its stay in Cuba was the control of yellow fever, and for this purpose we paid great attention to the improvement of the hygienic conditions all over the island. But Habana being the only endemic focus in the island, and, for that matter, anywhere else in North America, the energies of the military government were concentrated at this point.

None who knew anything of yellow fever had any clear idea how its eradication was to be accomplished, but there was a general belief and hope that by improving the sanitary conditions the disease here could be greatly decreased, and possibly in the course of a number of years gradually gotten rid of, as has been the case in the cities of the United States. But no one, I think, who knew anything of yellow fever practically would have ventured to predict that much could have been done in this line in the course of three years.

In Habana the government went vigorously to work, rapidly organizing street cleaning, disposal of garbage, and the cleaning of premises. In a very few months the streets were as clean as those of any modern city and the garbage regularly disposed of. But the internal sanitation of houses and the organization of the sanitary department for the reporting and control of contagious and infectious diseases, and similar matters, took a longer time.

In the early part of 1899, the first year of the military occupation, very little yellow fever occurred. The preceding five years had been years of war, and for the last few months the American blockade had practically put an end to immigration into Habana, and the nonimmune population was pretty well exhausted, so that there were few left capable of having this disease. In January, there was one death; in February, none; in March, one; in April, two; in May, none; in June, one, and in July, two. That is, in the first seven months of 1899 there were only seven deaths from yellow fever. The military governor of the city, Gen. Ludlow, felt sure that the measures which were being taken had pretty well eradicated it.

But about the 1st of August, Spanish immigration began to pour into Habana, and between August and December some 12,000 immigrants arrived in the city, about 60 per cent of whom settled in Habana. This at once started up yellow fever, and by December of 1899 we were having a severe winter epidemic. This continued right along through 1900, during which year we had a very sharp epidemic, having in all some 1,400 cases.

The general sanitary conditions had improved, as indicated by the falling death rate, in a very satisfactory manner; but our work was evidently having no effect upon yellow fever. This disease was under control everywhere else in the island, but the principal means of reducing it, the deportation of the nonimmune population, so successful everywhere else, was not practicable in Habana.

By the beginning of 1901 the sanitary department was pretty well satisfied that ordinary sanitary measures were having no immediate effect upon yellow fever. The city during the year 1900 was as clean and in as good sanitary condition as it was possible for labor to make it, and affairs could not be gotten into better condition until after the completion of a sewer system.

In the summer of 1900 a commission of Army medical officers headed by Maj. Walter Reed, United States Army, had been sent to Cuba for the investigation and study of yellow fever. Due to the financial assistance given by the military governor to this commission, they were enabled to experiment on the human subject. They took up the theory advanced by Dr. Carlos Finlay of Habana, in the year 1880, that the *Stegomyia* mosquito was the sole means of the transmission of yellow fever. Dr. Finlay had maintained this theory for some 20 years, and had done considerable experimental work in this direction.

The commission, through elaborate and careful experimentation, proved this to be correct, and in February, 1901, Dr. Reed read a paper before the International Sanitary Congress, in Habana, giving the results of their work. This idea was so new and so entirely contrary to all former theories on the subject, and, apparently, to all former experience, that the paper was received with scant belief. I myself had seen the work, and was convinced that the mosquito could convey yellow fever, but I was hardly prepared to believe that it was the only way, or even the ordinary way, of conveying the disease.

But all ordinary sanitary measures for the preceding two years had been flat failures. Yellow fever at the beginning of 1901 was about as bad as it had ever been in Habana at that time of the year. The city was infected in every part, and there was present probably the largest nonimmune population that had ever before been in Habana.

I had very little hope of accomplishing much; it seemed to me that even if the mosquito did convey yellow fever, he could not be gotten rid of, and, apparently, from all past experience, the mosquito was not the only way, or even the principal way, of conveying the disease; but, as he evidently could convey the disease, it was our duty to take precautions in this direction.

The military governor readily granted the necessary appropriation and authorized the employment of as large a force as needful for mosquito work. Work was commenced on this line February 4, 1901, and pushed in every direction. The results soon began to be apparent. In January there were seven deaths from yellow fever; in February, the first month of mosquito work, five deaths; in March, one death; none in April, May, or June; one in July; two in August; and two in September, and for the nine months following September, 1901, not a single case nor a death has occurred from this disease. This result convinced the sanitary department that the mosquito not only could convey yellow fever, but that it was the ordinary way, and the only way, at least in Habana, for the conditions in Habana during 1901 were as favorable for a yellow fever epidemic as they had ever been. The city had the largest nonimmune population, probably, that it had ever contained. Infection was scattered in every part of the city; not only so, but the small towns surrounding the city were thoroughly infected, and were constantly sending cases into the city. We continued the same sanitary measures that had been taken during the preceding year, and which had not had the slightest effect upon the march of yellow fever; but, in addition, we took measures looking to the Stegomyia mosquito as the means of conveying the disease. Immediately after the adoption of these measures, yellow fever began to decrease, and by September had been entirely eradicated from the city.

The demonstration is the more effective in Habana from the fact that in all other cities of North America yellow fever lasts for a greater or lesser number of years, and then disappears from natural causes, to reappear again when conditions are favorable. In Habana the conditions have been different. For 150 years yellow fever has been constantly present in the city. From September, 1901, to July, 1902, not a single case nor a death has occurred. In the 150 years referred to, not any year, probably, can be picked out in which during the same period there were less than 100 deaths.

This, it seems to me, is a practical demonstration, given in the only endemic focus for yellow fever in North America, and in a year when the conditions were most favorable for the development of the disease, of the fact that the Stegomyia mosquito is the only method of transmitting it—a fact proved by the Army commission.

Under Army administration the death rate in Habana has decreased in a marked degree. In 1898, the number of deaths was 21,252, giving a rate of 91.03; in 1899, the first year of our occupation, we had 8,153 deaths, giving a rate of 33.67; in 1900, we had 6,102 deaths, giving a rate of 24.40; in 1901, we had 5,720 deaths, giving a rate or 22.11; for the first four months of 1902 there occurred 1,896 deaths, which if kept up for the year would give 5,688 deaths, a rate of 20.68 for the year.

Thus it can be seen that under the military government, in a little over three years the death rate was reduced from 91.03 to 20.68. The latter rate would be a favorable one for the better class of cities in Europe or the United States. And this has come about without making any permanent sanitary installations, such as sewage. The city was kept as clean as it was possible for labor to make it, with regard to the streets, disposal or garbage, and the interior of the houses. But every house in Habana, somewhere under the house, still has a cesspool, the flow from which sinks into the surrounding ground, and as this has been going on for 400 years, the ground itself is as thoroughly saturated with organic matter as is possible.

The authorities had hardly hoped for such marked improvement until this system of cesspools has been done away with by a good system of sewage. But apparently the condition referred to has no very great effect upon the general health of the city; the improvement has come about from a careful street cleaning, disposal or garbage, internal sanitation of houses, and rigid control of infectious and contagious diseases.

Our work down here has been a useful lesson in municipal sanitation. The same thing could be accomplished by any community anywhere else, if they were willing to spend money and labor upon it. No elaborate machinery of any kind is necessary; merely men and brooms.

The primary object of the war with Spain was the liberation of Cuba from Spanish domination, but, at the same time, the United States had hoped to accomplish a good deal in improving the sanitary condition of the island. In this she has succeeded beyond her utmost expectations, and the results in Cuba have been a new departure in military conquest. The only other people who bear comparison with us in attempting to improve the sanitary conditions of a tropical country are the English, and neither in Jamaica nor in India have they been very successful in this respect.

Much to our surprise, we find that not only can a native city like Habana be made as healthy as the better class of cities in the United States, but that our own troops, with proper care, thrive just as well in the Tropics as they do in the Temperate Zone. With the troops, the health conditions have steadily improved, until at the evacuation of Cuba the health rate was better among them than the average of troops in the United States.

Our first year in Cuba, 1898, with an average of 8,345 men, we had a death rate from disease of 67.94 per thousand. The health conditions steadily improved during the four years of our occupation, and for the last three months of 1902, with an average strength of 5,000 men, we had a death rate from disease of 1.76 per thousand. This means that the first year of our life in the Tropics we lost 67 men out of every thousand, from disease; the last year of our stay, we had profited by our experience to such an extent that we lost only 7 men per thousand.

From our experience in Cuba, several useful lessons can be deduced. We find that the native in the Tropics, with the same sanitary precautions that are taken in the Temperate Zones, can be just as healthy and have just as small a death rate as the inhabitants of the Temperate Zone; that to bring this about, no elaborate machinery of any kind is needed; that it can be attained by any community, no matter how poor, if they are willing to spend sufficient labor in cleaning, and observing well-known rules with regard to disease; that the North American Anglo-Saxon can lead just as healthy a life and live just as long in the Tropics as in the United States.

But by far the most important sanitary lesson is with regard to yellow fever—that this disease is only conveyed by the stegomyia mosquito; that the disease can readily be eradicated, even when it has gotten a firm hold, and easily kept from establishing itself by taking measures looking to the mosquito as its cause.

I look forward in the future to a time when yellow fever will have entirely disappeared as a disease to which mankind is subject, for I believe that when the yellow fever parasite has once become extinct it can no more return than the dodo or any other species of animal that has disappeared from the earth.

Source: Gorgas, William. (1911). "Report of Maj. W. C. Gorgas, Medical Corps, United States Army." In *Yellow Fever, A Compilation of Various Publications*, James Carroll, William Crawford Gorgas, Robert Latham Owen, and Walter Drew McCaw. Washington, DC: Government Printing Office, 234–238.

ANALYSIS

Popular culture of the early 20th century created a new type of hero: the medical scientist. Claude Bernard and Rudolf Virchow would have been astonished to find experimental medicine glorified in newspaper articles, novels, and in a brand new medium, "motion pictures," that is, movies.

Louis Pasteur was the first international scientific hero. In 1885, shortly after Joseph Meister was pronounced clear of rabies, four boys from Newark, New Jersey, were attacked by a mad dog. Money was raised for them to travel to Paris in order to be treated by the great Pasteur. As everyone knew, time was of the essence: would the boys make it to Pasteur before the virus traveled its deadly route through their nervous system? The *New York Times* gave a day-by-day account of the trip, the treatment, and the continued health of the boys, who were, in fact, successfully treated and returned home. A few curmudgeons raised the point that the Newark dog might not, actually, have been mad and that in any case the boys had not been severely bitten, nothing like young Meister. The *Times'* reading public did not care. Pasteur was the hero of the hour, "full of gentleness and sympathy for the children," while maintaining the strictest scientific standards in his laboratory.

The *Journal of the American Medical Association* celebrated Pasteur in 1915, but a more widely read celebration of the medical scientist came 10 years later, with the publication of *Arrowsmith* by Sinclair Lewis (1885–1951). Lewis's collaborator was the American scientist Paul DeKruif (1890–1971), whose 1926 book *The Microbe Hunters* remains, like *Arrowsmith*, a classic of medical literature. Many prominent researchers of the late 20th century attested to the impact of both books on their decision to study science.

Movies further spread the image of the medical scientists as benefactors to humankind, often portraying them struggling against ignorance or political power. William Dieterle's *The Story of Louis Pasteur*, starring Paul Muni, was the first film biography to focus on a scientist, rather than a political or military figure. Frank Nugent, reviewing the film in the *New York Times*, called Pasteur's own life "warm and vital, of itself," and the movie "a monument to a life of a man." Robert Koch's life was never accorded the full Hollywood treatment, but he appeared in another of Dieterle's film biographies, *Dr. Ehrlich's Magic Bullet*. Paul Ehrlich (1854–1915) was another medical hero, renowned for developing treatments for syphilis and diphtheria, "possibly the greatest mind in modern medical Germany," as he was described in the excerpt above.

Walter Reed was portrayed in the 1934 play *Yellow Jack*, followed by a movie of the same name in 1938. The screenplay was written by Sidney Howard (1891–1939) and Paul De Kruif, based on the chapter on Walter Reed in *The Microbe Hunters*. Many of those associated with both the play and the movie are famous for other things. Howard went on to write the screenplay for *Gone with the Wind* and to win a posthumous Oscar for it. Private John O'Hara, who volunteered for the yellow fever experiment, was the first dramatic role for James Maitland "Jimmy" Stewart (1908–1997), one of the most beloved movie stars of the century. And Lewis Stone (1879–1953), who played Major Walter Reed in the film version of *Yellow Jack*, is best known as Judge James Hardy, Andy Hardy's father in the Mickey Rooney series.

FURTHER READING

Bucchi, Massimiano. (1997). "The Public Science of Louis Pasteur: The Experiment on Anthrax Vaccine in the Popular Press of the Time." *History and Philosophy of the Life Sciences* 19: 181–209.

De Kruif, Paul. (1926). *The Microbe Hunters*. New York: Harcourt Brace and Company.

Dr. Ehrlich's Magic Bullet. (1940). Directed by William Dieterle. Warner Brothers.

Hansen, Bert. (2004). "Medical History for the Masses: How American Comic Books Celebrated Heroes of Medicine in the 1940s." *Bulletin of the History of Medicine* 78: 148–191.

Nugent, Frank. (1936, February 10). "Review of *The Story of Louis Pasteur*." *New York Times*.

The Story of Louis Pasteur. (1936). Directed by William Dieterle. Warner Brothers.

Yellow Jack. (1938). Directed by George Seitz. MGM.

VACCINATION MADE COMPULSORY IN THE GERMAN EMPIRE

- **Document:** German Vaccination Law of April 8, 1874
- **Date:** 1874
- **Where:** Berlin, Germany
- **Significance:** By the second half of the 19th century, many European countries had introduced vaccination for smallpox, though it was not compulsory. The result was a striking decline in smallpox epidemics and an equally striking decline in mortality from the disease in the few outbreaks that did occur. Smallpox seemed to be a thing of the past, at least as far as middle-class patients were concerned. If anyone were to get smallpox, it would be the poorer classes, living in cramped, unhealthy conditions. Why, then, should they bother to vaccinate their own clean, well-fed children?

The answer came when France and Prussia went to war in 1870, and the movements of troops and civilians led to a major smallpox epidemic across Western Europe. Everywhere, the disease followed the path of the most vulnerable, that is, least vaccinated, population. As the Prussian troops marched across France to victory in Paris, they left devastation in their wake, for only 59% of the French population had been vaccinated, while all Prussian soldiers were vaccinated when they enlisted. One thousand and two hundred French soldiers died of smallpox in Paris during the final siege, over five times as many deaths as in the entire Prussian army.

When the increasingly militaristic German government issued the Vaccination Law in 1874, not only physicians but also military leaders throughout Europe paid close attention.

DOCUMENT

We Wilhelm, by the Grace of God German Emperor, King of Prussia etc., decree in the name of the German Empire and by the assent of the Federal Council and the Imperial Diet, as follows:

§ 1. Vaccination is compulsory for:

1. Every child before the end of the year following the year of its birth; provided, it has not been medically certified (§ 10) to have previously already suffered from natural small-pox.

2. Every pupil of a public educational establishment, or of a private school, with the exception of Sunday and evening schools, before the end of the twelfth year of the pupil's life; provided, it has not been certified by a medical man, that he

has been afflicted with natural small-pox once during the five preceding years, or that he has not already been successfully vaccinated.

§ 2. A person, liable to vaccination (§ 1), who cannot, according to medical testimony be vaccinated without his life or health being endangered, must be subjected to vaccination within a year after the cessation of the cause of such danger.

In cases of doubt as to whether that danger still exists, the competent official doctors (§ 6) opinion is decisive without further appeal.

§ 3. If, according to the opinion of the doctor (§ 5), the vaccination has been unsuccessful, it must be repeated at the latest during the following year; and in the event of its again being unsuccessful again in the third year.

The competent authorities have authority to order the last repetition of the vaccination to be performed by the vaccinating doctor (§ 6).

§ 4. If vaccination should have been omitted without any legal reason (§ 1, 2), it must be carried out within a period, to be fixed by the competent authorities.

§ 5. Every person vaccinated must show himself to the vaccinating doctor for re-examination at the earliest on the sixth day, and at the latest on the eighth day after having been vaccinated.

§ 6. Vaccination districts, each one under the supervision of a vaccinating doctor, must be established in every Federal State.

The vaccinating doctor has to vaccinate the inhabitants of the district free of charge between the beginning of May and the end of September of each year, in localities and on dates which must be made known previously. The localities, where the vaccination is to be performed and where those to be vaccinated have to appear for examination, must be chosen in such a manner, that no place in the district is further distant than five kilometres from the nearest vaccinating station.

§ 7. A list of the children liable to vaccination (§ I No. 7) must be prepared by the proper authorities before the commencement of the vaccination period. The directors of educational establishments concerned, must also prepare a list of the children to be vaccinated, who come under § 1 No. 2.

The vaccinating doctors should state in the list, whether the vaccination was successful or a failure, or why it has been quite or temporarily omitted.

The lists must be handed to the authorities after the end of each calendar year.

The arrangement of the lists is determined by the Federal Council.

§ 8. In addition to the vaccinating doctors, only medical men are authorised to vaccinate.

They must keep lists, similar to the forms prescribed in § 7, of all vaccinations performed; the lists must be handed in to the competent authorities after the end of each year.

§ 9. The governments of the different Federal States according to detailed regulations of the Federal Council have to provide for the fitting up of a suitable number of vaccination stations for the preparing of the vaccine.

The vaccination stations must supply public vaccinating doctors with vaccine lymph free of charge, and must keep lists of the source and supply of the same.

The public vaccinating doctors are obliged, when requested to do so, to supply other doctors free of charge with vaccine lymph, as far as their store suffices.

§ 10. A certificate of vaccination has to be drawn up by the doctor concerning the result (§ 5) of every vaccination. The certificate must state the Christian and surname, as well as the year and the day of birth of the child vaccinated, and also certify whether the law has been complied with by the vaccination, or whether the vaccination must be repeated again in the next year.

In the medical certificate which is given for the purpose of showing an absolute or temporary exemption from vaccination (§ J, 2), the reason and period of such exemption must be stated, in addition to a description of the person, for whom it is made out.

§ 11. The Federal Council has to determine the form to be used for the above mentioned certificates (§ 10).

The first certificates are made out free of cost and stamp duties.

§ 12. Parents, foster parents and guardians are bound, if officially called upon to do so, to prove by means of the prescribed certificates (§ 10), that their children, foster children or wards have been vaccinated, or that lawful reasons have prevented vaccination from being carried out.

§ 13. The directors of those educational establishments, whose pupils are subject to compulsory vaccination (§ 1 No. 2), must ascertain, when receiving pupils, whether obligatory vaccination has been complied with, by asking for the certificates prescribed.

It is their duty to see, that pupils, who become liable to vaccination (according § 1 No. 2), comply with the regulations regarding the same during their stay in the institute.

Should vaccination have been omitted without a lawful excuse, they must insist on its being carried out.

They are obliged to lay a list before the competent authorities, four weeks before the close of the school year, of those pupils who cannot prove that they have been vaccinated.

§ 14. Parents, foster parents and guardians, who are unable to produce the certificate required by § 12, will be punished by fines not exceeding twenty marks. Parents, foster parents and guardians, whose children and wards remain unvaccinated, or who omit to present themselves for re-examination (§ 5), without any valid excuse when officially called upon to do so, will be punished by fines not exceeding fifty marks, or by imprisonment, not exceeding three days.

§ 15. Doctors and headmasters of schools, who do not comply with their duties, as laid down in § 8 No. 2, § 10 and § 13, are liable to a fine not exceeding one hundred marks.

§ 16. Any one vaccinating without authority to do so will be punished by a fine not exceeding one hundred and fifty marks, or with imprisonment not exceeding fourteen days.

§ 17. Any person acting without the necessary care when vaccinating, will be punished by a fine not exceeding five hundred marks, or with imprisonment not exceeding three months, provided that the penal code does not prescribe a severer punishment.

§ 18. This law becomes valid on the 1st April 1875.

The individual Federal States will take the necessary steps for the proper carrying out of this Law.

The existing regulations in the individual Federal States with regard to compulsory vaccination in the event of a small-pox epidemic, are not affected by this Law.

Given under our hand and seal.
Berlin, 8th April 1874.
Wilhelm.
v. Bismarck.

Source: German Empire. (1904). *Vaccination Law of April 8, 1874.* Berlin: B. Paul, 1–6.

- **Document:** Decrees of the Federal Council dated June 28, 1899, concerning vaccination
- **Date:** 1899
- **Where:** Berlin, Germany
- **Significance:** This revision of the Vaccination Law of 1874 shows the practical experience gained by 25 years of legislation. It takes for granted the value of the law and focuses on the mechanisms needed to enforce it.

DOCUMENT

Resolutions and outlines of regulations for enforcing the vaccination law.
1. Resolutions concerning the physiological and pathological state of the vaccination question.
   1. Persons who have been once attacked by small-pox are, with rare exceptions, immune from a second attack.
   2. Inoculation with vaccine has the effect of bringing about a similar immunity.
   3. The duration of the protection from smallpox by means of vaccination varies within wide limits, but averages 10 years.
   4. In order to obtain a sufficient immunity by means of vaccination, one well developed vaccination pustule is at least necessary.
   5. A second vaccination is necessary ten years after the first vaccination.
   6. Vaccination of the entourage of a single individual, increases his relative immunity, and vaccination therefore confers not only an individual but also a general benefit in regard to the danger from smallpox.
   7. Vaccination can under certain circumstances be attended with danger for the person vaccinated.
   In vaccinating with human lymph the danger of transmission of syphilis is not completely excluded, although very slight. Other injury resulting is confined to slight wounds, as has been proved.

All these dangers may be limited by careful performance of the vaccination to such a small extent, that the benefits of vaccination infinitely outweigh any possible injury.

8. Since the introduction of vaccination no increase of certain illnesses or general mortality, that could be attributed as a consequence of vaccination, has been scientifically proved.

2. Resolutions concerning the general introduction of vaccination with animal lymph.

1. No essential facts have been established up to the present which would point to a causal-nexus between the known germs contained in animal lymph and the inflammatory symptoms, which appear after vaccination.

2. Vaccination should be performed with animal lymph. Human lymph may only be used exceptionally for public or for private vaccination.

3. Animal lymph for all vaccinations may only be used, if obtained from government vaccination institutes or their branches, or from such private institutes, which are under State supervision.

4. Special regulations are drawn up for the fitting up and working of State institutes.

5. The following regulations apply for the sale of animal lymph in apothecary's shops:

a) The lymph must have been obtained from government vaccination stations, their branches, or from such private establishments which are under State supervision.

b) The lymph must be kept in a cool place and protected against light.

c) The lymph should only be supplied in wrappers of the vaccination station, and such wrappers must be accompanied by the name of the station with details of the number of the order-book, of the day, on which the lymph was taken, of the amount of lymph contained inside the wrapper, as well as with directions for use. The latter should be worded according to §§ 13–19 the regulations laid down for doctors for the performance of vaccination.

d) Lymph should not be supplied, which is over 3 months old.

e) Entries should be made of the lymph received and supplied, and of the day of receipt, the name of the institute, in which the lymph was prepared, the day on which it was supplied, and of the name and address of the person when has been supplied.

3. Outline of regulations, to be complied with by doctors when they are vaccinating.

A. General Regulations.

§ 1. It is desirable that the vaccinating doctor should perform public vaccinations in every locality in his district.

In places where contagious illnesses, such as scarlet fever, measles, diphtheria, croup, whooping cough, spotted typhus or erysipelas are very prevalent, public vaccination should not be performed during the duration of the epidemic.

Should the vaccinating doctor become acquainted with the existence of such complaints in the localities concerned only after having commenced the vaccinations, or should even isolated cases of vaccination erysipelas occur, he must immediately stop vaccinating in the locality and notify hereof the proper authorities.

If the vaccinating doctor is treating individual cases of contagious sicknesses, he must prevent in a suitable manner their spreading through himself, when vaccinating.

It is advisable to avoid public vaccinations during the time of the greatest heat (July and August).

§ 2. The vaccination doctor together with the local police authorities must see that the necessary order is maintained on the vaccination days.

The overcrowding of the rooms set apart for vaccinating must be avoided and sufficient ventilation provided for.

The simultaneous presence of children undergoing first vaccination and of those being vaccinated for a second time must be avoided where possible.

B. Supply and production of Lymph.

I. When Animal Lymph is used.

§ 3. Vaccination doctors receive all the lymph, they require for public vaccinations gratis and carriage paid, from government vaccination stations.

§ 4. The vaccinating doctor should enter the name of the vaccination station from which and the time, when he has obtained lymph, in his stock book.

II. When Human Lymph is used.

§ 5. The vaccinated child, from whom lymph is to be taken for further vaccination must have its whole body previously examined, and must be found to be perfectly healthy and well nourished. It must be descended from parents who do not suffer from hereditary disease; children of mothers who have gone through several abortions or miscarriages should under no circumstances be made use of for obtaining lymph.

The children from whom lymph is to be obtained must be at least 6 months old, legitimate and not the first child of their parents. These requirements are only to be deviated from in rare exceptions, and only if not the slightest doubt exists as to the good health of their parents.

Such children must be free from boils, scars and eruptions of all kinds, from condylomes on the gluteal parts, lips, or under the arms and navel, from swollen glands, chronic affections of the nose, eyes or ears, as well as from swellings and inflections of the bones, and must also show no symptoms of syphilis, scrofula, rhachitis, or any other constitutional weakness.

§ 6. The lymph of revaccinated children must only be used in cases of necessity and never for first vaccinations.

The examination of the state of health of a revaccinated child, from whom lymph is to be obtained must be carried out with particular care, and in conformity with the views expressed in § 5.

§ 7. Every vaccinating doctor must keep a record where and when he obtained his lymph. Particularly is he bound to make a note of the name of the vaccinated child, from whom the lymph is obtained, and also the date when he obtained it, whether he desires to store the lymph for his own use later on, or for supplying other doctors. The lymph itself must be marked in such a manner that no mistake can occur later on as to its origin.

Such notes must be kept until the end of the following calendar year.

§ 8. Lymph must not be taken later than the same day in the week after the vaccination.

The pustules serving for the purpose of lymph extraction must be clean and uninjured, and only situated on a moderately inflamed base.

Pustules which have formed at the beginning of erysipelas, must under no condition be used for obtaining lymph.

At least one pustule must remain unopened on the person vaccinated.

§ 9. The pustules must be opened by puncturing or cutting. All squeezing of the pustule or its surrounding in order to obtain more lymph must be avoided.

§ 10. Only such lymph may be used, which exudes of itself and in which neither blood nor pus can be detected by the naked eye.

Bad smelling or very thin lymph must not be used.

§ 11. Only the purest glycerine may be mixed with lymph, and mixing must be performed by means of a clean glass rod.

C. The carrying-out of vaccination and re-vaccination.

§ 12. The children to be vaccinated must be inspected by the vaccinating doctor before the operation; the relatives accompanying them must also be asked about the state of health of such children.

Children who are suffering from serious acute or chronic illnesses, or such, which are detrimental to nourishment, or which alter the humours of the body, should as a rule, not be vaccinated or re-vaccinated.

Exceptions are permissible (especially in the case of natural small-pox) and are left to the discretion of the vaccinating doctor.

§ 13. Vaccination must be regarded as a chirurgical operation, and all precautionary measures necessary to prevent illnesses through an inflamed wound must be taken; the vaccinating doctor must pay special attention to the cleanliness of his hands, vaccinating instruments and of the vaccination locality; the store of lymph must be kept covered over whilst vaccination is being performed, so as to prevent its becoming polluted.

§ 14. Animal lymph should be used for vaccination as soon as practicable after its receipt, and must be kept in a cool and dark place until used. Lymph must not be diluted by the addition of glycerine, water or other substances.

§ 15. Only instruments that have been rendered free from germs by moist or dry heat (by thorough heating or boiling), or by treating them with alcohol may be used for vaccinating each child.

The lymph required each time can be either taken direct from the lymph vessel with the vaccinating instrument, or placed on a little glass saucer on which there are no germs. In using hair tubes, it may be dropped directly out of them on to the instrument.

§ 16. As a rule vaccination is performed on the upper arm; for the first vaccination on the right, and in the case of revaccination on the left one. Four cuts at the most, not more than 1 cm in length are sufficient. The single vaccination incisions must be at least 2 cms apart. Loss of blood is to be avoided in vaccinations. It is generally not necessary to rub the lymph more than once into the wound which is held open by stretching the skin. It is forbidden to paint the lymph in with a brush.

Surplus lymph must not be replaced in the vessel or used for later vaccinations.

§ 17. First vaccinations are to be regarded as successful, if at least one pustule develops uniformly. In the case of revaccination the formation of little knots or blisters on the vaccinated spots is sufficient.

§ 18. The vaccinating doctor is bound to determine exactly, if possible, any disturbances in the course of the vaccination and every real or supposed after illness, and to immediately notify the same on such becoming known to him, to the proper authorities . . .

6. Regulations with reference to a selection of suitable vaccinating doctors.

1. The vaccinating doctors are appointed by the state authorities.

2. The duties of public vaccination are to be entrusted by preference to official doctors.

3. A special swearing-in of vaccinating doctors takes place before they enter on their duties.

4. The remuneration of vaccinating doctors requires the confirmation by the state authorities.

7. Regulations concerning the technical training of doctors for their vaccination duties.

1. Concerning the technical training of doctors for their vaccination duties the following is to be required:

a) During the clinical training of students they should be instructed particularly how to vaccinate, as well as given opportunities of learning vaccinating practically at the public vaccination and revaccination stations.

b) In addition, every doctor who desires to vaccinate publicly or privately must be able to prove, that he has been present at least at two public vaccinations and revaccinations, and has acquired the necessary knowledge concerning the extraction and preservation of lymph.

A knowledge of the theory of vaccination and its attendant duties is required by the medical examination.

8. Regulations concerning the institution of the permanent technical supervision of vaccination by officials from the medical civil service.

1. The supervision of vaccinating doctors should be entrusted to an official doctor, and in case the medical official is a vaccination doctor himself, to a superior medical official.

2. The supervision consists in an inspection, carried out on the spot, of one or several public vaccinations.

3. The books of the vaccinating doctor should be inspected once in every 3 years.

4. The inspecting officials should chiefly occupy themselves in inspecting the execution of the process of vaccination, the results, the keeping of lists, the selection of vaccination localities, number of children vaccinated, etc.

5. Vaccinations performed by private doctors are also open to inspection, provided they are not performed by doctors in their capacity as family doctors.

6. Likewise, a technical supervision of state and private stations for obtaining animal lymph is also necessary, and must be carried out by repeated inspections at suitable intervals.

7. The attention of the official supervising vaccination should also be directed to the commerce, or trade with lymph . . .

Source: German Empire. (1904). *Vaccination Law of April 8, 1874.* Berlin: B. Paul, 20–41.

ANALYSIS

During the 1860s and 1870s, as German scientists like Robert Koch were at the forefront of medical research, the German states, led by Prussia, were expanding their political and military power. The defeat of France in 1871 led to the creation of the German Empire, with Wilhelm I (1797–1888) crowned in the Hall of Mirrors in Versailles as emperor. The new German federation became the dominant power of central Europe, a position it would hold through World War 1 (1914–1918).

During the same period, Germany became a model of innovative medical practices. Students around the world flocked to its universities and research institutes. In 1883, the chancellor, Otto von Bismarck (1815–1898), promoted the first national insurance system to provide health care to workers. Legislation ensuring accident insurance—an early form of worker's compensation—and old age pensions followed. Bismarck's goal was to undercut the growth of workers' political parties by co-opting part of their platform. Public health reformers from other nations watched the German state with admiration for its policies, mixed with fear that their soldiers and citizenry might suffer the consequences if they did not adopt similar strategies.

Great Britain also passed a compulsory vaccination act in 1874, but this led to widespread opposition and the development of an active anti-vaccine movement. The act was modified in 1898 so that parents who believed vaccination was detrimental to their children's health could gain an exemption. This was a compromise that pleased no one: anti-vaccine activists argued that the exemptions were too difficult to obtain, and those in favor of compulsory vaccination argued that individual exemptions put the wider community at risk. A writer in the *British Medical Journal* used data from the German documents, above, to provide answers to British objections to vaccination. To the argument that vaccines were just ways for doctors to make money off of their patients' suffering, he pointed out that doctors worldwide were paid very little for vaccination and that their patients would suffer much more from smallpox. To the argument that compulsory vaccination is an attack on personal liberty, he said that patients have the right to choose their doctors and to demand the highest standards of health and safety—more liberty, in fact, than they had about whether to pay their taxes or send their children to school. To the argument that smallpox, like plague and cholera, was disappearing, he presented the data marshaled by statisticians in Germany and confirmed all over Europe: that smallpox was disappearing precisely because of compulsory vaccination and that without it, smallpox outbreaks were as contagious and as deadly as ever.

The writer's most forceful arguments came from the statistics. In Germany, Hungary, and Italy—all countries which had compulsory vaccination—smallpox had decreased to negligible amounts. In Great Britain, alone among Western

European nations, smallpox outbreaks and the mortality rate had increased. He would have agreed with the statement made by the British politician David Lloyd George (1863–1945) in his support of the National Insurance Act of 1911: Great Britain should be "putting ourselves in this field on a level with Germany; we should not emulate them only in armaments."

FURTHER READING

Anderson, Warwick. (2007). "Immunization and Hygiene in the Colonial Philippines." *Journal of the History of Medicine and Allied Sciences* 62: 1–20.

Blanplain, Jan. (1978). *National Health Insurance and Health Resources: The European Experience*. Cambridge, MA: Harvard University Press.

Hau, Michael. (2000). "The Holistic Gaze in German Medicine, 1890–1930." *Bulletin of the History of Medicine* 74: 495–524.

Hennock, Ernest. (1987). *British Social Reform and German Precedents: The Case of Social Insurance, 1880–1914*. Oxford, England: Clarendon Press.

"National Health Service." *The National Archives*. http://www.nationalarchives.gov.uk/cabinetpapers/themes/national-health-insurance.htm.

POLITICAL WARFARE OVER SMALLPOX TREATMENT IN MILWAUKEE, 1894

- **Document:** Milwaukee Common Council Public Health Ordinance
- **Date:** 1894
- **Where:** Milwaukee, WI
- **Significance:** In 1894, a worldwide smallpox epidemic traveled to the United States. From a public health point of view its effects were comparatively mild: the virus was not the virulent *Variola major* but a much milder strain. Although an estimated 164,000 people contracted the disease, only 5,627 died. This was a death rate of approximately 3%, rather than the 30% that might have been expected from earlier, more virulent strains of smallpox.

  Unfortunately, prevention efforts were hampered by the fact that the disease appeared to be mild. Parents insisted that the disease could not be smallpox and refused to listen to public health authorities. Family members were especially adamant that their sick relatives be cared for at home and not confined to smallpox hospitals, generally known as "pesthouses." In Milwaukee, public outcry was so great against the public health officials who tried to enforce public health ordinances that city authorities revised the statute, allowing residents to remain in their homes.

DOCUMENT

The mayor and common council of the city of Milwaukee, do ordain as follows:

Section 1. Section 3 of the ordinance entitled "An ordinance to amend section 199 of the general ordinances of the city of Milwaukee relating to the city hospital and the duties of the commissioner of health in connection therewith" is hereby amended so as to read as follows: "It shall be the duty of the commissioner of health to place in said hospital, under the care of competent nurses any person who may be found in the city of Milwaukee laboring under any of the following diseases, viz.: Small-pox, diphtheria, scarlet fever, measles, typhus fever or any other dangerous, contagious or infectious diseases, when such person is a non-resident of this city, a traveler, a guest at a hotel, or has no residence of his own in this city where he can be taken of. But the commissioner of health shall not remove to any Isolation Hospital in said city any child or person suffering from any such disease who can be nursed and cared for during such illness in his or her home during the continuance of the disease except upon the recommendation and advice of the said commissioner of health or one of the assistant commissioners of health, and the physician, if any, attending upon such child or person, not being a member of the health department of said city; and in case such commissioner, or assistant commissioner and such physician shall be unable to agree as to the advisability of removing such child or person, then they shall call in and appoint another physician not a member of the health department , and the decision of the majority of such physicians and commissioner or assistant commissioner shall be decisive to the question.

The third physician called in, as above provided, shall not receive or be entitled to any fees from the city for consultation or service in the decision of the case submitted to such board of physicians. . . .

Any person suffering with small-pox who shall be removed to any Isolation Hospital in said city shall be conveyed there in an ambulance which shall be used for the purpose of removing persons suffering with small-pox only, and such persons shall not be taken to said hospital in any other vehicle of conveyance whatsoever. Whenever any person who may have recovered from any of said contagious diseases shall be dismissed from said hospital it shall be the duty of said commissioner of health to cause such person to be conveyed to his place of residence in said city of Milwaukee, in a proper vehicle to be kept and used, or hired for such purpose. The commissioner of health shall keep daily record of the condition of each patient confined in any Isolation Hospital in said city, and whenever he shall be requested thereto by any parent, guardian, relative or friend of such person, he shall furnish them with a copy of said report, verified by the signature of the secretary of the health department. Whenever any person who may have been removed to any Isolation Hospital in said city shall be so dangerously ill that his recovery is doubtful the commissioner of health shall at once notify the parents, guardians, relatives or friends of such person, and if any one of them shall desire to be admitted to said Isolation Hospital for the purpose of nursing and caring for said patient the commissioner of health shall give them a permit to enter and remain in said hospital for such purpose.

Source: "137—An Ordinance." Milwaukee Common Council Proceedings, 1894–1895. Ordinances Appendix, 22–23.

DID YOU KNOW?

Vaccine Salesmanship

The development of vaccines contributed to the transformation of drug companies—which might produce and market anything from cosmetics to patent medicines to flavors for soda water—to modern pharmaceutical companies, which create products for medical consumption. Nowadays these products are very carefully regulated. But in the 19th century, the only regulation was by market forces: if doctors or hospitals or veterinarians thought a product was safe and effective, they would buy it. Pharmaceutical companies therefore spent considerable sums on specialty advertising in pharmaceutical, medical, and veterinary journals. They hosted dinners at medical and veterinary conventions and arranged special tours of their laboratories for visiting medical personnel.

The H. K. Mulford Company, based in Philadelphia, was particularly active in the production of vaccines. They exemplified the new medical business approach by controlling all the materials necessary for production, from the animals needed to produce the vaccine, to the syringes needed to administer it, to advertising and distribution needed to market it. They published full-page advertisements in medical journals, explaining "How Mulford's Vaccine Is Made," showing bucolic, white-washed buildings in a park-like setting with paved walkways and mowed lawns. "They were constructed," the advertisement continues, "after careful inspection of the leading vaccine establishments in Europe. The buildings embody all the latest features of sanitary construction with the details observed in modern hospitals and hygienic laboratories." The stables, containing the calves from which the vaccine was derived, were "of cement, slate, and porcelain finish and are frequently and thoroughly flushed and disinfected." Each animal had its own compartment and was well cared for by veterinarians, "in constant attendance." Most important, at least, highlighted in bold letters, "the virus from absolutely healthy animals is used exclusively."

This information, accompanied by photographs, was followed by another full-page depiction of "How Mulford's Vaccine Is Made." The operating room in which the calves were treated "is maintained so rigidly aseptic that in it abdominal operations upon the human being could be safely performed." The filling tubes were filled by a vacuum apparatus and then "hermetically closed." Their syringe was designed "for simplicity and accuracy—no parts to get out of order" and was kept completely clean, "no contamination possible". More information was always available directly from the company or from druggists in "every American city." Remember, the advertisements concluded, Mulford's products "Save More Lives."

Advertisements like these helped build the modern pharmaceutical industry. Yet they came at a cost in public confidence. Patients throughout the history of medicine have been concerned that personnel in the health-care industry might get rich at their expense. As modern business practices became commonplace in medicine, consumers began to question the role of what came to be known as "Big Pharma." Those questions are still with us, as pharmaceutical companies are inextricably linked with modern vaccine development.

Source: H. K. Mulford Company. (1902). "How Mulford's Vaccine Is Made" and "How Mulford's Antitoxin Is Made." *Detroit Medical Journal* 2: xxiv–xxvi.

ANALYSIS

The United States, like European countries, enacted a series of statutes requiring smallpox vaccination in the last quarter of the 19th century. As in Britain, these statutes provoked opposition, leading to anti-vaccination activism. Some of the anti-vaccination leaders came from prosperous urban families, for whom smallpox seemed a relic of the dark ages. Their children were healthy and active, the public health regulations of the preceding 50 years having ensured that they were more likely to grow to adulthood than any earlier generation. Enlightened young parents would no more think of injecting them with something dangerous than feeding them rancid meat or bathing them in dirty water.

There were, however, some distinctive features of public health policies in the United States that contributed to its being, in the words of a contemporary writer, "the least vaccinated of any civilized country" (cited in Willrich, 2011, 14). One was that laws having to do with vaccination were at the level of state and local governments, rather than at the national level. That meant they were more likely to be influenced by local politics. Another was that American public health officials generally did not have the authority or staff to enforce their statutes, as they did in other countries. That means they were largely dependent on law enforcement officials to carry out public health policies in the face of public opposition.

In the excerpt above, what began as an implementation of public health laws became bound up in partisan politics, when Walter Kempster, a new health commissioner of English descent, clashed with influential aldermen representing wards of residents with German descent. Kempster, being notified of several cases of smallpox in one of the wards, made energetic attempts to stop it, including removing infected children to the city's smallpox hospital. Parents and neighbors were outraged and refused to allow the child to be moved. It made matters worse that the isolation hospitals set aside for smallpox patients were located in the city's undesirable South Side, uncomfortable, understaffed, and associated with poverty and disease.

But the city council's attempt to placate its residents by allowing them to care for smallpox patients in their own homes did no good. Quarantine officials, assigned to prevent people from entering houses of smallpox patients, were attacked by local residents. Health-care workers transporting patients to hospitals faced angry crowds. Kempster complained that he had been stripped of his most valuable weapons against smallpox, and he warned the epidemic would only get worse. His political opponents responded by impeaching him. The subsequent investigation highlighted the split between his English-speaking political supporters and German-speaking political opponents. The split was further emphasized when the city council voted to dismiss Kempster, and state officials reinstated him a year later. It seems likely that the opposition to public health policies exacerbated Milwaukee's sufferings from smallpox: there were 894 reported cases and 244 deaths, an unusually high death rate for this epidemic.

Other factors besides political infighting and ethnic division hindered vaccination efforts in the United States. The medical profession was split between "regular" or "allopathic" doctors and homeopathic or other alternative treatments. While many physicians on both sides of the divide advocated vaccination as a public health measure, the pharmaceutical companies that supplied their medications did not. Companies that provided lymph for cowpox vaccination took full advantage of modern sales and advertising techniques to promote their product. Companies that provided homeopathic remedies took full advantage of the same techniques to attack vaccination as unsafe compared to their own, gentler remedies.

By the turn of the 20th century, most state and city governments were sufficiently concerned about the vulnerability of their own population to institute compulsory vaccination for students attending public and parochial schools. That brought the federal government in as arbitrator of quality control, as we will see in the next chapter.

FURTHER READING

Colgove, James. (2004). "Between Persuasion and Compulsion: Smallpox Control in Brooklyn and New York, 1894–1902." *Bulletin of the History of Medicine* 78: 349–378.

Durbach, Nadja. (2002). "Class, Gender, and the Conscientious Objector to Vaccination, 1898–1907." *Journal of British Studies* 41: 58–83.

Leavitt, Judith Walzer. (1996). *The Healthiest City: Milwaukee and the Politics of Health Reform*. Madison, WI: University of Wisconsin Press.

Starr, Paul. (1984). *The Social Transformation of American Medicine*. New York: Basic Books.

Willrich, Michael. (2011). *Pox: An American History*. New York: Penguin Press.

SMALLPOX EPIDEMIC IN MUNCIE, INDIANA

- **Document:** Hugh Cowing, "Notes on the Epidemic of Smallpox in Muncie," read before the Academy of Medicine of Cincinnati
- **Date:** 1895
- **Where:** Cincinnati, OH
- **Significance:** Not all cities faced the same political turmoil as Milwaukee in the face of smallpox. After some initial upheaval, the residents of Muncie, Indiana, made it through the epidemic with a comparatively low death rate and their public health staff still in office.

DOCUMENT

Population of Muncie, 22,000. Duration of epidemic, August 19 to November 4, 1893.

Total number of cases, 150.

Number vaccinated, 10,000.

Total number of deaths, 22.

Number of houses infected, 70.

Expense of epidemic, $23,217.00.

LESSONS OF THE EPIDEMIC.

1. Domiciliary quarantine is ineffective in preventing the spread of small-pox, especially during an epidemic.

2. It is economy, in the beginning of an epidemic, to provide the most comfortable and commodious hospital quarters, with the best medical and nurse skill obtainable.

3. Then let the authorities and the medical profession unite to secure the removal of all afflicted to the pest-hospital.

4. As a rule, a well-appointed hospital, with faithful medical and nurse service, offers better conditions for recovery than if the patient remains at home.

5. By the early removal of patients from the home the danger of infection to others is greatly diminished.

6. The details connected with the removal of the diseased to the hospital, the burial of bodies, the disinfection of houses and personal quarantine of infected persons and persons exposed to infection, and the liberation of the infected from quarantine, should all be under the supervision of the health officials.

7. During an epidemic of small-pox all public meetings should be discontinued, and persons should be warned from entering houses where sickness is known to exist until the character of the disease is clearly defined. Fool-hardy and criminally careless persons should be prosecuted to the full extent of the law.

8. Railroad quarantine should require not merely a disinfection of baggage, but also a change of all clothing possibly exposed, or a thorough disinfection of the same.

9. To suppress epidemic small pox there must be a mutual and intimate bond of harmony and support among health officials, physicians and citizens.

10. An unusual prevalence of varicella [chicken pox]; especially of a severe type, should be reported by the attending physician. Under such circumstances the health authorities should take all precautions. The history of small-pox epidemics shows that in many instances they have been preceded by epidemics of varicella.

11. The history of this and former epidemics proves that vaccination, isolation and disinfection are the three important factors in stamping out an epidemic of small-pox, and, when necessity arises, there should be no hesitation on the part of the authorities in enforcing all of these measures.

12. Aseptic bovine lymph should always be used. All care and attention should be thrown around the vaccinated subject, and every precaution should be taken to protect the vaccine wound against infection.

At the beginning of the epidemic there were at least eight infected homes. We had enough to encounter to appall the heart of any health officer. The conditions were peculiar, because of the fact that the diagnosis of the disease at first was in doubt. It seems to be the unfortunate tendency among physicians and among the people that when a number of cases of small-pox develop in any locality there are enough Thomases around to throw cold water on the efforts of the officials. The health officers were met at the door, usually by the head of the house; vaccination was refused, quarantine was denied, and all opposition was thrown in the way at the outset. This is the history of the incipiency of the disease, and what may seem to you a very small blaze was fanned into a fierce flame.

Doubtless there was a mistake made right at the first, but it was the natural result of conditions. The mistake I mean was domiciliary quarantine. In attempting to control the disease it was suggested by some that a hospital be provided, and that that was the only true way to control it; yet the very fact that many doubted the disease was small-pox made it utterly impossible to remove the infected persons until public opinion came to our support. On the 19th of August, at the beginning of the epidemic, we had these conditions to meet in the homes, principally because the people had been told the cases were not small-pox, but varicella; and I might say, too, there were some cases of varicella in connection, so that it gave color to the diagnosis of varicella, even at the beginning of the epidemic.

Secondly, it is the best method, and it is economy, to provide the most comfortable and most commodious hospital quarters, with the best nurses obtainable. At the beginning we had to fight not only the disease, but we had to fight the surroundings and the people. After working along with domiciliary quarantine from the 19th of August until the 8th of September, Hospital No. 1 was opened up at Muncie, and it was the result of experience that house quarantine was an utter failure. Right at the beginning of the epidemic guards were appointed to guard each house, to let no one go out or in, and nothing should pass into the house except through the guards. By the time we had seventy houses affected there were 140 guards, at one time 150. That made an enormous expense. Then the guards themselves were taken from among the people, and were not always responsible. They had to be taken where we could get them. One guard refused to be vaccinated and refused to obey the rules, and was afterwards taken to the hospital with the disease. So you can see how ineffective house quarantine is in preventing small-pox. To provide the most commodious hospital quarters at the beginning of the epidemic, and then to remove all patients thereto, is the best plan.

The hospital used at Muncie was built for a hotel, and had never been occupied. The first patients were taken there on the 8th of September. A superintendent and a physician were provided at the outset, and no expense was spared to do everything to make it comfortable for the patients. That did a great deal toward breaking down the prejudice which for some time was entertained against the hospital. But it was not until a number of our best citizens came, with their families, into the hospital that the public understood the wisdom of the action of the authorities and physicians in charge. A lady, the wife of one of our leading dentists, took her own child and went to the hospital, and with persons of that character coming, and because the Sisters of Charity were provided as nurses, gave countenance and respectability to the hospital. Unless this is done I believe that hospital quarantine will fail. That was a time, too, when many men were out of work, loafing on the streets, idle, talking and criticising. Loitering and talking should be avoided as much as possible.

As to the qualifications of the health officers, they must be firm, intelligent, and at such a time as this the health officer must not expect to attend to the details, as he is the general who is to conduct the campaign; he is not supposed to go hither and thither, to do this and that; if he attempts to enter into the details he will make a failure. While he is watching one loop-hole there will be another opened, and he will find the disease spreading under his eyes.

We learned in the epidemic that, as a rule, a well-appointed hospital is better for the patient than to remain at home. The difficulty of securing nurses in the homes is often encountered. In the hospital they are selected because of their special fitness, while in the homes they are naturally the friends and relatives, who probably never had any experience. I said hospital all along; I believe it is better than to call it pest-house. Pest house means something horrible. If it is a hospital it ought to be all that the term implies. While you may not be able to get people to go to the pest-house, you may control their movements so as to get them in the hospital. Some of our physicians said the disease never began to spread until we began to quarantine. It was not until all the cases were in the hospital that the disease was in any way controlled. By early removal from the home the danger of infection to others is diminished.

Let me read you some of the points that should come under the supervision of the health officers. The details connected with the removal of the diseased to the hospital, the burial of the bodies, the disinfection of homes and personal quarantine of infected persons and persons exposed to infection, and the liberation of the infected from quarantine, should all be under the supervision of the health officials.

The removal of the diseased to the hospital in our epidemic occurred, usually, as soon after the case was discovered as possible. Sometimes people would not be willing to let the patients go, and sometimes offered resistance, and shot at the officials. One time a man who was conducting a removal was shot in the arm by one of the family; they stood out and stoned the officers. One young man met the officials at the door with a shot-gun, and said his father should not go; he was not removed except by death. Opposition, as you understand, was intense, yet all that is connected with the removal of the diseased must be under the supervision of the health officer; also burials, which are not to be attended except by those absolutely necessary.

Persons should be warned not to enter houses where sickness is known to exist. Fool-hardy and criminally careless persons should be prosecuted to the full extent of the law. One family had avoided the vigilance of the officials, concealing a case from them; this case was finally unearthed. One member of the family had, in the meantime, been going to his usual business. He was arrested and put in a box-car that was provided for tramps and others, possibly infected, who were not taken to jail; he was afterwards put in Hospital No. 2. Perhaps this example was wholesome to others who may have contemplated such fool-hardy conduct. But the extreme limit of moral depravity was reached when bundles of infected rags were thrown into back yards; and thus, I believe, the disease was spread intentionally.

Railroad quarantine should require not merely a disinfection of baggage, but also a change of all clothing possibly exposed, or a thorough disinfection of the same. We found it difficult to control passenger traffic. Many persons would drive out of town to some other railroad station, and there procure a ticket. This led to a quarantine against Muncie by adjacent towns. At one time at least fifteen hundred people had left our city, going to new homes or visiting among friends. Telegrams and letters would report: "Mr. A. is here with his family. What shall we do with him?" In each of our towns our local health officers were of great service to us, enforcing quarantine and disinfection.

The results from vaccination were all that its most earnest advocates could desire. The twenty-two persons who remained in the hospitals for weeks, and only protected by vaccination, all escaped small-pox. But in no instance did one not vaccinated and quarantined with small-pox cases escape the disease. Quoting from the excellent report of Dr. G. D. Leech:

"Of the twenty-two who died only four had been vaccinated. Two of these died of the hemorrhagic form; of the other two, one, a man fifty-two years old, died of phlegmonous erysipelas (complication), and the other one, a child nine months old, died of numerous abscesses in the seventh week of the disease. . . .

Of the thirty-six marked bad in this report, twenty-six had not been vaccinated. Of the thirty-nine cases marked mild in this report, thirty-one had been vaccinated. Of the sixty-three cases of the confluent form, only fourteen had been vaccinated. . . .

It should also be noted here that on the 19th of August, when I took charge as physician, we had eight cases of confluent small-pox in as many different houses; eight houses quarantined, with six on the average to the house, making forty-eight in all, who were at once vaccinated, and afterwards revaccinated, until thirty-five at least were successful. (The majority of these were already exposed to small pox before vaccination.) Crowded in quarantine with bad cases, all in small houses except one, and that did not furnish as many rooms as patients, explains why so many of these contracted the disease.

The occurrence of nine cases of the hemorrhagic form in this climate, and in warm weather, was sufficient of itself to mark the virulence of the epidemic. And yet within two and a half months (I think with great credit to the health boards and the council committee) this terrible epidemic was brought to a close. And to any one conversant with the history of the epidemic from its inception, considering the chances of infection and spread of the disease before the health officers took charge, and the many difficulties thrown in the way of the authorities by some citizens, it must seem remarkable that Muncie was rid of the scourge before the winter months."

Source: Cowing, Hugh. (1895). "Notes on the Epidemic of Smallpox in Muncie." *The Cincinnati Lancet-Clinic* 74: 9–12.

ANALYSIS

Isolation hospitals for epidemic diseases, often known as plague or pesthouses, have been generally shunned by their intended patients. Daniel Defoe's *Journal of the Plague Year* gives a graphic account of the lengths patients in 1666 in London would go to in order to avoid being shut up in either their houses, or hospitals, with other plague victims. A recent depiction of the same behavior can be found in the 1995 movie *Outbreak.* Prior to the 1920s, most patients who went to hospitals assumed they would die there, for the clear reason that conditions that were not life-threatening were treated at home. For wealthy patients, even surgery might be performed at home, since they had enough room and staff to provide sterile conditions.

Small wonder, then, that families confronted with the possibility that one of their household might be taken away to a hospital chose to conceal their disease rather than admit the diagnosis of smallpox. Local doctors, unused to smallpox, might reasonably misdiagnose it as the mild childhood disease of chicken pox (varicella) or might feel they were protecting the family by certifying it as chicken pox rather than smallpox. For that reason, as Cowing notes in the document, "At the beginning we had to fight not only the disease, but we had to fight the surroundings and the people." Only once it became clear that the disease was live smallpox and that home-based quarantine was not working to contain it, the public health authorities were able to start moving patients into isolation hospitals.

Cowing explained the conditions necessary for this to be effective. First, there had to be cooperation between city officials, the health officers, and residents. The last was often hard to come by, and many residents simply fled the city. That meant there had to be cooperation among public health officials along the railroad lines and among neighboring cities so that infected persons could be isolated and treated, no matter where they traveled. Second, the hospitals had to be pleasant, comfortable, and staffed with excellent nurses and doctors. They had to provide a superior level of care so that patients did not feel as if they had been sent to prison and given a death sentence. Third, there could not be one rule for the rich and another for the poor. All citizens, from "ladies" to poor "women," had to be confined to hospitals and treated with the same care and attention.

And finally, treatment of existing cases of smallpox had to be accompanied by active vaccination of all vulnerable residents. Vaccination alone could keep the disease away, whether the patient resided in or out of the hated hospitals. As Cowing said, "The results from vaccination were all that its most earnest advocates could desire. The twenty-two persons who remained in the hospitals for weeks, and only protected by vaccination, all escaped small-pox. But in no instance did one not vaccinated and quarantined with small-pox cases escape the disease."

FURTHER READING

Colgove, James. (2004). "Between Persuasion and Compulsion: Smallpox Control in Brooklyn and New York, 1894–1902." *Bulletin of the History of Medicine* 78: 349–378.

Mckiernan-Gonzaález, John. (2012). *Fevered Measures: Public Health and Race at the Texas-Mexico border, 1848–1942.* Durham, NC: Duke University Press.

Outbreak. (1995). Directed by Wolfgang Petersen. Warner Brothers.

Rosenberg, Charles. (1987). *The Care of Strangers: The Rise of America's Hospital System.* New York: Basic Books.

Stevens, Rosemary. (1999). *In Sickness and in Wealth: American Hospitals in the Twentieth Century.* Baltimore, MD: Johns Hopkins University Press.

6

VACCINES AND EVERYDAY LIFE
(1900–1940)

"THE PEOPLE INFORMING THE DOCTORS THAT THEY PREFERRED SMALLPOX TO TETANUS"

- **Document:** "Tetanus Following Vaccination," *The Medical News*
- **Date:** 1901
- **Where:** Camden, NJ
- **Significance:** By the early 20th century, childhood vaccination for smallpox had become a part of everyday life, and vaccination for other infectious diseases followed over the next 40 years. There were, however, no federal regulations setting quality and safety standards and only sporadic regulation by state and local boards of health. This matched the sporadic regulation of health and safety standards in other areas of American life: the production and marketing of food, including milk and agricultural products, of drugs used for a variety of ailments, and even, in many communities, clean drinking water. That meant that vaccines were produced like all other commercial products, by companies regulated only by their own health and safety policies. That was not enough, as became clear in a series of incidents where questionable vaccine quality led to unquestionable harm.

DID YOU KNOW?

Timeline of Human Vaccine Development, 1900–1940

Disease	Year
Diphtheria	1923
Tetanus	1926
Pertussis (Whooping cough)	1926
Tuberculosis	1927
Yellow fever	1935
Influenza	1936
Typhus	1938

Source: Plotkin, Stanley, Walter Orenstein, and Paul Offit, eds. (2013). *Vaccines.* Philadelphia, PA: Elsevier Saunders.

DOCUMENT

Tetanus Following Vaccination

The residents of Camden are becoming alarmed over the deaths from tetanus following vaccination and many of them are afraid to submit to the operation. Five deaths have occurred within the last ten days and several other cases have been treated. At least one death has occurred in this city. Physicians have no hesitancy in ascribing the cases to carelessness in caring for the wounds, but it is exceedingly difficult to convince the laity of that fact. It is thought that the unusually dry weather of the past two months has caused the tetanus bacilli to be disseminated through the air to an unusual degree. One fatal case, a boy of seven years, was reported by his physician as having dropped the scab from his arm into the street. The boy replaced the scab and afterward developed tetanus. But one fatal case of smallpox has occurred in Camden.

Source: "Tetanus Following Vaccination." (1901). *The Medical News* 79: 829.

- **Document:** "Smallpox in New Jersey," *The Philadelphia Medical News*
- **Date:** 1901
- **Where:** Philadelphia, PA

DOCUMENT

Smallpox in New Jersey

Smallpox, which has been prevalent in Hudson County, has broken out in the jail and almshouse at Snake Hill. The Pennsylvania Railroad station at Colonia has been quarantined and no trains stop there, on account of a case of smallpox in the station-master's family. Cases are reported in Trenton, and Camden has had 49 cases since December 15. The Camden Public Schools will not open until January 13. Free vaccination is not at all encouraged, the people informing the doctors that they prefer smallpox to tetanus. Smallpox hospitals are to be constructed at Bridgeton and Gloucester. There are forty cases of smallpox in Hackettstown, and the place has been isolated by the direction of the local Board of Health, the members of which have acted under the advice of the State Board of Health. The large number of cases is said to be due to the ignorance of the local physicians, who had been treating numerous cases, but did not know the disease was smallpox until it spread to twenty people. Experts on the disease came from New York and pronounced the cases to be smallpox.

Source: "Smallpox in New Jersey." (1901). *The Philadelphia Medical Journal* 9: 50.

- **Document:** Official Report of the Camden Board of Health, printed in *The Sanitarian*
- **Date:** 1902
- **Where:** Camden, NJ

DOCUMENT

Official Report of the Camden Board of Health Concerning Cases of Tetanus which Occurred in Patients Who had been Vaccinated

We have thoroughly investigated the cases of tetanus occurring in Camden, and beg to present to the public the following facts and conclusions:

1. Samples of all the different makes of vaccine employed in Camden have been tested for tetanus germs by the State Bacteriologist of New Jersey, and have been found pure and entirely free from tetanus germs; hence, tetanus could not have been caused by the virus employed. (See report of Dr. Mitchell, Secretary of New Jersey State Board of Health.)

2. The history of each case of tetanus has been carefully collected from the attending physician, and in every instance vaccination was practiced in a correct and cleanly manner; the infection of tetanus resulting from neglect on the part of the patients to present themselves to the attending physicians, so that their vaccination could receive proper attention.

3. One case of tetanus has occurred from gunshot wound, during the same period, in a boy who had not been vaccinated, proving that the tetanus germs were in the atmosphere.

4. Indisputable evidence of the fact that the tetanus germs were not introduced at the time of vaccination is that acute tetanus occurs in from 5 to 9 days after the introduction of the germs, whereas in every case acute tetanus occurred in from three to four weeks after the vaccination. If the virus had been contaminated, tetanus would have ensued within 9 days after vaccination. Tetanus developed in every make of vaccine used.

5. Further proof of the purity of the virus exists in the reports of the physicians in Cooper Hospital, who tested on animals samples of all makes of vaccine employed in Camden. If the virus had been contaminated, the animals would have developed tetanus because of their extreme susceptibility to this disease. (See animal experiments.)

6. During the past five weeks there have been vaccinated in Philadelphia a very large number of people with the same virus as employed in Camden. In not one of these cases did tetanus occur.

7. The tetanus cases in Camden are to be explained upon atmospheric and telluric conditions which have prevailed in Camden during the past six weeks. There has been a long period of dry weather with high winds, so that tetanus germs, which have their normal habitat in the earth dust, dirt of stables, etc., have been constantly distributed in the atmosphere. It is noticeable in all the cases, after careful examination as to the cause, that the wound had been exposed by the scab being knocked off or removed, or else the arm had been injured and infection resulted; frequently children scratched the vaccinated area with their dirty fingers and nails and infected the wound.

8. That vaccination should be regarded as a surgical operation and should be performed in an aseptic or clean manner, and in every instance the physician should be consulted for advice if any unusual inflammation should develop.

9. It is the unanimous opinion of the Board of Health, as well as of their committee of experts, that, inasmuch as vaccination is harmless, it should be insisted upon by physicians as an absolutely necessary procedure for the prevention of smallpox. Tetanus, or any other infection, can never occur if the vaccination is properly protected from contact with the atmosphere or with soiled clothing, bandages, etc.

Henry H. Davis, M.D., President.

Joel W. Fithtan, M.D.

S. G. Bushey, M. D.

Committee Board of Health.

State House, Trenton, N. J., Nov. 26, 1901.

Dr. H. H. Davis, President Camden Board of Health:

Laboratory examinations of vaccine forwarded by your Board of Health show that no tetanus bacteria were present.

Henry Mitchell, M.D.,

Secretary New Jersey State Board of Health.

The Cooper Hospital, Camden, N. J., Nov. 26, 1901.

We report herewith the results of our experiments with the vaccine virus employed in Camden:

The virus was purchased from fifteen different pharmacies in Camden, and represented those brands of vaccine with which the patients who died of tetanus were vaccinated. All of these samples of vaccine were purchased in the open market without any person's knowledge that they were to be tested for the presence of tetanus germs.

These experiments were conducted in the Cooper Hospital, so that constant and careful observations could be made. White rats were selected because they are extremely susceptible to tetanus and because in these animals tetanus develops within twenty-four hours after infection. A large number of white rats were inoculated with all the samples of vaccine and kept under observation for five days. Not a single one of the animals has, at any time since their inoculation, manifested the slightest symptoms of tetanus.

The results of our experiments enable us to state positively that the vaccine virus was pure and free from tetanus germs, thus proving that the cases of tetanus which occurred in Camden were not caused by the vaccine employed.

This investigation should remove all fear from the public mind and should encourage people toward vaccination as a preventive to a disease which is imminent as an epidemic.

Alexander Scanlin Ross, M.D.

S. Edward Fretz, M.D.

Philadelphia, PA., Nov. 27, 1901.

Henry H. Davis. M.D., President Board of Health, City Hall, Camden, N. J.:

Dear Doctor:—In answer to your inquiry of even date, I desire to state that our vaccine physicians have vaccinated nearly one hundred thousand persons in the past three months, and during the same period it is safe to state that at least 700,000 persons in Philadelphia have been vaccinated, without a single case of tetanus having been reported to this office.

Yours truly,
J. Lewis Good.
President Philadelphia Board of Health.

Source: "Vaccination, Antitoxin, and Tetanus." (1902). *The Sanitarian* 48: 32–34.

ANALYSIS

Between 1901 and 1902, residents in the populous state of New Jersey experienced the first smallpox epidemic in 16 years. For the most part, the cases presented the milder form, but some were virulent and deadly. The epidemic spread along the many railroad and tram lines that formed a dense transportation network across the state, south and east, from the major population centers of New York, Philadelphia, Newark, and Trenton to Vineland, the Jersey Shore, and Cape May. The New Jersey Board of Health issued a warning about smallpox, calling for general vaccination. In Camden, public authorities built a smallpox hospital, and the Camden Board of Education announced that it would enforce the law requiring all school children to be vaccinated. Private doctors and local druggists carried out the bulk of the vaccinations, but municipal authorities also provided vaccination free of charge at local dispensaries. By October, almost a third of the city's residents, including some 5,000 schoolchildren, had been treated with state-of-the-art vaccine, manufactured from cow lymph and treated with glycerin as preservative and germicide.

On November 11, 1901, disaster struck: 11-year-old Thomas Hazelton became ill while playing in the street. Within a day, he was dead of the agonizing disease, tetanus, popularly known as lockjaw. Within the next few weeks, other cases surfaced. During the month of November, nine otherwise healthy children died horribly of tetanus. Parents made the immediate link between vaccination and tetanus and refused to vaccinate their children, fearing the vaccine would be tainted. As Document 2 indicates, they "preferred smallpox to tetanus." Panic gripped the city, and as the cases of smallpox mounted, Camden closed public schools until January. As news of the Camden deaths spread to other cities, so did fear of smallpox vaccination. In city after city, parents refused to vaccinate their children, and school after school was "closed for want of attendance" (Willrich, 2011, 178).

The Camden Board of Health mounted a prompt and effective investigation into the cases, led by three prominent researchers with considerable experience in public health. They found that there was little common ground among the affected children and their families. They lived in different parts of the city and had been vaccinated by different practitioners. None had any previous condition or recent injury that could account for their developing tetanus. The only thing they had in common was the company that had produced their vaccine: the H. K. Mulford Company, a highly respected manufacturer of vaccines and other medical materials. Yet, as described in Document 3, when researchers purchased samples of vaccine from Mulford as well as other companies they could find no evidence that the vaccine was contaminated. Indeed, if it had been, the cases of tetanus would have been far more widespread. They, therefore, concluded that each of the cases was local and individual: it was simply coincidence that they had occurred after the children had been vaccinated.

This explanation may well have reassured parents, though it is likely that they were more reassured when cases of smallpox receded, schools reopened, and they could ignore calls for smallpox vaccination. But, in fact, they were right to raise the outcry, for later investigation showed that vaccine manufacturers in the United States were by no means as careful as their European counterparts to maintain sterile conditions. It was common practice to assume that the glycerin added to the vaccine would kill all germs, with the result that tainted vaccines were potentially much more common than anyone knew. The nine children who died of tetanus, out of the 27,000 Camden residents who were vaccinated, could be considered a measure of the level of impurity of the vaccine. By modern standards, Camden residents were right to consider that level as unacceptably high. Indeed, most would argue, a rate of even one patient death caused by avoidable manufacturing error was unacceptably high.

FURTHER READING

Durbach, Nadja. (2005). *Bodily Matters: The Anti-Vaccination Movement in England, 1853–1907*. Durham, NC: Duke University Press.

Leahy, Ellen. (2003). " 'Montana Fever': Smallpox and the Montana State Board of Health." *Montana: The Magazine of Western History* 53: 32–45.

Liebenau, Jonathan. (1987). *Medical Science and Medical Industry: The Formation of the American Pharmaceutical Industry*. London: Macmillan.

Pratt, Joan Klobe. (2002). "The Free Economic Society and the Battle against Smallpox: A 'Public Sphere' in Action." *The Russian Review* 61: 560–578.

Willrich, Michael. (2011). *Pox. An American History*. New York: Penguin Press.

QUALITY CONTROL AND DAMAGE CONTROL

- **Document:** "Tetanus Following Vaccination and Injection of Anti-toxin," *North American Journal of Homeopathy*
- **Date:** 1901
- **Where:** New York, NY
- **Significance:** The early 20th century is often known as the Progressive Era in American history, with many groups working for social and legislative reform. The following excerpts show the importance of medical journalism in raising awareness of unsafe practices. The outbreaks of tetanus in Camden came at the same time as an outbreak in St. Louis, where it was conclusively linked to tainted diphtheria antitoxin. Antitoxin is given as a treatment to people who have already contracted diphtheria, that is, it is not a preventative vaccine. Outraged residents and observers were more interested in the similarities than the differences, however, pointing out that both outbreaks were clearly linked to faulty manufacturing processes.

DOCUMENT

Tetanus Following Vaccination and Injection of Antitoxin.

During the past few weeks fatal results have followed vaccination in Camden, N. J., Philadelphia and Bridgton, N. J. In St. Louis the use of antitoxin has been followed by no less than fourteen deaths, and more are expected. There seems no question but that the cases of tetanus, some twenty in number, in St. Louis, are directly due to the use of anti-diphtheritic serum furnished by the Health Department of that city. The report of the City Bacteriologist discloses some interesting facts. The horse from which the antitoxic serum was taken was kept at "the poor house stables." On August 24 he was bled and the serum so obtained was duly prepared and distributed. This was the fatal preparation that has already caused fourteen deaths.

Nothing is said in this somewhat curious report concerning the care taken of the horse used for the production of the serum. The condition of the stable is not stated, and the surroundings are not described. The ice chest used to receive the blood from the horse is "three hundred yards" from the stable. That is all the information that is vouchsafed concerning the care of the horse or of the precautions taken to prevent contamination of the blood. On October 1 the horse was pronounced ill with tetanus and killed. August 30, six days after the blood had been placed in "the ice chest three hundred yards" from the stable, it was brought to the laboratory and duly prepared. Ten cubic centimeters were drawn off and tested on six guinea pigs.

After this, on September 10, small bottles holding 10 cc. were filled "by our careful janitor" and the distribution proceeded. Shades of Lister! Filled by our careful janitor! Why not the bottles washed by "our careful scrubwoman," and the corks put in by the "careful office boy"! And then a little later twenty-two cases of tetanus. Criminal carelessness? Why how could it be with "our careful janitor"? Just a mysterious visitation of providence. But a careful review of the report shows pretty conclusively that proper precautions were not taken with the horse either as to cleanliness or as safeguarding against tetanus; that neither blood nor serum were adequately protected from contamination; that the tests upon guinea pigs were hasty and inconclusive and that the employment of "our careful janitor" was an offense so gross as to be without palliation.

But it is very likely that the men directly connected with the preparation of this death-dealing serum are not the most to blame. The final censure should rest upon a rotten and criminally corrupt political system. Ignorant and insolent "bosses" would not provide the money to decently run the health department. That is why the janitor appeared, and that is why no health department in any city should be allowed to furnish antitoxin. Politics and science will not mix, and when ring politicians control laboratories the public and science are both betrayed.

Source: "Tetanus Following Vaccination and Injection of Antitoxin." (1901). *North American Journal of Homeopathy* 49: 748–749.

- **Document:** "The Diphtheria Antitoxin and Tetanus Outbreak in St. Louis," *The Sanitarian*
- **Date:** 1901
- **Where:** New York, NY

DOCUMENT

The Diphtheria Antitoxin and Tetanus Outbreak in St. Louis

Drs. B. Meade Bolton, C. Fisch and E. C. Walden, the commission appointed to investigate the cases of tetanus following the administration of diphtheria antitoxin in St. Louis, have reported (St. Louis Medical Review of November 23, 1901) as follows:

"As a result of our investigations we draw the following conclusions: "The diphtheria antitoxin prepared by the Health Department of the City of St. Louis, and dated September 30, and some of the serum dated August 24, was the cause of the recent deaths from tetanus in the cases where this antitoxin was used. This antitoxin was sterile, but contained the toxin of the tetanus bacillus in considerable amount.

"There were two different sera issued under the date of August 24; one portion not containing the tetanus toxin and characterized by other properties, while the other contained the tetanus and was identified with the serum bearing the date of September 30.

"The most important result we have arrived at is the positive demonstration that the toxic serum dated August 24 and that dated September 30 are identical. From this we conclude that the serum of September 30 was issued without having been tested by the proper methods, and that a part of it was filled into bottles bearing the date of August 24, and furnished with labels having previously been stamped with this date. We are justified in drawing this conclusion from two observations. First, that the serum of September 30 was issued before there was time to have performed the simple tests necessary to determine the antitoxic potency of the serum. Second, in the same way, serum dated October 23 came into our possession on November 1. This serum had been issued to physicians by the Health Department, and by them returned to the coroner. It is obvious from this that no animal experiments could have been made with this antitoxin. As this was the case with the serum of October 23, it is the natural inference that the serum of September 30 was issued in the same way.

"We must deny any possibility of latent tetanus having existed in the horse 'Jim' from August 24 to September 30, as no well-authenticated cases have been reported in which the incubation period extended over seven days, in experiments directed to test this point. The period of incubation cannot be determined from clinical observation, from the nature of the case. It therefore follows from this that the serum drawn on August 24 was free from tetanus, but that the serum of September 30 was drawn during the period of incubation, and had it been tested upon animals it must necessarily have revealed its toxic properties.

"From the foregoing facts we are forced to conclude that the diphtheria antitoxin prepared by the City Health Department has been issued before it was possible to have obtained results from the absolutely necessary tests. Had these tests been performed, the results upon animals would have been such that the serum would not have been dispensed, and the cases of tetanus forming the basis of this report could not have resulted."

Source: "The Diphtheria Antitoxin and Tetanus Outbreak in St. Louis." (1902). *The Sanitarian* 48: 32–34.

ANALYSIS

Homeopathic medicine was first introduced into the United States as an alternative to the harsh treatments often prescribed in the early 19th century, especially bloodletting and drugs that produced sweating, purging, or vomiting. It became a kind of medical counterculture, focusing on small doses of gentler herbal remedies, and its practitioners often advocated for social justice causes, such as abolition, women's education, and voting reform.

It was especially favored by well-to-do families for women and children; many of its principles were adopted by the new specialty of pediatrics. During much of the

19th century, homeopathic physicians were trained in homeopathic medical schools, like Hahnemann Medical College in Philadelphia, while "regular" or "allopathic" physicians were trained in the more traditional schools, like the University of Pennsylvania medical school. Professionally, the two types of physicians were fierce rivals, each with its own city, state, and national associations. On a personal level, though, there was often collaboration, including family practices in which a male allopath physician treated the men in a household, while his wife, a homeopathic physician, treated the women and children.

After the acceptance of the germ theory, the training at both types of medical schools began to converge. The harsh therapies of previous generations were regarded by both sides as barbaric and unscientific; the original homeopathic theories of disease gave way to study of microorganisms. By 1900, the curriculum of Hahnemann medical school looked very similar to the curriculum at the University of Pennsylvania medical school. But physicians influenced by the homeopathic tradition still tended to be more interested in social justice and more likely to publicly criticize unsafe professional or business practices.

The author from the *North American Journal of Homeopathy* was especially clear about the need for health officials to take responsibility for their own poor management and not to fall back on the age-old excuse, "accidents happen." As the article noted, "A verdict has been rendered against the St. Louis Board of Health finding it negligent in the preparation of the antitoxin used." Expert bacteriologists had concluded "that the diphtheria antitoxin prepared by the City Health Department had been issued before it was possible to have obtained results from the absolutely necessary tests. Had these tests been performed, the results upon animals would have been such that the serum would not have been dispensed and the cases of tetanus forming the basis of this report could not have resulted."

This negligence not only led to unnecessary deaths from tetanus but also injured this and future public health efforts. "It is very probable," the author pointed out, "that these most unfortunate occurrences will influence the public mind against both vaccination and antitoxin. But if we are to have the confidence of the public we should make it impossible for such catastrophies to happen" (752). This was a lesson destined to be all-too-closely interwoven with the technological advances of the 20th and 21st centuries.

FURTHER READING

Buerki, Robert. (1971). "Reception of the Germ Theory of Disease in The American Journal of Pharmacy." *Pharmacy in History* 13: 158–168.

Daemmrich, Arthur and Mary Ellen Bowden. (2005). "A Rising Drug Industry." *Chemical and Engineering News* Special Issue 83. http://pubs.acs.org/cen/coverstory/83/8325/8325intro.html.

Geist, Edward. (2012). "When Ice Cream Was Poisonous: Adulteration, Ptomaines, and Bacteriology in the United States, 1850–1910." *Bulletin of the History of Medicine* 86: 333–360.

Kaufman, Martin. (1971). *Homeopathy in America: The Rise and Fall of a Medical Heresy.* Baltimore, MD: Johns Hopkins University Press.

Young, James Harvey. (1995). "Federal Drug and Narcotic Legislation." *Pharmacy in History* 37: 59–67.

U.S. GOVERNMENT REGULATES
VACCINE PRODUCTION

- **Document:** Biologics Control Act
- **Date:** 1902
- **Where:** Washington, DC
- **Significance:** One of the most famous outcomes of Progressive Era reforms was the Pure Food and Drug Act, enacted in 1906. Not many realize that it was based on the 1902 Biologics Control Act, the first law to provide federal regulation of manufacturing practices in industries that affected the public health. Any company that wished to produce vaccines had to obtain a license from the U.S. government, issued only after inspection of the manufacturing facilities. The Biologics Control Act brought U.S. vaccine manufacturing standards up to the same level as those in European countries. In fact, from the 1920s, American medical companies came to dominate the pharmaceutical research and production industry.

DOCUMENT

An Act to Regulate the Sale of Viruses, Serums, Toxins, and Analagous Products

Be it enacted . . . That from and after six months after the promulgation of the regulations authorized by . . . this Act no person shall sell, barter, or exchange, or offer for sale, barter, or exchange . . . any virus, therapeutic serum, toxin, antitoxin, or analogous product applicable to the prevention and cure of diseases of man, unless (a) such virus, serum, toxin, antitoxin, or product has been propagated and prepared at an establishment holding an unsuspended and unrevoked license, issued by the Secretary of the Treasury . . . nor (b) unless each package of such virus, serum, toxin, antitoxin, or product is plainly marked with the proper name of the article contained therein, the name, address, and license number of the manufacturer, and the date beyond which the contents can not be expected beyond reasonable double to yield their specific results . . .

That no person shall falsely label or mark any package or container of any virus, serum, toxin, antitoxin, or product aforesaid; nor alter any label or mark . . .

That any officer, agent, or employee of the Treasury Department, duly detailed by the Secretary of the Treasury for that purpose, may during all reasonable hours enter and inspect any establishment for the propagation and preparation of any virus, serum, toxin, antitoxin, or product aforesaid . . .

That the Surgeon-General of the Army, the Surgeon-General of the Navy, and the supervising Surgeon-General of the Marine-Hospital Service, be, and they are hereby, constituted a board with authority, subject to the approval of the Secretary of the Treasury, to promulgate from time to time such rules as may be necessary in the judgment of said board to govern the issue, suspension, and revocation of licenses . . .

That the Secretary of the Treasury be, and he is hereby, authorized and directed to enforce the provisions of this Act . . .

That no person shall interfere with any officer, agent, or employee of the Treasury Department in the performance of any duty imposed upon him by this Act . . .

That any person who shall violate, or aid or abet in violating any of the provisions of this Act shall be punished by a fine not exceeding five hundred dollars or by imprisonment not exceeding one year, or by both such fine and imprisonment, in the discretion of the court . . .

Approved July 1, 1902.

Source: Biologics Control Act, Public Law 57-244, 57th Congress, 1st session, July 1, 1902.

IMPACT OF FEDERAL REGULATION

- **Document:** Federal Control of Vaccine Virus, *Western Druggist*
- **Date:** 1905
- **Where:** Chicago, IL
- **Significance:** The impact of federal regulation was immediate and profound, as were the challenges faced by the U.S. Public Health Service. This article in the *Western Druggist* appears to be in favor of the new law, but not all industry professionals would have agreed.

DOCUMENT

Federal Control of Vaccine Virus

Dr. John F. Anderson, of the U. S. Public Health and Marine Hospital Services, states as the result of the new federal law regulating interstate traffic in viruses, serums and toxins, four firms were found manufacturing vaccine virus by obsolete methods, and, being unable to comply with modern requirements of asepsis and laboratory control, preferred to retire from business.

Dr. Anderson goes on to relate that on account of certain insanitary conditions and faulty methods of laboratory control of some of the firms, the inspectors found it necessary to recommend that their establishments and methods of manufacture be considerably improved before the issuance of a license could be recommended, the license being withheld until these faults were corrected ...

A description of the manner in which the inspections are made will show the thoroughness with which this part of the law is carried out. The officer detailed for this purpose calls on the head of the establishment without notice, stating the object of his visit. Then, in company with the expert having supervision of vaccine production, a rigid inspection is made of all portions of the establishment, including the stables, barns, warehouses, records and animals, especial attention being given to sanitary conditions, the water supply, the screening of stables to protect animals against insects, disposal of refuse, character of food supplies, and proximity to stables used for housing horses (danger of tetanus contamination).

Close attention is given to laboratory methods, especially those of disinfection and bacteriologic control, in order to insure freedom from outside contamination. The inspector also observes the method of glycerinating the pulp, the process of grinding and mixing the virus, the distribution into tubes and the preparation of points. The inspector then observes the vaccination of a calf and the collection of virus from a "ripe" vaccination. All this is done in order to insure the inspector that the technic of the manufacture is safe and effective. The inspector purchases on the open market vaccine made by the concern and it is forwarded to the

Hygienic Laboratory of the service, situated in Washington, where it is examined for purity and potency.

In accordance with the law, monthly purchases of vaccine virus are made on the open market and the product is examined in the Hygienic Laboratory. This examination is two-fold, for purity and for potency. The person buying the vaccine virus forwards it to the laboratory with a memorandum giving the retailer's name, date of purchase, conditions under which it was kept in the drug store, and any other facts that he may think pertinent.

When received in the laboratory the package is first examined to see whether the regulations have been complied with in that the name and address of the manufacturer, his license number and the date of manufacture and of return are plainly stated on the label . . .

Cultures of cocci and certain other organisms are made from the plates and their pathogenicity ascertained by animal inoculation. Within the past year streptococci have been found on but rare occasions. Seldom has a virulent staphylococcus been found. Streptothrices have been found in the product of almost every manufacturer, though not virulent for laboratory animals. No evidence of tetanus has been found in any vaccine examined in the Hygienic Laboratory.

The product is finally tested for potency by primary vaccinations on children, using two tubes or two points taken from packages the remainder of which has been examined bacteriologically. The case is kept under daily observation and special attention is given to the character of the "takes." If any faults are discovered, especially bacteriologic contamination of a serious nature or a lack of potency, the facts are reported to the surgeon-general, who calls the attention of the manufacturer to them.

Vaccine has been examined in the laboratory almost continuously since early in the winter of 1901–2 and the following figures will convey an idea of the degree of contamination before the attention of manufacturers was directed to the large amount of contamination and since the passage of the act approved July 1, 1902. Vaccine virus examined during the winter of 1901–2 gave a general average of 4,698 bacteria per tube and 4,809 per point, the highest count for a tube being 30,080 and for a point 20,828. In the examinations conducted since the act went into effect the general average of the tubes has been 309, for points 1,223; the highest for a tube being 1,501, and for a point 8,860.

We cannot but feel that this decided improvement has been due to the rigid inspection and control of the manufacture of vaccine virus by the federal government.

While commercially it may be impossible to place a virus on the market that is absolutely free from microbial contamination, it is not too much to ask that no vaccine be placed on the market unless it is free from pathogenic cocci and other dangerous bacteria . . .

Source: "Federal Control of Vaccine Virus." (1905). *Western Druggist* 27: 433–434.

ANALYSIS

Theodore Roosevelt (1858–1919) is well known as a reforming president, but one of his most effective legislative measures, the Biologic Control Act, is often overlooked in his list of accomplishments. It was passed without debate in both Houses of Congress and signed into law on July 1, 1902, the very day that Congress adjourned for the summer. Roosevelt spent much of the rest of the day finishing up legislative enactments so that he, too, could leave Washington to spend the summer with his family in New York.

Once signed, the Biologics Control Act did not produce any of the controversy that would be a hallmark of Roosevelt's tumultuous two terms in office. The *New York Times* spelled out the reason for the unusual degree of bipartisan cooperation, stating that the bill "would involve a dangerous expansion of Federal Authority were it not aimed to correct an evil yet more dangerous as directly and immediately affecting the public health" (Willrich, 2011, 206). The dead children in Camden and Jim, the infected horse in St. Louis, had provided graphic illustration that tainted vaccines and medications were emphatically a greater evil than federal government.

Administration of the act devolved upon the U.S. Laboratory of Hygiene, an already established part of the Marine Health Service. The laboratory was tasked with inspecting and issuing licenses to pharmaceutical companies for the production of vaccines as well as other materials used in the prevention and treatment of disease. As the second excerpt shows, the mandatory inspections succeeded in enforcing quality where voluntary self-policing had failed. Vaccine supply firms that could not meet federal standards were refused licenses or simply shut themselves down. Even well-established firms, like H. K. Mulford and Parke-Davis found their licenses suspended when they put tainted products on the market.

Laboratory staff expanded from 1 full-time scientist in 1902 to 13 in 1904, and it continued to expand with the growth of the science and administration of public health. In 1912, the Marine Health Service was renamed the Public Health Service. The Laboratory of Hygiene is best known in American medicine by the name it acquired in 1948, the National Institutes of Health.

FURTHER READING

Bren, Linda. (2002). "The Road to the Biotech Revolution—Highlights of 100 Years of Biologics Regulation." *About FDA*. http://www.fda.gov/AboutFDA/WhatWeDo/History/FOrgsHistory/CBER/ucm135758.htm.

Kondratas, Ramunas. (1982). "The Biologics Control Act of 1902." In *The Early Years of Federal Food and Drug Control*, edited by James Harvey Young. Madison, WI: University of Wisconsin Press, 6–12.

Milstien, Julie. (2004). "Regulation of Vaccines: Strengthening the Science Base." *Journal of Public Health Policy* 25: 173–189.

"Regulations for the Sale of Viruses, Serums, Toxins, and Analogous Products." (1909). *Public Health Reports* (1896–1970) 24: 629–633.

A Short History of the National Institutes of Health. https://history.nih.gov/exhibits/history/index.html.

Willrich, Michael. (2011). *Pox. An American History*. New York: Penguin Press.

VACCINES IN WORLD WAR I

- **Document:** "Keeping the Army Fit," *Harper's Pictorial Library of the World War*
- **Date:** 1920
- **Where:** New York, NY, and London, United Kingdom
- **Significance:** There were about 7 million deaths among military personnel in World War I, but it was the first war in history where more were killed by weapons than by disease. New, horrific methods of war took their toll: machine guns, exploding shells, and poison gas. But the widespread adoption of vaccination and sanitary measures spectacularly reduced the deadly epidemics of previous centuries, among both soldiers and civilians.

DOCUMENT

Keeping the Army Fit
The Wide Field of Sanitation and Disease Prevention over Which the Activities of the Medical Service Now Extend

In the days when contagious disease was looked upon as a scourge from God or a visitation from the devil, it would hardly have been considered fair to hold the doctor responsible for the health of an army. It is, however, surprising to note to what a late date this viewpoint has, at least implicitly, been held—and by the same token, to what a degree the course of wars has been governed by epidemic.

Campaigns which by all military prognostication should have succeeded have failed because cholera, plague, typhoid, typhus, smallpox, malaria, dysentery and yellow fever have surpassed the powers of shot and shell to destroy. Thus the returns show that in the brief war with Spain, our dead from sickness—mainly typhoid and yellow fever, as will be remembered—were seven times more numerous than the direct casualties of fighting. In the Balkan War which served as preliminary to the vast conflict of all nations, the Bulgarian campaign broke down largely because of epidemics. There were 30,000 cases of cholera in one day! ...

DID YOU KNOW?

Influenza Pandemic of 1918

In 1918, just as World War I drew to a close, a dreadful, virulent strain of influenza or "flu" erupted, leading to many more casualties than the war itself. An estimated 1/5 of the world's population was infected during the flu pandemic of 1918–1919, and from 2% to 3% died—between 20 million and 40 million people. Most influenza epidemics affect the very young or very old, who generally have the weakest immune systems. But the 1918 pandemic disproportionally attacked young, healthy adults. Influenza was responsible for 80% of U.S. war casualties and for the 1/3 of the deaths of all physicians. The death rate was unthinkably high throughout the world but nowhere more than in the islands of the South Pacific. Influenza carried off over 20% of the population of the islands of Samoa, Fiji, and Tahiti. In reports that echo documents from the bubonic plague epidemic in Europe in 1348, government officials wrote that "it was impossible to bury the dead ... Day and night trucks rumbled throughout the streets, filled with bodies for the constantly burning pyres" (cited in Oldstone, 1998, 174).

Scientists now think that the high mortality was one reason why the pandemic only lasted a year: like bubonic plague and other deadly epidemics, influenza simply killed off most of the vulnerable population. Modern researchers have used tissue samples from influenza victims to try to figure out where the virus came from. Influenza occurs regularly in birds, pigs, and other mammals. As a particular viral strain moves from one species to another, it can undergo genetic change. Whether this change makes it more or less deadly depends on the specific interaction between virus and species. Scientists believe that the 1918 influenza could have started out as a milder disease in pigs, chickens, or even people, before evolving into the pandemic virus.

Though the first influenza vaccine was developed in 1936, that was only the start of the scientific process. Each time a new strain of influenza appears, scientists in pharmaceutical research laboratories must analyze its composition and develop a vaccine precisely adapted to block it from infecting the body. Every annual flu shot is the product of an enormous effort in medical surveillance, that is, tracking the existing strains of the disease worldwide, and in medical research, adapting existing vaccine expertise and technology to anticipated new strains. The goal is to stay one step ahead of the microbe, to make sure the 1918 flu epidemic will never happen again.

Sources:

"Influenza 1918." *The American Experience.* http://www.pbs.org/wgbh/americanexperience/films/influenza/.

Oldstone, Michael. (1998). *Viruses, Plagues and History.* New York: Oxford University Press.

Preventing Infection

The agency through which the army surgeon meets and defeats disease is of course inoculation. He makes a better showing than the surgeon in civil life only because of his greater power to learn correctly all pertinent facts, and his greater authority to deal with his patients. Given the researches of Pasteur and his successors, plus the technique of sanitary engineering as developed in Cuba, Panama and the Philippines by the American military, and organized immunity from disease is reduced to very simple terms. This is amply illustrated by the record of the British Army in the World War. In the first six months, only 421 cases of typhoid had occurred on all the fronts and in all home camps; and of these cases 305 were in men who had not been inoculated within two years. Among those who had been inoculated there had been but a single death, and this was of a man who had received only one inoculation in place of the regular two. This record stands out in sharp contrast with that of the British in the Boer War, where they had 58,000 cases, of which 8,000 terminated fatally. The difference was simply a matter of inoculation.

Source: "Keeping the Army Fit." (1920). In *The Inventive and Industrial Triumphs of the War, Harper's Pictorial Library of the World War,* edited by Austin Lescaboura and J. Bird. 12 vols. New York and London: Harper & Brother's Publishers, 8: 392–393.

ANALYSIS

World War I—the Great War, as it was called until World War II—had been over barely two years when Harper & Brother's, publishers of a widely read journal, *Harper's Magazine,* produced their handsome, 12-volume *Pictorial Library of the World War.* Volume 8 was devoted to the "inventive and industrial triumphs of the war," using clear language and high-quality imagery to depict military, transportation, and medical innovations. The war had produced "no towering military figure," the volume editor wrote, "no Napoleon, no Wellington, no Grant, no Lee." Instead, it was a war of technology, the "aeroplane and the observation balloon, with the camera and the telescope, the powerful searchlights, and illuminating bombs, the telephone and radio, the long range guns, the tank, the deadly gasses" as well as the professionals who created or managed them, like chemists and engineers.

Key to this new, inventive war were the people Harper's referred to as, Sanitary Engineers, whose job was to provide an effective fighting force by keeping military personnel healthy. They could be compared to public health officials in civilian life, with certain points of distinct contrast. Military medical authorities had much more control over their patients than public health officials: they could simply issue orders to enforce compliance to health standards, where a city public health officer might have to beg and cajole. They could screen out obviously unhealthy recruits, particularly any with contagious disease. They could enforce healthy eating and exercise habits. And they could enforce vaccination. An army training camp in 1914 may well have been one of the most healthful environments in the world.

Of course, all that changed when soldiers went into the extreme conditions of battle. Food, sleep, cleanliness, and dry clothing disappeared. A single gunshot wound was not necessarily lethal, but multiple trauma wounds perpetrated by machine gun fire almost certainly was. Shrapnel with its jagged edges almost always led to serious infection in the wounded area, even if the initial injury was relatively minor. And the new technological advances, particularly in transportation, made it possible to deploy armies on the field much longer than ever before. The Battle of the Somme, which lasted from July through November 1916, had over a million casualties. It is considered one of the bloodiest battles in world history. This is in part because never before in world history had it been possible to keep two large armies on the field for four months without fear of a major epidemic.

FURTHER READING

Allen, Arthur. (2007). *Vaccine: The Controversial Story of Medicine's Greatest Lifesaver*. New York: W. E. Norton & Company.

Barnes, David. (2006). *The Great Stink of Paris and the Nineteenth-Century Struggle against Filth and Germs*. Baltimore, MD: Johns Hopkins University Press.

Dyer, R. E. (1944). "The Role of Immunization in Wartime Advances in Medicine." *Proceedings of the American Philosophical Society* 88: 182–188.

Linton, Derek. (2010). "'War Dysentery' and the Limitations of German Military Hygiene during World War I." *Bulletin of the History of Medicine* 84: 607–639.

Magowska, Anita. (2014). "The Unwanted Heroes: War Invalids in Poland after World War I." *Journal of the History of Medicine and Allied Sciences* 69: 185–220.

VACCINATION ON VACATION

- **Document:** "Prevent Tetanus by Using Tetanus Antitoxin" and "Anti Typhoid Vaccination for Vacationists," Weekly Report of the Department of Health of the City of New York
- **Date:** 1921
- **Where:** New York, NY
- **Significance:** During the 1920s, vaccination and antitoxins became a routine part of urban life, as protection against Fourth of July accidents or germs picked up when traveling abroad.

DOCUMENT

Prevent Tetanus by Using Tetanus Antitoxin

On June 9th, last, a fourteen year old boy of this city sustained what was considered an extremely trivial injury to the palm of the left hand, as a result of an explosion of a blank cartridge. Little attention was paid to the wound until a week later, when the boy complained of a severe pain in the back of the neck, and developed convulsions and other symptoms characteristic, of the justly dreaded disease, tetanus. He died on June 18.

For years, the Department of Health has been bringing to the attention of the public the necessity of treating every wound inflicted by a blank cartridge or by fireworks of any description, promptly and thoroughly, with a view to immunizing the patient against tetanus. A perfectly harmless injection of tetanus anti-toxin, promptly administered in every case of the kind cited, is practically sure to prevent the disease.

The Department takes occasion on the eve of July 4th, to urge a sane celebration, eliminating all fireworks, so as to maintain the record of previous years in this city when, as a result of safe and sane celebrations, the deaths from tetanus became few and far between. Further, it urges upon the public generally, and physicians in particular, that every patient injured by fireworks should promptly receive an immunizing dose of tetanus anti-toxin. In each of the main offices of the Department a supply of tetanus anti-toxin is kept on hand for emergency, and any physician who has to treat a patient, injured by fireworks, can have tetanus anti-toxin sent to him at once by special messenger, if he reports the case by telephone to the Department headquarters. This notice, if heeded, may be the means of saving the lives of persons who, contrary to our advice, or through accident, are exposed to injury by fireworks.

Anti-Typhoid Vaccination for Vacationists

The summer, and with it the vacation season, is upon us, bringing with it the certainty that many will expose themselves to typhoid fever in out-of-town resorts. Therefore, physicians throughout the city are urged to persuade their patients to submit to immunization against typhoid fever. The vaccine may be obtained, free of charge, at the Department of Health for use by physicians, or the Department will immunize any individual, free of charge, at any of its clinics.

The value of typhoid immunization has been shown to be indisputable, and was proven by universal experience in the recent war. The history of typhoid fever in France shows that, in previous wars, the typhoid mortality was 1,120 to 2,100 out of each 100,000 soldiers. During the World War, and prior to February, 1915, immunization was not extensive nor systematic, and there were 678 cases, and 98 deaths per 100,000 soldiers. Later, in 1917, when immunization was generally and systematically done, there occurred only 57 cases and only 4 deaths per million of military strength.

The history of typhoid fever in Japan shows that, before vaccination became compulsory, the morbidity in the army was 800 per 100,000; and since compulsory vaccination, the morbidity was 70 per 100,000. The civilian population, shows no similar decrease in the prevalence of typhoid fever.

The history of typhoid fever in the United States shows that, in the Civil War, 50 per cent of the deaths were due to typhoid fever; in the Spanish War, 1 death from typhoid fever occurred among every 71 soldiers; in the World War, 1 death from typhoid fever occurred among every 25,641 soldiers. The civilian population, in 1917, showed 1 death from typhoid among 7,143 civilians. Therefore, improvement in sanitary conditions is not alone responsible for the continued and great reduction in typhoid fever incidence. Immunization has played a great part in producing these results.

Doctors and newspaper editors can do a great service through their co-operation in spreading this information, in eliminating the needless suffering, the economic losses, and the sacrifice of life which becomes pronounced each year because of the failure of summer vacationists to avail themselves of the three harmless injections of typhoid vaccine, given seven days apart, to prevent typhoid fever.

Source: "Prevent Tetanus by using Tetanus Antitoxin" and "Anti Typhoid Vaccination for Vacationists." (1921, July 2). *Weekly Report of the Department of Health of the City of New York* 10 (27): 209–210.

ANALYSIS

Between 1900 and the outbreak of World War II in 1939, much of what we think of as modern American life emerged. In 1900, very few homes used any form of mechanical energy; by 1950, 94% of homes had electricity, 80% had refrigerators, 76% had flush toilets, 50% had central heating, and 47% had washing machines. The percentage of the population living in cities and suburbs steadily increased, while the percentage of those living in rural areas declined. In 1900, there were 8,000 cars on the road; by 1910, there were 500,000; by 1920, there were nearly 10 million. For many Americans, real income increased, with the result that they had more leisure and more discretionary income to spend on it.

These excerpts indicate the way 20th-century health hazards had also become modern. As summer approached, New York City officials did not have to worry about deadly cholera outbreaks, as their predecessors had 50 years previously. Instead, they could concentrate on accidents associated with children out of school for the summer: fireworks, unsupervised swimming, and reckless driving. Many families decided to spend their disposable income on that staple of modern life, summer vacation travel, and that, too, posed health hazards. Sanitary standards varied around the United States, and increased mobility for people, as always, meant increased mobility for microorganisms. From the 1920s, "shots" were firmly established as an essential part of planning for vacation travel, like packing the picnic basket and filling up the car with gas.

In the era before commercial plane travel, only a comparative handful of Americans traveled overseas—approximately 160,000 per year, many of them on luxury cruise liners. Though novels like Henry James's *Daisy Miller* emphasized the possibility of dying from fever (in the novel, *Roman Fever* or malaria), by the 20th century, most common infectious diseases were preventable through vaccine or sanitary precautions. The leading cause of preventable deaths to travelers, then and now, was road-traffic injuries.

FURTHER READING

Caplow, Theodore, Louis Hicks, and Ben Wattenberg. (2001). *The First Measured Century: An Illustrated Guide to Trends in America, 1900–2000.* Washington, DC: AEI Press.

Cross, Gary and John Walton. (2005). *The Playful Crowd: Pleasure Places in the Twentieth Century.* New York: Columbia University Press.

Jarvis, Eric. (2011). " 'Secrecy Has No Excuse': The Florida Land Boom, Tourism, and the 1926 Smallpox Epidemic in Tampa and Miami." *The Florida Historical Quarterly* 89: 320–346.

Rothstein, William. (2012). "The Decrease in Socioeconomic Differences in Mortality from 1920 to 2000 in the United States and England." *Journal of the History of Medicine and Allied Sciences* 67: 515–552.

Sleet, David, David Ederer, and Michael Ballesteros, eds. (2016). "Injury Prevention." *CDC Health Information for International Travel* (CDC Yellow Book). http://wwwnc.cdc.gov/travel/yellowbook/2016/the-pre-travel-consultation/injury-prevention.

VACCINES AND CHILDREN'S LITERATURE

- **Document:** Carl Sandburg, *Rootabaga Stories*
- **Date:** 1922
- **Where:** New York, NY
- **Significance:** By the 1920s, vaccinations were part of the everyday experience of children. This fanciful excerpt from Carl Sandburg's popular children's book, *Rootabaga Stories*, puts the authority of head vaccinator of the vaccination bureau of the health department somewhere above the ward alderman and the street cleaning department but below the weather bureau. This cleverly reflects a young child's view of the world, where a person who could make the wind change was much more exciting than a person who gave an injection, let alone a person who cleaned streets or sat in an office all day.

DOCUMENT

How Bimbo the Snip's Thumb Stuck to His Nose When the Wind Changed

Once there was a boy in the Village of Liver-and-Onions whose name was Bimbo the Snip. He forgot nearly everything his father and mother told him to do and told him not to do.

One day his father, Bevo the Hike, came home and found Bimbo the Snip sitting on the front steps with his thumb fastened to his nose and the fingers wiggling.

"I can't take my thumb away," said Bimbo the Snip, "because when I put my thumb to my nose and wiggled my fingers at the iceman the wind changed. And just like mother always said, if the wind changed the thumb would stay fastened to my nose and not come off."

Bevo the Hike took hold of the thumb and pulled. He tied a clothes line rope around it and pulled. He pushed with his foot and heel against it. And all the time the thumb stuck fast and the fingers wiggled from the end of the nose of Bimbo the Snip.

Bevo the Hike sent for the ward alderman. The ward alderman sent for the barn boss of the street cleaning department. The barn boss of the street cleaning department sent for the head vaccinator of the vaccination bureau of the health department. The head vaccinator of the vaccination bureau of the health department sent for the big main fixer of the weather bureau where they understand the tricks of the wind and the wind changing.

Source: Sandburg, Carl. (1922). "How Bimbo the Snip's Thumb Stuck to His Nose When the Wind Changed." *Rootabaga Stories.* New York: Harcourt, Brace and Company, Inc., 124.

DIPHTHERIA GOES TO SCHOOL

- **Document:** Wilfred Kellogg, "Immunization against Diphtheria" and Louis Olsen, "Palo Alto Enlisting Parents' Cooperation"
- **Date:** 1923
- **Where:** California, CA
- **Significance:** In 1905, the U.S. Supreme Court ruled in *Jacobson v. Massachusetts* that states could enforce compulsory vaccination laws for the common good. This ruling was reinforced in 1922, in *Zucht v. King*, which upheld the authority of a school system to refuse admission to a student who had not received the required vaccinations.

    As a result of immunization and the development of an effective treatment, deaths from diphtheria fell dramatically between 1900 and 1940. In 1900, there were 40 deaths from diphtheria per 100,000 populations each year. By 1940, the death rate was down around 5 per 100,000. By 1960, improved vaccination and treatment had reduced the number to zero.

DID YOU KNOW?

No More Diphtheria

In the 1920s, a new and enthusiastic supporter joined the ranks of vaccine advocates: the Metropolitan Life Insurance Company of New York City. "Insurance today is really a great social institution," declared one MetLife executive. "The insurance company is simply a medium through which aggregations of individuals protect themselves against the risks and contingencies of life" (cited in Colgrove, 2006, 88). And what better way to preserve the health and longevity of its patients than by encouraging vaccination? According to the company's chief statistician, Louis Dublin (1882–1969), childhood illnesses like diphtheria cost the country $200,000,000 in medical costs and lost wages for parents.

MetLife donated money and advertising materials to New York State's "No More Diphtheria" campaign promoting diphtheria vaccination and partnering with community organizations like the Boy Scouts. "Lucky Babies" announced the headline in their advertisement in *Boys Own Life*: "Lucky indeed is the baby who has a mother wise enough to follow the doctor's advice—'Bring the baby to me when he is six months old and let me vaccinate him against diphtheria. That is one disease he need never

DOCUMENT

Immunization against Diphtheria

The steady increase in the prevalence of diphtheria in California, together with the fact that the mortality from this disease continues high in spite of our possession of a specific treatment in antitoxin, prompts the following brief consideration of the subject.

With the introduction of antitoxin about twenty-five years ago there was a remarkable fall in the percentage of cases that resulted fatally. This drop was from an average case fatality rate of forty per cent to about ten per cent, which percentage, since that time, has not been reduced. The reasons for this failure of antitoxin to completely suppress the death rate from diphtheria are several and to a considerable extent unavoidable. They include such things as delay in recognition of the condition by both parents and physicians, delay in calling the physician in cases of throat trouble and sometimes inadequate dosage of antitoxin. Diphtheria, therefore, continues to be one of the terrors of childhood and it is responsible for from twenty to thirty thousand deaths of children each year in the United States. The usual control measures available to the health officer have been the quarantine of cases of diphtheria and the search for and isolation of healthy carriers of the diphtheria bacillus. Owing to the existence of many cases of true diphtheria that are so mild as to escape identification as such and to the great difficulty of finding and controlling carriers, diphtheria continues to be practically as common and widespread as ever.

The most effective control measure for any communicable disease would be a method of immunizing individuals against it; such as vaccination against smallpox, which has resulted in reducing this disease from the dreaded plagues of the middle ages and from the universal destroyer of even a century ago to a state of comparative abeyance, a condition that accounts for the large number of persons who honestly believe that smallpox is not a disease to be dreaded.

There are very few diseases in which we have such a specific preventive, only three in fact, and these are smallpox, typhoid fever and diphtheria. The preventive measure for the latter disease is the most recent and the most spectacular advance that has been made in preventive medicine. It is not a vaccination, as in the case of smallpox, but a subcutaneous administration of a very small quantity of diphtheria toxin made from cultures of the organism and practically neutralized by antitoxin so that it gives little or no reaction and does not produce a sore on the arm as does the inoculation of vaccine virus. This toxin-antitoxin as it is usually called, or diphtheria prophylactic as it would better be known on account of the confusion in names when the other term is used, should come into general use; should be advocated by all physicians; and should be demanded by mothers of the children who are the prospective victims of this dread

have.'" Forbidding disease statistics were domesticated to make the point. "Last year more than 100,000 who had not been inoculated had diphtheria. About 10,000 of them died—an average of more than one every hour of any day in the year." Fortunately, the advertisement continued, "Diphtheria can be prevented by simple, painless inoculation which is lasting in its effect." If your child was not yet vaccinated, "call up your doctor now and make an appointment."

MetLife advertisements combined their serious message with attractive images of middle-class family life. The "Lucky Babies" advertisement depicted a world of loving, attentive mothers, healthy sons, and doctors who were only a phone call away. The *ABC Book of Health for Children* includes happy, well-fed children drinking milk ("You need plenty/But not tea or coffee/Before you are twenty"), bathing ("Each day in a tub/Followed at once/By a brisk body-rub"), and generally enjoying good health ("That is built day by day/By the Habits you form/In your work and your play").

These advertisements shrewdly addressed the changing nature of public health. Many American families no longer had direct experience of dangerous diseases and could not easily be persuaded to vaccinate their children through fear of epidemics. They could, however, be encouraged to think of health as a consumer good, like the food, clothes, and books they provided for their families.

Sources:

Colgrove, James. (2006). *State of Immunity: The Politics of Vaccination in Twentieth-Century America.* Berkeley, CA: University of California Press.

Metropolitan Life Insurance Company. (191–). *The ABC Book of Health for Children.* New York: The Company. HathiTrust Digital Archives. https://babel.hathitrust.org/cgi/pt?id=mdp.39015080463816.

Metropolitan Life Insurance Company. (1929). "Lucky Babies." *Boys Own Life.* November: 32.

disease. In every community where this prophylactic measure against diphtheria has been adopted generally, diphtheria has ceased to exist absolutely and the parents of children no longer have the dread of infection hanging over them nor are they harassed by the necessity and inconvenience of quarantine and isolation.

Palo Alto Enlisting Parents' Cooperation

In order that the parents of children in Palo Alto may be advised of any known exposure to a communicable disease, Louis Olsen, city health officer, is making use of the form reproduced here. Parents are glad to receive the official notification of exposure and cooperate in preventing further spread of the disease ...

To Parents or Guardians:

You are hereby notified that the child presenting this notice has been exposed in school to the disease marked below. Kindly keep the child under close observation.

If symptoms of the disease develop, keep the child at home and notify the Health Officer at once. Your cooperation in this matter is strongly desired to prevent the further spread of the disease.

Respectfully,

Louis Olsen, Health Officer.

- Scarlet Fever—Early symptoms: sore throat, sudden and projectile vomiting, and high fever. Incubation period 1 to 7 days, usually 2 to 4.
- Diphtheria—Early symptoms: sore throat, headache, listlessness. Incubation period variable, usually from 2 to 5 days.
- Measles—Cold in head, inflamed eyes, cough, Koplik spots in mouth, followed by rash on 13th to 15th day after exposure.
- Chickenpox—A crop of blisters, slight fever. Incubation period about 2 weeks.
- Mumps—Swelling at the angle of the jaw, resembling a sock, heel below ear and toe toward chin. Incubation period variable, from 1 to 3 weeks.
- Whooping Cough—A cough which develops into a spasmodic coughing followed by long crowing inspiration. Incubation period 1 to 2 weeks.
- Smallpox—Vomiting, terrific headache and backache. Incubation period 5 to 20, usually 10 to 12, days.

The following diseases are required by law to be reported immediately to the Health Office: Chickenpox, diphtheria, German measles, malaria, measles, mumps, plague, pneumonia, poliomyelitis, rabies, scarlet fever, smallpox, tuberculosis, typhoid fever, whooping cough.

Date of exposure: _____

Date when first symptoms may be expected: _____

Source: Kellogg, Wilfrid, "Immunization against Diphtheria" and Olsen, Louis, "Palo Alto Enlisting Parents' Cooperation." (1923, November 10). *California State Board of Health Weekly Bulletin* 2 (39).

ANALYSIS

In 1900, about 55% of Caucasian students between the ages 5–19 and about 30% of African Americans and other groups were enrolled in school. By 1940, the percentages had gone up, to approximately 75% for Caucasians and 65% for African Americans and other groups. American students of all races and ethnicities and of all genders stayed in school longer and were more likely to graduate high school, as the century progressed. This educational trend has been conclusively linked to the increase in technological innovation and national income levels over the 20th century.

Like other 20th-century developments that brought together large groups of children for longer periods of time, improved education was dependent on keeping them healthy. That meant it was dependent on local, state, and national infrastructure that provided clean water, sanitation, and a system of public health to monitor and protect against infectious diseases. In the 1920s, as these excerpts make clear, a great deal of monitoring was necessary, because there were only three diseases for which vaccinations were available: smallpox, typhoid fever, and diphtheria. Diphtheria, "one of the terrors of childhood," was still "responsible for from twenty to thirty thousand deaths of children each year in the United States," despite the existence of antitoxin. The other diseases specified in the checklist for parents issued by the Palo Alto health officer were familiar enough in the children's literature of the 1920s and 1930s, as childhood killers: measles, whooping cough, and scarlet fever.

In modern debates, state-mandated vaccination requirements are sometimes presented as infringements on civil rights. In fact, the current schedule of vaccinations for preschool-aged children is much less intrusive than the early 20th-century system of surveillance for infectious diseases among school-aged children. It also means that children do not have to undergo the bullying or outright ostracism suffered by children who were known to have had an infectious disease. Even in the 21st century, there have been incidents in which children coming to school with head lice or AIDS have been badly treated by other students and families. Most school boards and parent-teacher associations would prefer not to think about the controversy that could erupt if some of their students were the unwitting carriers of vaccine-preventable diseases.

FURTHER READING

Duffy, John. (1978). "School Vaccination: The Precursor to School Medical Inspection." *Journal of the History of Medicine and Allied Sciences* 33: 344–355.

Fairchild, Amy, Ronald Bayer, James Colgrove, and Daniel Wolfe. (2007). *Searching Eyes: Privacy, the State, and Disease Surveillance in America*. Berkeley, CA: University of California Press.

Mondale, Sara, ed. (2002). *School: The Story of American Public Education*. Boston, MA: Beacon Press.

Snyder, Thomas, ed. (1993). *120 Years of American Education: A Statistical Portrait*. National Center for Education Statistics. http://nces.ed.gov/pubs93/93442.pdf.

Steele, Volney. (2005). "Fear in the Time of Infantile Paralysis: The Montana Experience." *Montana: The Magazine of Western History* 55: 64–74.

Woolworth, Stephen. (2004). " 'The Warring Boards': Sanitary Regulation and the Control of Infectious Disease in the Seattle Public Schools, 1892–1900." *The Pacific Northwest Quarterly* 96: 14–23.

DOG TEAMS SAVE THE CHILDREN OF NOME

- **Document:** Dr. Curtis Welch, Telegram
- **Date:** 1925
- **Where:** Nome, AK
- **Significance:** While middle-class American children in urban areas in the 1920s had ready access to modern medical care, it was not true of poor children or those in remote areas. The famous story of Balto bringing diphtheria antitoxin to Alaskan children shows the fragility of distribution networks and the dangers to public health when they were disrupted.

DOCUMENT

Telegram from Dr. Curtis Welch, Nome, Alaska to U.S. Public Health Service, Washington DC:

An epidemic of diphtheria is almost inevitable here STOP I am in urgent need of one million units of diphtheria antitoxin STOP Mail is only form of transportation STOP I have made application to Commissioner of Health of the Territories for antitoxin already STOP There are about 3000 White natives in the district.

Source: National Library of Medicine. https://www.nlm.nih.gov/nativevoices/ timeline/435.html?tribe=Inupiaq/Inupiat.

- **Document:** *Report of the Governor of Alaska to the Secretary of the Interior*
- **Date:** 1925
- **Where:** Juneau, AK

DOCUMENT

During the first part of January diphtheria appeared at Nome, 34 cases with 5 deaths. No provision had been made for supplying antitoxin in isolated communities, and the scant amount on hand in the office of the assistant commissioner of health was 5 years old. However, it had not lost its potency and was used with good effect until exhausted. An additional supply was dispatched from Fairbanks by special dog team, with no further deaths reported after its arrival. Great credit is due Doctor Welch for the extremely efficient manner in which the situation was managed, under the most difficult and trying circumstances . . .

Alaska never has had anything approaching a sanitary survey except in localities adjacent to the more populous centers. Each year emergencies arise which demand, or seem to demand, immediate attention, and it costs many thousands of dollars annually to meet these situations. Much of this expenditure is wasted because of imperfect knowledge of conditions in isolated districts, and for want of cooperation between such relief measures as are at hand. No one knows the number of hospitals in the Territory nor their equipment; the number and location of physicians, nor even approximately the number of people, whites and natives, depending on them for relief. Areas containing thousands of natives never have seen a physician and in matters of sanitation are still in the stone age.

Many examples could be cited showing the need of definite knowledge of our medical facilities and their coordination to a common purpose. For instance, about one month ago we received a report through one of the large packing companies in Bristol Bay stating that an epidemic of influenza was raging through the district. The Territorial department of health was not officially notified for several days, and the governor's office never received notice except through the press . . . The recent epidemic of diphtheria at Nome is another. Centralized responsibility would have assured a supply of antitoxin. After the loss of valuable lives thousands of dollars were spent in an effort to remedy a situation which should not have occurred. The cost of these belated efforts to relieve some urgent call for assistance can not be ascertained, but it is safe to say that it is greater than would be the cost of investigating and consolidating our resources for medical relief in the Territory.

Source: Report of the Governor of Alaska to the Secretary of the Interior. (1925). Washington, DC: Government Printing Office, 75–76.

ANALYSIS

In January, 1925, Dr. Curtis Welch recognized that the outbreak of severe sore throats that he had been treating among the children of Nome was not tonsillitis, but rather diphtheria. He had antitoxin on hand but not very much, and it was five years old. He sent telegrams to the U.S. Public Health Service, to the governor of the Alaska territories, and to all the Alaska towns desperately searching for more antitoxin. What happened next became known at the time as the "Great Race of Mercy." Diphtheria antitoxin was flown from Seattle, Washington, to Anchorage, Alaska. It was then taken by train to Nenana, Alaska, from which it was transported along the Iditarod Trail by dogsled teams, working in relays, the remaining 674 miles to the snowbound community. "We who live in a climate such as we have in the United States," Senator Clarence Dill of Washington said to his colleagues, "cannot possibly realize what that trip meant. It is a trip of 650 miles which, made regularly by the mail teams, takes from twenty-five to thirty days. By the use of relay teams they covered it in five and a half days. It is an accomplishment that will be talked about in Alaska, not only through this Winter, but for many years to come."

The teams worked in blizzard conditions. In the first few days, mushers were Alaskan natives, well aware of the devastating effect of diphtheria on their own communities. The longest and most dangerous part of the run was carried out by Leonhard Seppala (1877–1967), a dogsled champion from Nome whose eight-year-old daughter was at risk for diphtheria. He and his lead dog, Togo, successfully transported the serum 260 miles across treacherous ice and steep snow-covered trails. The final run of 78 miles was completed by Gunnar Kaasen (1882–1960) with his lead dog, Balto. The serum arrived on Monday, February 2, at 5:30 am. It was frozen solid but was thawed and ready for use by 11 am.

Newspapers worldwide picked up the story, and lead dog Balto became a national celebrity. President Calvin Coolidge awarded each of the mushers a gold medal and $25, at that time a large sum of money in the territories. The sculptor Frederick Roth (1872–1944) was commissioned to create a statue of Balto for New York's Central Park. The Citizens' Medical Reference Bureau, an organization claiming that the germ theory was a "medical fad," tried to block the statue, arguing that there was no evidence that diphtheria antitoxins were effective. "This is an organization that has been putting forward the most horrible statements and lies," responded Dr. William Hallock Park (1863–1939), director of New York's public health laboratories and a world-renowned authority on diphtheria. Balto's statue was unveiled on December 17, 1925, on the path leading to the Children's Zoo.

Yet, as the excerpt from the governor of Alaska makes clear, while the story of Togo, Balto, and their human handlers is heartwarming, it should never have happened at all. As Senator Dill told his colleagues, "The Public Health Service ought to see to it that never again shall a great ice-locked Northern port ... be left with antitoxin that was from four to six years old." Alaska needed a sanitary survey, the report clearly stated, and it needed more coordination across its vast territories. There was no central authority keeping track even of what healthcare was available, let alone the extent of the population and its public health needs. As a result, Alaska residents suffered what in any other part of the rapidly modernizing United States would be considered a major public health disaster: "After the loss of valuable lives thousands of dollars were spent in an effort to remedy a situation which should not have occurred."

Senator Dill was right that the event would be talked of for many years to come. In 1973, the Iditarod Trail dogsled race was created to celebrate the historic contributions of mushers and dogs. As of 2014, the record for the more than 1049 mile race was 8 days and 13 hours. In 1995, the story of the Great Race of Mercy was retold in an animated film, *Balto*, starring the voice talents of Kevin Bacon, Bob Hoskins, and Bridget Fonda.

FURTHER READING

Fortune, Robert. (1989). *Chills and Fever: Health and Disease in the Early History of Alaska.* Fairbanks, AK: University of Alaska Press.

Houdek, Jennifer. "The Serum Run of 1925." *LitSite Alaska*, University of Anchorage. http://www.litsite.org/index.cfm?section=Digital-Archives&page=Land-Sea-Air&cat=Dog-Mushing&viewpost=2&ContentId=2559.

Phebus, George. (1995). *Alaskan Eskimo Life in the 1890s: As Sketched by Native Artists.* Fairbanks, AK: University of Alaska Press.

Salisbury, Gay and Laney Salisbury. (2005). *The Cruelest Miles: The Heroic Story of Dogs and Men in a Race against an Epidemic.* New York: W. W. Norton & Company.

Wolfe, Robert. (1982). "Alaska's Great Sickness, 1900: An Epidemic of Measles and Influenza in a Virgin Soil Population." *Proceedings of the American Philosophical Society* 126: 91–121.

LICE AND TYPHUS

- **Document:** *Code of Federal Regulations of the United States of America*, Title 35: Panama Canal
- **Date:** 1939
- **Where:** Washington, DC
- **Significance:** Typhus, known through the centuries as "jail fever" or "hospital fever" because it so often occurred in those institutions, is transmitted by body lice. By the beginning of the 20th century, its incidence had declined in Western Europe and the United States due to improved hygiene that eliminated lice. There were major outbreaks in Eastern Europe, however. In Russia, the combination of the Revolution of 1917 and the ensuing civil war led to more than 3 million deaths. In Poland, 4 million cases were reported in an epidemic in 1922. U.S. immigration authorities often assumed anyone entering from Eastern Europe was a typhus carrier and insisted on harsh disinfectant measures.

DOCUMENT

Typhus fever. A vessel arriving from a port infected with typhus fever may be considered free from infection if passengers and crew are free from lice of all kinds; it will be considered suspected if passengers or crew are infested with lice, and infected if cases of typhus fever have occurred on board. Suspected vessels will be detained until put in good sanitary condition, this to include fumigation of such living quarters as may harbor lice; passengers and crew, together with their effects, may be detained and freed from lice. The same treatment will be given infected vessels, after removal and isolation of the sick, and in addition persons found infested with lice may be detained for 12 days after delousing. (Rule 9, E.O. 4314, Sept. 25, 1925 (§ 24.78)) [Reg. 116.6, Regs. Gov., Aug. 1, 1931]

Source: Code of Federal Regulations of the United States of America. (1939). "24.64. Typhus Fever." Title 35: Panama Canal, 932.

ANALYSIS

In the 1930s, Rudolf Weigl (1883–1957) developed the first vaccine for typhus in his laboratory in Lviv (Lwow), then in Poland, now in Ukraine. It involved growing healthy lice by means of specially designed clamps that could be strapped on the legs of human volunteers, keeping the lice in place while allowing them their preferred diet, human blood. After 12 days, the lice were injected with rickettsia, microorganisms that cause typhus. The lice were then grown for an additional five days. At that point they were removed from the clamp, and their guts were extracted and ground into paste. The result was a vaccine that could be injected into humans to prevent typhus.

By that time, neither the method nor the disease was at the forefront of scientific medicine. Carbolic soap and other fumigating agents were highly effective in destroying lice in jails and hospitals, and no public health officials anywhere expected the recurrence of the killer epidemics of the 1920s. In New York, the bacteriologist Herald Cox (1907–1986) found that rickettsia could be grown in egg membranes, a more sustainable research method that led to the modern vaccine in 1938.

Had World War II not broken out, Weigl's vaccine might have been forgotten. But in September, 1939, Soviet troops occupied Lviv. In June, 1941, they withdrew, and the Nazis took over, ordering Weigl to produce typhus vaccine for the German military. Weigl, nearly 60, decided to save his laboratory and his staff by hiring as many people as possible as lice breeders. Since his method required lice to feed on human blood and since the war effort required large-scale industrial production, Weigl was able to employ over a thousand Lviv residents, including most of the university community. Lice feeders were paid a small monthly stipend and were issued additional rations—not very much but enough to make up some of the loss of blood and allow them to survive the war. They smuggled some of the vaccine to the resistance and even the Jewish ghetto.

After the war, Weigl was criticized for supplying vaccines to aid the German war effort, but his employees felt his lice had saved their lives. "It was understood that the vaccine was barely adequate for the Germans, but good enough," one remembered, "That was the price you had to pay. You had to be careful, because if the Germans didn't like the vaccine, they'd kill. Every few days I'd . . . see people hanging from the streetlights with signs around their necks. We didn't want to end up like that. So you compromised to survive. You seldom get 100 percent in life, especially during a Nazi occupation" (cited in Allen, 2014, 231).

In 2003, Weigl's name was added in the Garden of the Righteous among Nations in Israel's Yad Vashem, the international memorial to the Holocaust.

FURTHER READING

Allen, Arthur. (2014). *The Fantastic Laboratory of Dr. Weigl.* New York: W. W. Norton & Company.

Lindenmann, Jean. (2002). "Typhus Vaccine Developments from the First to the Second World War (On Paul Weindling's 'Between Bacteriology and Virology . . .')." *History and Philosophy of the Life Sciences* 24: 467–485.

Stapleton, Darwin. (2005). "A Lost Chapter in the Early History of DDT: The Development of Anti-Typhus Technologies by the Rockefeller Foundation's Louse Laboratory, 1942–1944." *Technology and Culture* 46: 513–540.

Weindling, Paul. (1995). "Between Bacteriology and Virology: The Development of Typhus Vaccines between the First and Second World Wars." *History and Philosophy of the Life Sciences* 17: 81–90.

Zinsser, Hans. (1934; revised edition 2007). *Rats, Lice, and History*. Piscataway, NJ: Transaction Publishers.

7

DO WE TRUST OUR DOCTORS? VACCINATION, PATIENTS' RIGHTS, AND CONSUMER ADVOCACY (1940–PRESENT)

ORIGIN OF THE MARCH OF DIMES

- **Document:** Franklin Delano Roosevelt, "Radio Address for the Fifth Birthday Ball"
- **Date:** January 29, 1938
- **Where:** New York, NY
- **Significance:** Though not the deadliest disease of the 20th century, polio—short for poliomyelitis, also known as infantile paralysis—was one of the most frightening ones. In an irony of the history of medicine, polio became an epidemic because of improved sanitation. For much of the world's history, polio existed as an endemic disease, which children would contract very young, when they were between 18 months and five years old. It would appear as just another virus, and the vast majority would recover with no ill effects and immunity to subsequent infection. Improved sanitation meant that fewer young children caught the disease, but it also meant that if they did catch it, they would be at much greater risk of paralysis.

  The disease was mysterious and frightening. Otherwise healthy children would wake up one morning, suddenly unable to walk. Grown, active men could be completely immobilized. And even wealthy, powerful men like Franklin Delano Roosevelt (1882–1945) found themselves disabled for life.

DOCUMENT

My friends, my heart goes out in gratitude to the whole American people tonight—for we have found common cause in presenting a solid front against an insidious but deadly enemy, the scourge of infantile paralysis.

It is a very glorious thing for us to think of what has been accomplished in our own lifetime to cure epidemic diseases, to relieve human suffering and to save lives. It was by united effort on a national scale that tuberculosis has been brought under control; it was by united effort on a national scale that smallpox and diphtheria have been almost eliminated as dread diseases.

Today the major fight of medicine and science is being directed against two other scourges, the toll of which is unthinkably great—cancer and infantile paralysis. In both fields the fight is again being conducted with national unity—and we believe with growing success.

Tonight, because of your splendid help, we are making it possible to unite all the forces against one of these plagues by starting the work of the new National Foundation for Infantile Paralysis. The dollars and dimes contributed tonight and in the continuing campaign will be turned over to this foundation, which will marshal its forces for the amelioration of suffering and crippling among infantile paralysis victims wherever they are found. The whole country remains the field of work. We expect through scientific research, through epidemic first aid, through dissemination of knowledge of care and treatment, through the provision of funds to centers where the disease may be combated through the most enlightened method and practice to help men and women and especially children in every part of the land.

Since the first birthday celebrations in 1931, many splendid results have been accomplished so that in literally hundreds of localities facilities for combating the disease have been created where none existed before.

We have learned much during these years and when, therefore, I was told by the doctors and scientists that much could be gained by the establishment of this new National Foundation for Infantile Paralysis, I was happy, indeed, to lend my birthday to this united effort.

During the past few days bags of mail have been coming, literally by the truck load, to the White House. Yesterday between forty and fifty thousand letters came to the mail room of the White House. Today an even greater number—how many I cannot

---

DID YOU KNOW?

Timeline of Human Vaccine Development, 1940–1999

Disease	Year
Polio, injected	1955
Polio, oral	1963
Measles	1963
Mumps	1967
Rubella	1969
Meningococcus	1974
Pneumococcus	1977
Adenovirus	1980
Hepatitis B	1981
H influenzae type b	1985
Typhoid	1989
Japanese encephalitis	1992
Varicella	1995
Hepatitis A	1996
Rotavirus	1999

Source: Plotkin, Stanley, Walter Orenstein, and Paul Offit, eds. (2013). *Vaccines*. Philadelphia, PA: Elsevier Saunders.

---

tell you—for we can only estimate the actual count by counting the mail bags. In all the envelopes are dimes and quarters and even dollar bills—gifts from grownups and children—mostly from children who want to help other children get well.

Literally, by the countless thousands, they are pouring in, and I have figured that if the White House staff and I were to work on nothing else for two or three months to come we could not possibly thank the donors. Therefore, because it is a physical impossibility to do it, I must take this opportunity of thanking all of those who have given, to thank them for the messages that have come with their gifts, and to thank all who have aided and cooperated in the splendid work we are doing. Especially am I grateful to those good people who have spread the news of these birthday parties throughout the land in every part of all the big cities and the smaller cities and towns and villages and farms.

It is glorious to have one's birthday associated with a work like this. One touch of nature makes the whole world kin. And that kinship, which human suffering evokes, is perhaps the closest of all, for we know that those who work to help the suffering find true spiritual fellowship in that labor of love.

So, although no word of mine can add to the happiness we share in this great service in which we are all engaged, I do want to tell you all how deeply I appreciate everything you have done. Thank you all and God bless you.

Source: Roosevelt, Franklin Delano. (1938, January 29). "Radio Address for the Fifth Birthday Ball." *The American Presidency Project*. http://www.presidency.ucsb.edu/ws/?pid=15584.

ANALYSIS

During the summer of 1921, former vice presidential hopeful Franklin Delano Roosevelt was relaxing with his family at Campobello Island in New Brunswick, Canada. While out on his yacht, he unexpectedly lost his balance and fell into the Bay of Fundy. He assumed the freezing waters were responsible for the soreness he felt the next day. But by the third day, he could no longer stand up. He and his wife, Eleanor Roosevelt (1884–1962), consulted the best physicians. On August 25, Roosevelt was diagnosed with infantile paralysis. At that time, there was no known cure: all doctors could do was prescribe physical therapy like massage and targeted exercise. Roosevelt pushed himself to recover his strength and the use of his legs. He especially concentrated on swimming, which became a standard part of polio therapy. Since the water helped support the weight of the body, patients could focus on building up muscle strength, improving circulation, and stimulating the nervous system. Roosevelt learned to stand upright with special leg braces and to go downstairs by supporting himself on his arms. He was determined to walk and set himself the goal of walking by himself from one end of the driveway to the other. Sadly, he was never able to meet that goal.

At the time that Roosevelt contracted polio, he was working as a lawyer in a private firm, but it had always been his intention to go back into politics. The question was, could he do it confined to a wheelchair? Americans expected their political leaders to be strong, masterful men: would they vote for someone who could not even stand on his own two feet? Both Eleanor and his political strategists urged him to run for office, which he did with spectacular success, becoming governor of New York State from 1928 to 1932 and serving as president of the United States from 1932 to 1945. An exemplary politician, Roosevelt was well aware of his public image, and he made a point of standing whenever he was called upon to speak at public events. He requested that the press not photograph him in his wheelchair or maneuvering in and out of his car, and the Secret Service had orders to stop anyone photographing him at those moments. Fortunately, for the historical record, some observers managed to take pictures anyway so that we can see Roosevelt at some of his bravest and most determined moments.

From early in his career, Roosevelt recognized the power of radio as a medium of communication, and his "fireside chats" broadcast from Washington made every American feel as though they had a personal friend in the White House. He also made use of radio to raise support for medical research on polio and support for patients stricken with the disease. The excerpt above documents the official launch of the National Foundation for Infantile Paralysis, the organization later known as the March of Dimes. In its first year, the organization raised $1,800,000; by 1955, it had raised $233 million. The name "March of Dimes" had been coined by the radio personality Eddie Cantor (1892–1964) and is one of the earliest examples of celebrity advertising for a cause. The March of Dimes campaigns are considered to mark the beginning of modern fundraising, in which many small contributions add up to large sums. Children were urged to donate a dime to help other children, and the March of Dimes collected as many as 7 billion dimes.

In acknowledgment of President Roosevelt's contribution to this effort, his face now appears on the U.S. dime.

FURTHER READING

Berish, Amy. "FDR and Polio." *Franklin D. Roosevelt Presidential Library and Museum.* https://fdrlibrary.org/polio.

Clausen, Christopher. (2005). "The President and the Wheelchair." *The Wilson Quarterly* 29: 24–29.

"FDR Timeline." *Franklin D. Roosevelt Presidential Library and Museum.* http://www.fdrlibrary.marist.edu/archives/resources/timeline.html.

Minchew, Kaye. (1999). "Shaping a Presidential Image: FDR in Georgia." *The Georgia Historical Quarterly* 83: 741–757.

Rogers, Naomi. (1992). *Dirt and Disease: Polio before FDR.* New Brunswick, Canada: Rutgers University Press.

"THE ONLY WAY YOU CAN KEEP GOING IS IF YOU'VE GOT A SENSE OF HUMOUR"

- **Document:** Marshall Barr, interviewer, "The Iron Lung—A Polio Patient's Story"
- **Date:** 2008
- **Where:** Berkshire Medical Heritage Centre, Reading, United Kingdom
- **Significance:** This patient, identified as Miss A. W., recovered from childhood polio but experienced medical challenges throughout her life. Though many "polios"—the slang term for poliomyelitis patients—dreaded the iron lung, her account highlights the way in which humor and a strong family support network allowed patients to lead productive lives. This interview is transcribed from an oral history carried out by the Berkshire Medical Heritage Centre, part of the Royal Berkshire Hospital Medical Museum.

DOCUMENT

Getting polio

I developed polio in 1949 when I was about 7 years old. I remember not feeling very well and not being able to get out of bed. It then transpired that I was paralysed down the left side. The doctor came and I was taken to the Royal Berkshire Hospital. I was in hospital over Christmas which I remember quite fondly because it was quite fun really, although I couldn't sit up. I know my parents spent Christmas Day with me. After that I cannot remember the details but I was taken to Oxford, I think it was to the Churchill. At that time it was thought a good idea to put patients out in the cold. I remember being pushed out of the veranda windows in the bed in February. I was sent home still unable to walk fully. I did not have callipers or anything like that but I was too weak down the left side. When I went back to school for half-days I had to be taken in a wheel-chair. But by the time I got to about 10, I was 'normal' apart from the fact that my back had started to curve: my spine was curved, but it did not stop me doing anything.

Breathing problems due to curved spine

I didn't really have any ill-effects, or at least I didn't realize it at the time. It wasn't until I was in my 20s in 1971 that I began to have breathing difficulties, but without realizing it. I just thought I was weary, until it got to the point that I couldn't walk up the street. I had been involved in the Woodley Carnival which did mean quite a bit of walking, and probably I'd been overdoing it. I finished up in the Royal Berkshire Hospital in intensive care. A doctor came from Oxford and then the next thing I knew was the bell ringing on the ambulance and I was being taken to Oxford.

I don't remember anything for about a week. I had a respirator mask when I came round and it was really uncomfortable.

Into the iron lung

Then they said they were going to put me into an iron lung and I went 'Oh!!!' I did not know what an iron lung was, and had never seen one. But the relief of not having a respirator on my mouth and just laying flat on my back with the breathing taken over was quite relaxing. It was restful because there wasn't much for you to do in the iron lung. There was a mirror in front of you so that you could see what was going on behind. There was a frame over the top where they could put a book or a newspaper, but you had to have someone to turn the pages so not much point really; you would usually just shut your eyes and go to sleep, it was quite relaxing.

The bit that you lay on actually pulls out like a tray. You would lay on it and get pushed inside. The mechanics are underneath the machine so you're laying on the pump. And of course you get the vibration underneath. Like: … breathing, bump; breathing, bump … It was not quite like a smooth breath.

You can eat in the iron lung because your head is outside but the rest of your body is inside, although since you are flat on your back you really need to be careful when you swallow; you have to swallow in rhythm with the machine because it's pulling your diaphragm in and then pushing it out again. You just wait until it's breathing out and then you swallow. Coughing was a bit more difficult because you don't cough in rhythm with the iron lung. It was something you had to work round. But that was just sort of a down side. You cannot turn over or anything. The iron lung had port holes on the side which came in useful for physiotherapy. They had a rubber seal so you could open them on the down breath and put a hand in, to do physiotherapy or anything inside.

It is a pity that when I was in the Royal Berkshire I can't remember Dr Price and the intensive care staff, because from the minute I arrived I really did not come round until I was in Oxford. While vaguely recollecting the ambulance and the siren going, I didn't really believe I was so sick because I was not in pain; you associate being really ill with pain. The fact that you can't breathe is neither here nor there. At Oxford I do recall Dr Spalding and Dr Small. Dr Small, in his 70s, was quite a modern doctor: he was in jeans and without a white coat. To me that was like it just wasn't a doctor. The doctors were normally quite austere people but he was nice, and it was a small unit … a nice little unit with about six beds and only one iron lung. I am still friends with one of the nurses on the unit when I was in there.

They used to come and say, 'You can come out for a little while,' and I used to sit up perhaps to have a cup of tea, but then they would have to keep an eye on me because my fingers would go blue and in about 15 minutes I would have to go back in again. When I say in, I mean lay down again. Gradually, the 15 minutes became 20, and 20 became 30, and then you could come out of the iron lung and sit in the chair. Everything was a lot of effort, even like getting dressed or having a wash, but gradually it improved. I was probably in the iron lung for about three weeks.

The iron lung at home

I came home about September time assuming that I was OK. But a week of being without the iron lung was absolutely impossible. It was just so silly and I was back in again. I needed one at home! Fortunately we lived in a bungalow so the iron lung was put into my bedroom. It was a bit daunting at first having it in the room because the pump was rather large and it did take up quite a bit of room. But it kept my breathing going at night and kept me doing quite normal things by day. I have a brother and sister and if we had not had humour in the house I think it would have been a bit dire. My parents were probably worse off because my mother had to shut me in every night. But it was fine and we just got into a routine. When she used to put the lid down the only down side was, with your head outside and your arms inside, if you had an itch on your nose you couldn't scratch it. My mother's last job was usually to sort out any itches that I'd got. It was 'left, right, up, down, and yes, that's right'. If you laughed and made your eyes have tears they would trickle down into your ears and that was annoying because there was nothing you could do about it. Having just shut me in, if my mother came back to say something she had forgotten, she would almost wake me up: in about 2 minutes I would be asleep.

With the iron lung at home it was really accepting that I only slept in it at nights. Once I got the idea that the iron lung was just something that happened at night then I went back to work in about November. Fortunately I could drive. I think my confidence might have been a little bit different if I hadn't been able to drive, because obviously it meant that I was able to get about more. I just went back to work and sleeping in the iron lung at night.

There were some funny sides to it. One night I decided to go to bed early. At the time the Royal Berks Hospital was servicing the pump. It had been taken away for service but the pump it had been exchanged for was set on positive instead of negative. When I got in, instead of drawing breath in the pump did the opposite! This was about 10:30 at night so my mother phoned the hospital and spoke to the technician. He said my own pump had actually been serviced but the problem was transport to bring it back because it was so heavy. He said, 'Leave it with me and I will see what I can do.' At about 1 o'clock the phone rang and he said he had got transport and they would be with us soon. Next thing came a fire engine and two firemen bringing the pump back. There were my Mum and Dad sitting in the living room at 2 in the morning having a cup of tea with the firemen. The neighbours wondered what on earth was going on. I was just laying in the iron lung quite happily.

A few weeks later at work in the Abbey National in Reading, I was behind the counter and this man came in and said, 'How is your machine?' As I said, sleeping in the iron lung at night was something that I really forgot during the day, and I had just bought a new sewing machine. So I thought, 'Machine? How does he know I bought a sewing machine?' 'Don't you remember,' he said, 'the last time I saw you it was midnight and you were in bed.' This was in the public area of the Abbey National! I do remember a lot of these funny things because the only way you can keep going is if you've got a sense of humour.

Newer breathing machines

I have never stopped using breathing machines. The iron lung, the 'old one' as I called it, I had from 1971 to 1986. The pump was getting worn out and by that time somebody had invented a smaller type which I could operate myself. My mother obviously was getting older so I had that one instead. It was not as comfortable because it was much smaller, but it was convenient to be able to do it myself.

I came to go to St Thomas' Hospital because in the early 70s after I had the iron lung and was back to work, it was apparent that my parents were the losers because they couldn't go on holiday. They had to shut me in the iron lung. I thought if there was a hospital in the country which had iron lungs I could perhaps go and stay and they could have a holiday. So I wrote to the Central Disabled Council who very kindly sent my letter on to St Thomas' Hospital, saying there was somebody knowledgeable there and they had iron lungs. I was quite amazed really. I had a phone call from the hospital saying that people there could make a jacket that might possibly be OK and would I like to go up. I went in the week. Dr Spencer, an amazing man, said 'How have you come to be here?' because you normally go to the hospital through another doctor or something or somebody. But luckily he knew Dr Price (Dr David Price, in charge of Reading's Intensive Care Units) who was the very kind doctor that I had seen here. Dr Spencer actually knew him, they communicated and it was fine, and I have been going to St Thomas' ever since. They have kept me really fit, as fit as I can be.

St Thomas' were all geared up with iron lungs and such things. It was certainly beneficial from my point of view. They did make me this cuirass jacket. It was a shell-like thing that fits over your body and you just have a little pump that drives it. In the early days the world was wonderful. For short periods I could be without the iron lung. Anything was possible! And I did actually take it to Jersey. I flew over to Jersey to stay with a friend. There was trouble at the airport but some kind passenger carried the pump for me. It weighed about 35 lbs. I enjoyed being with my friend, but just the normal daily things you do wore me down and I quite looked forward to getting back into the iron lung. But it was worth it at the time. And I was able to visit relations using this cuirass jacket at night.

Because I normally could only do things during the day, I went on a day trip on Concorde. There was an advert in the paper. I thought 'I fancy that' and sent off the money. Then I thought 'Oh! Would my breathing be alright for that?' So I rang Dr Spencer. Yes, he said that will be fine; you will enjoy it. And it was really really good. The only thing I was a bit worried about was when they started to talk about what we would do with the oxygen if there was anything disastrous because I wasn't at that time supposed to have oxygen. But then I thought if it got to the point we needed oxygen there was not much use in worrying because it would be too late anyway. It was really wonderful.

Then in 1991 St Thomas' got me another type of breathing machine which I still use now. It's called a 'Nippy' which is positive pressure. Just with a little thing over my nose and a black box about as big as a portable television, and it *is* portable. I mean, I have taken it away to stay with friends. Unfortunately now I need oxygen as well so it isn't so convenient but it's nice to be able to sleep in a bed. From 1991 I have been able to sleep in a bed, rather than laying flat on my back, although I do still find that I am laying on my back when I sleep. The iron lung was probably better from the point of view of taking over your breathing but the advantage of the one I've got now is sleeping in a bed.

Retirement and reflection

I retired in 1994 on ill-health grounds. At the time I was looking after my mother who was really not very well. It was quite taxing because as I slept on the ventilator at night if I heard her I had to interrupt my sleep. I was also on oxygen at the time, 16 hours a day which meant that by 3 in the afternoon I was plugged into the oxygen for the rest of the day. It obviously restricted what I did, and I couldn't carry on going into work. I didn't miss work; I probably missed the company, but I felt so much better when I stopped work because the day then took its own routine.

My mother then went into a home, and I used to go and see her every day. I don't mind my own company; I have hobbies and things that I do so it doesn't really worry me. And fortunately with my Nippy breathing machine I am independent. When I had the iron lung I used to think that I would eventually be somewhere where I would have to be looked after.

I used to wonder what would happen if I needed to go into hospital: London is a long way from Reading if you're in a dire situation. But I have been in the Royal Berks twice recently, and Castle Ward was very welcoming and very caring. I don't think people realize that if you have a medical condition, it's an advantage to keep a diary of what happens and when, because you get asked questions so many times that it all gets blurry.

Once I go down with my breathing it takes a long time for it to build back up again and there was no urgency to send me home from Castle Ward. So I am not so bothered now. I can't fault the medical profession. I know people get bad deals but I have never in my life had any bad deals. I have never asked for anything; whatever medical equipment I have been given has just been given because I need it. I am a bit cynical in some cases; people sometimes expect too much.

What is normal is doing what you can. You only have one life. OK, when I do go down I am ill. It is hard and it is difficult and sometimes you sort of think is it worth carrying on. But I must say polio people have got that stubbornness; perhaps stubborn isn't the right word but they've got it. You have to get on with it you know. But I do get tired quickly and you have to stop. That is why I have to balance out what I do. I can just stop, sit in a chair and watch TV for half an hour or read a book and then start over again; you just need to recharge. My friends know that. If I plan to go out somewhere and can't manage it I just don't go.

I don't think about the fact that I had polio, to be honest. It is only when I go through a door or have a bath and I think 'Oh silly, you should know that's the size you are'. There are some worse things about now.

I mean at St Thomas' Lane Fox Unit on my outpatient days I always feel that I am the lucky one because there are people in wheelchairs and paraplegic persons and things like that. In the early days you met people you had known in the ward. But I always used to feel a bit unsure about getting up and walking across the room to go and get a magazine, because everybody else was in bed or in wheelchairs and it used to take me a little while to get over that. But now the hospital is used for many other problems and, therefore, you can't say that the people you're meeting are polio. They could have other disabilities. I consider I have been lucky. OK, it's not always easy to get clothes, and shoes are a bit of a problem, but I don't have to worry about callipers and things like that. The only thing is that I am short. I wouldn't mind being a bit taller.

The Royal Berkshire Hospital is now so big and quite daunting. But the Museum is in a convenient corner and very accessible. It's fascinating to see all the medical equipment, although it seems a bit strange to see something you slept in. I am fairly sure I have slept in that actual machine. Early on I once had a week in the Royal Berks sleeping in the iron lung while my parents were on a holiday. It was very good of the hospital and Dr Price was a very kind man. It is not exactly the best place to have a holiday, in intensive care, but it meant my parents could go away. I used to go home for a little while in the day and come back into the iron lung at night.

Hospitals really don't worry me because I have had quite a bit to do with them. I just find it quite interesting. If you are in intensive care although actually really all right, you see how busy the nursing staff are and their responsibility. As a 6-year-old I was in Maidenhead Hospital in isolation with scarlet fever, and then a year later came the Royal Berks and Oxford with the polio. So hospitals have no fear for me. I mean things like being afraid of needles and things, I find really stupid. I say if someone is sticking a needle in you they are doing it for your benefit; why worry about it? You really just have to get on with it.

Source: Barr, Marshall, ed. (2010). "The Iron Lung—A Polio Patient's Story." *Journal of the Royal Society of Medicine* 103: 256–249. Used by permission of SAGE Publications.

ANALYSIS

Polio is best known as a disease of children, and fundraising efforts often featured adorable, smiling children in braces to tug at donors' heartstrings and wallets. Less well known is the impact it had on adults, who had jobs and, in many cases, families to support. Polio patients could face lifelong challenges, and providing healthcare could create challenges for their families and social services as well.

In this interview, Miss A. W. recognized that she was fortunate. As she said, "I have never in my life had any bad deals. I have never asked for anything; whatever medical equipment I have been given has just been given because I need it." She was especially fortunate because her medical treatment was paid for by the National Health Service, a national health insurance system established in Great Britain after World War II. In contrast, the U.S. government in the 1940s and 1950s had rejected any proposals for national health insurance. There were a few, scattered private health insurance plans available. But for the most part, patients were expected to pay for their own healthcare out of their own pocket. Federal programs providing health insurance for senior citizens and low-income groups—Medicare and Medicaid respectively—only became available in 1965. A full national health insurance system was only implemented in 2010.

What, then, became of American families in which the primary wage earner became too ill to work? And who required lengthy, expensive hospital treatment to regain any mobility at all, let alone be well enough to work? As Turnley Walker, a New York executive, wrote in his first-person account *Rise Up and Walk*, "Your hospital bed is your only place in the world, and in polio's first stages you resent all advances across its borders. Any handling of your useless body enrages you. Your loneliness is all you have . . ." Walker makes clear how devastating polio could be for men of his generation, who lived through World War II only to find what should have been a bright future apparently wiped out by the disease. Fortunately, the National Association for Infantile Paralysis—the March of Dimes—came to Walker's aid, as it did for many families. The March of Dimes covered much of the cost of hospital treatment and rehabilitation for polio patients, and it also provided support for their families.

In the end, many polio patients found the inner resources they needed to persevere. As Miss A. W. said, "Polio people have got that stubbornness; perhaps stubborn isn't the right word but they've got it . . . You really just have to get on with it."

FURTHER READING

Schell, Marc. (2005). *Polio and Its Aftermath: The Paralysis of Culture*. Cambridge, MA: Harvard University Press.

Silver, Julie and Daniel Wilson. (2007). *Polio Voices: An Oral History from the American Polio Epidemics and Worldwide Eradication Efforts*. Westport, CT: Praeger.

Steele, Volney. (2005). "Fear in the Time of Infantile Paralysis: The Montana Experience." *Montana: The Magazine of Western History* 55: 64–74.

Walker, Turnley. (1950). *Rise up and Walk*. New York: E.P Dutton.

Wilson, Daniel. (2007). *Living with Polio: The Epidemic and Its Survivors*. Chicago: University of Chicago Press.

KISSING ELVIS

- **Document:** Joanne Kelly, Interview with the Elvis Information Network
- **Date:** 2007
- **Significance:** After the development of the Salk polio vaccine in the 1950s, the March of Dimes shifted its focus to encouraging parents to give the vaccine to their children. Poster children like Joanne Kelly were important advocates for the value of vaccination to prevent the disease in healthy children.

DOCUMENT

Elvis Information Network (EIN): The role of the March of Dimes organisation has changed since the 1950s. What is its main roles or roles today?

Joanne Kelly (JK): Today the MOD raises money for research into Birth Defects. A lot of polio survivors are disappointed that they aren't much help to those of us who now have come down with Post Polio Syndrome. We need to go back into braces and use motorized wheelchairs and that's expensive.

EIN: How prevalent in the US today are diseases such as polio?

JK: There are still outbreaks of polio in the USA today! There are cults/communes/sects who don't believe in immunization and there have been cases of polio out west.

EIN: It must have been a real honor being the March of Dimes poster girl. How did you become the poster girl?

JK: I was 18 months old when I caught the polio virus. It was the summer of 1952. I was put in isolation for 3 weeks and then spent the next nine months in the hospital's nursery. My crib was at the end of the large room and in the corner.

One day several debutantes, one of whom was Maria Riva, Marlene Dietrich's daughter, visited. They were doing charity work for the MOD (March of Dimes) and came into the nursery. I was a bit of a tomboy so I bounced up and down calling and waving

---

DID YOU KNOW?

Ed Roberts, Disability Rights Activist

Edward Roberts (1939–1995) contracted polio at the age of 14. He survived but was paralyzed from the waist down. For the rest of his life, he slept with an iron lung at night and rested in it during the day.

The Americans with Disabilities Act was only passed in 1990: before that time, even public schools were not required to accept disabled students. Roberts's mother advocated for him when an administrator claimed he could not receive his diploma, because he could not complete the gym and driver's education requirements. He went on to San Mateo Community College, where a professor recommended that he apply to the University of California at Berkeley (UC Berkeley). "I knew I was ready to go on," Roberts remembered later. "... I realized ... that the path to my future and to my working or whatever was going to be education, totally. Because nobody was going to hire me the way I was. There was so much prejudice about disability" (Roberts, 1994, 4).

To attend Berkeley, though, he had to confront two challenges. The first came from the California Department of Vocational Rehabilitation, which refused to pay for his college fees, stating that it was not medically feasible that he would ever get a job. The second came from UC Berkeley, where, it was reported, one of the deans said, "We've tried cripples before and it didn't work" (cited in Silver and Wilson, 113).

With support from his family and more sympathetic administrators, Roberts made it work. He had difficulty finding housing that would accommodate his 800-pound iron lung, but he received permission to live in an empty wing of the Cowell Hospital. At first, Roberts remembered, "I didn't have high hopes about this. But . . . [Henry Bruyn, the Director of Student Health Services] was so friendly . . . He knew a lot about polio, and he looked at me, and . . . he said out loud—I remember it was one of the first things he said—'There must be a lot of people your age from these old polio epidemics that are ready to go on now to college, and they don't have much help' " (Roberts, 1994, 6).

Other disabled students, hearing of Berkeley's accommodations, applied and were accepted. As all Berkeley students became increasingly involved in activist politics, the "Rolling Quads" of Cowell took advocated for the civil rights of disabled Americans.

Roberts received his BA in 1962, but he remained in Berkeley as a graduate student, teaching political science and continuing his advocacy. In 1970, his group at Berkeley received a federal grant to establish the Physically Disabled Students Program, and in 1972, they created a similar program for nonstudents, called the Center for Independent Living. In 1975, he was appointed director of the California Department of Rehabilitation, where he advocated for consumer rights and protection. Among his many subsequent awards was a MacArthur "genius" fellowship.

Edward Roberts's legacy of "working towards our preferred future" is honored in the Ed Roberts Campus, a universally designed facility located by the Ashby BART station in Berkeley.

Sources:

Roberts, Edward. (1994). Oral History Interview. State Government Oral History Program. *California State Archives.* http://archives.cdn.sos.ca.gov/oral-history/pdf/roberts.pdf.

Silver, Julie and Daniel Wilson. (2007). *Polio Voices: An Oral History from the American Polio Epidemics and Worldwide Eradication Efforts.* Westport, CT: Praeger.

to them. They were looking for a child who smiled a lot and I fit the bill. They asked my Mom if I could pose for pictures to raise money for research on the polio vaccine. The only reason she agreed was because the pictures would be taken outside of the hospital and my Mom would be able to hold me and dress me in regular clothes.

Back then, visiting hours for parents were for one hour on Sunday. Your parents had to wear a white gown, mask and hat and were told to keep their hands off. My parents were also grateful the MOD because they paid for everything . . . surgeries, braces, crutches etc.

EIN: And for how long were you the poster girl?

JK: I was around two years old when I started. I was a poster child from 1953–1959. After the vaccine came out, they used my pictures to persuade other parents to get their children immunized.

EIN: Being the March of Dimes poster girl must have been a very exciting time for you. What were your main duties as poster girl?

JK: My main job was to smile and look happy when they wanted me too and also look sad when they wanted me too. The shoots always went fast so the photographers started to ask exclusively for me. My pic was in every NYC paper. I was on the Ed Sullivan show a couple of times and also the Sid Ceasar show. I've posed with Eleanor Roosevelt, Dr. Salk, Jack Benny, Otto Preminger, Tab Hunter, Elvis, Eddie Fisher, Michael Wilding, and lots of other radio, movie and TV celebrities. I had signed photos but they were stolen years ago. I do have some copies but they are unsigned.

EIN: And meeting Elvis, what do you remember about that? Were you excited?

JK: Not really. LOL I was around 6 or 7. I never knew who these people were. I just smiled for them. I liked to hang out with the elevator operators, the cooks in the kitchen or ride up and down on the camera dollies. I was an imp! Ed Sullivan gave me his dressing room to take a nap in. He really wanted me safely tucked away cause there were cables all over the studio floor and he was worried I'd fall.

EIN: Were you an Elvis fan when you met him?

JK: No and I didn't want to kiss him!! LOL Of course I never said anything and puckered up when the shot was taken. There's another pic of both of us licking the lollipop. I didn't get to take the huge lollipop home but I usually was given a doll or some toy to take home. My parents weren't fans either but Elvis spent over an hour with them. He offered all sorts of things to help me but my parents always refused these offers. They said he was the nicest celebrity they had ever met and Elvis was one of the last shoots I did because I was in school by then and my parents didn't want me to miss class.

When Eddie Fisher wanted to send a truck from FAO Swartz filled with toys and they said no. He spent a lot of time playing and singing for me. He put me up on a piano and when he finished each song, he'd ask who my favorite singer was. I told him over and over that it was Perry Como! ROFL Como was on TV early and Eddie Fisher's show was after I was in bed.

Otto Preminger offered to put me in a movie. He promised that I wouldn't be filmed walking, just sitting on a train and I would get royalties. They said no to that too. The MOD never filmed us walking. When I appeared on TV, I came out on stage during the commercial break and stood next to the mike. Sid Caeser was drunk and forgot who I was and what I was there for! LOL I asked him to lean over and I whispered to him "I'm Joanne. I have polio and I want some dimes." I had this plastic can and collected dimes from anyone I met.

EIN: How was the meeting arranged with Elvis' management?

JK: You'd have to ask the MOD about that. Both my parents have passed. I do know that the pic was taken on the afternoon of the day he appeared on Ed's show. He sang "You're Nothing But A Hound Dog." He was very young. I closed my eyes when I kissed him.

EIN: How did other young people react when they found out you had met Elvis?

JK: My relatives were impressed but the kids my age weren't buying records so he was just another reason I missed school to them.

EIN: Given many parents were against Elvis at the time, what did your parents think of you meeting him?

JK: My parents were surprised at how wonderful he was to them. Many other celebrities just show up for the pic and rush out as soon as they can. They said he seemed very concerned about my welfare and asked many questions about the surgeries I had had and what my future would be like.

EIN: What is your favorite Elvis song?

JK: Love Me Tender

EIN: And your favorite Elvis film?

JK: Jailhouse Rock

EIN: Did you ever get to meet Elvis again?

JK: No, I didn't. I never thought at 13 to contact Ed Sullivan when he had the Beatles on. I'm sure he would have remembered me and I was a big Beatles fan.

Source: Kelly, Joanne. (2007). "Interview, March of Dimes Poster Girl Who Kissed Elvis." http://www.elvisinfonet.com/interview_joannekelly.html. Used by permission of the Elvis Information Network (www.elvisinfonet.com).

ANALYSIS

The polio vaccine, developed by Jonas Salk (1914–1995) and Albert Sabin (1906–1993), coincided with the rise of television, and both transformed American life. In the 1950s and 1960s, variety shows featuring music, dance, comedy, and, above all, celebrity guest appearances were the mainstay of television programming. Two of the most famous hosts were Ed Sullivan (1901–1974) and Sid Caesar (1922–2014), and the March of Dimes was shrewd enough to realize that their shows provided the perfect opportunity to appeal to the hearts and minds of millions of viewers. People would remember a pretty little girl in braces, not to mention a kiss from Elvis Presley (1935–1977), much longer than a lecture on the advantages of vaccines.

Radio and television demonstrated that celebrities could "sell" vaccines to the public more effectively than the family doctor. At the time, doctors had no reason to be worried: both medical professionals and show-business celebrities were on the same side. It does not seem to have occurred to anyone that if celebrity endorsement was so effective at promoting vaccines, it could be equally effective at opposing them. A later generation of anti-vaccination advocates would make it clear that the power of mass media could be a curse as well as a blessing to medical science.

FURTHER READING

Gould, Tony. (1997). *A Summer Plague: Polio and Its Survivors*. New Haven, CT: Yale University Press.

Oshinsky, David. (2006). *Polio: An American Story*. New York: Oxford University Press.

Rogers, Naomi. (2013). *Polio Wars: Sister Kenny and the Golden Age of American Medicine*. New York: Oxford University Press.

Rose, David. (2003). *March of Dimes (NY): Images of America*. Charleston, SC: Arcadia Publishing.

Wilson, Daniel. (2009). *Polio: Biographies of Disease*. Westport, CT: Greenwood Publishing.

VACCINES' FINEST HOUR

- **Document:** Polio Vaccination Assistance Act
- **Date:** 1955
- **Where:** Washington, DC
- **Significance:** By 1953, Dr. Jonas Salk, then a prominent medical researcher at the University of Pittsburgh, had developed a vaccine for polio. After preliminary testing had indicated that it was safe and effective, the vaccine was delivered to Dr. Thomas Francis (1900–1969), director of the Poliomyelitis Vaccine Evaluation Center at the University of Michigan, for the most extensive and expensive series of field trials ever carried out on a new biological product. The polio vaccine trial was overseen by the National Foundation for Infantile Paralysis. It cost $17,500,000, employed 300,000 volunteers, and involved 1,800,000 children in grades 1–3. Of those children, 650,000 received Salk's vaccine, 750,000 received a placebo, and 430,000 received no treatment at all, to serve as a control. All the children received a certificate proclaiming them to be a "polio pioneer" and a piece of candy.

  The results were decisive: the new vaccine prevented polio. Salk's vaccine was licensed in 1955, and in the same year, Congress voted appropriations to ensure that all children and pregnant women could be vaccinated. The message from the U.S. government was equally decisive: vaccinations, like schools, were now a public good, and all American children had equal right to them.

DOCUMENT

S. 2501—A BILL to amend the Public Health Service Act to authorize grants to States for the purpose of assisting States to provide children and expectant mothers an opportunity for vaccination against poliomyelitis.

Be it enacted by the Senate and House of Representatives of the United States of America in Congress assembled, That section 314 of the Public Health Service Act, as amended (42 U.S.C. 246), is amended—

(a) by redesignating subsection (c) as subsection (c)(1) and by adding at the end of such subsection a new paragraph as follows:

"(2) To enable the Surgeon General to assist, through grants, the States to provide children (under the age of 20) and expectant mothers an opportunity for vaccination against poliomyelitis, there are hereby authorized to be appropriated for the period beginning July 1, 1955, and ending December 31, 1956, such sums as may be necessary to carry out the purposes of this paragraph. At the request of any State the Surgeon General may use all or any portion of any monetary grant authorized to be made to such State under this paragraph for the purchase of poliomyelitis vaccine to be furnished to the State in lieu of such grant (or such portion thereof). Vaccine so furnished shall be subject to the same requirements as to use as vaccine purchased from monetary grants to States under this paragraph. The Surgeon General may, in his discretion and in accordance with regulations designed to assure the most effective and equitable distribution of available supplies of poliomyelitis vaccine, specify certain categories of children and expectant mothers to be accorded priority in receiving an opportunity for vaccination against poliomyelitis, and during any period in which any priority group has been so established and is in effect all vaccine acquired by any State through assistance provided pursuant to this paragraph shall be made available only to persons within any such group. As used in this paragraph, the term 'State' means a State or the District of Columbia, Hawaii, Alaska, Puerto Rico, the Virgin Islands, Guam, American Samoa, and the Canal Zone."

Source: Senate Bill S. 2501 authorizing grants to the states to assist in providing children and expectant mothers with the vaccination against poliomyelitis. Report no. 839. 84th Congress, 1st Session, July 13, 1955.

ANALYSIS

In the movie, *The Story of Louis Pasteur*, the script had Pasteur describing the vaccine development process very simply: "Find the microbe, kill the microbe." In real life, vaccines are as complicated as the microbes they are intended to block. Most of the vaccines developed in the late 19th and early 20th centuries protected people against diseases caused by bacteria, because bacteria were large enough to be found, that is, to be seen under the microscopes available to scientists. Since they are living organisms, bacteriologists could develop an array of tools for studying their life cycles and for growing them outside of their host organism.

Viruses were much smaller, and scientists continue to debate whether they should be classed among "living organisms." The most basic facts of virology, such as their chemical composition and their means of reproduction, were not well established until after World War II. And not until the 1950s, when the electron microscope was developed as state-of-the-art laboratory equipment, could scientists actually see what viruses looked like and how they behaved.

Salk's work on polio vaccine, then, was on the cutting edge of medical research, as were Francis's clinical trials. And at that cutting edge came one of the most notorious accidents of modern vaccination history. Known as "The Cutter Incident," though perhaps a better description would be "The Cutter Tragedy," it occurred in 1956, the first year that Salk's vaccine was widely administered to children by doctors and special vaccination centers. Some of the vaccine manufactured by Cutter Laboratories was found to have contained live polio virus; that virus ultimately infected 4,000 children, primarily in California and Idaho. Most recovered, but approximately 200 were severely and permanently paralyzed, and 10 died of the infection.

Subsequent analysis showed that "The Cutter Incident" was not one accident but a set of distinct missteps on the part of the company as well as the U.S. government regulators at the Laboratory for Biologics Control. Two of the companies involved in manufacturing the polio vaccine, Eli Lilly and Parke-Davis, had produced the vaccine for the polio field trials, and they had learned from their experience. They had the highest internal testing standards of all the vaccine manufacturers, and as a result, they had no problems with contaminated vaccines. Of the three companies that had not been involved in the field trial, Cutter was the least experienced. They used the most virulent strain of the polio virus, the least reliable filtration method, and the least internal testing to ensure that the virus was completely inactivated.

Most troubling was the lack of communication between Cutter and the federal regulatory officials. Cutter scientists knew that they were having problems producing vaccines that were completely inactivated, but they never brought it to the attention of the U.S. Laboratory for Biologics Control. To compound the problem, the regulatory officials had dropped one of the key requirements that had been set for the field trial the previous year: that manufactures had to make at least 11 consecutive lots of vaccine that could pass safety testing before their vaccines could be administered to humans. Cutter never even made four consecutive lots of vaccine that could have passed the safety tests, but since that requirement had been dropped by federal regulators, no one knew about it until too late. "It was an error of professional judgment," noted a spokesperson from the National Institutes of Health, in what seemed to many an egregious understatement. "In retrospect," the surgeon general stated, "we should have received all the protocols" (Offit, 2005, 113). Most of the federal officials responsible for vaccine regulation lost their jobs.

Cutter Laboratories never admitted responsibility, and when sued by families of children who had contracted polio, the company took the case to trial. The jury came back with a mixed verdict: Cutter was not judged negligent when making the vaccine, as they had followed all existing protocols, but they were nonetheless required to pay affected families for the damages their vaccines had inflicted. The complexity of the verdict's legal implications matched the complexity of the polio vaccine, and from that point onward, vaccine manufacturing has been beset with legal challenges.

At the time, most parents saw the Cutter tragedy as an isolated case of industrial accident, and it did not prevent the widespread adoption of polio vaccine. There were 35,000 cases of polio in the United States in 1953. By 1961, the number had shrunk to 161.

FURTHER READING

Jacobs, Charlotte. (2015). *Jonas Salk: A Life*. New York: Oxford University Press.
Meldrum, Marcia. (1998). "'A Calculated Risk': The Salk Polio Vaccine Field Trials of 1954." *BMJ: British Medical Journal* 317: 1233–1236.
Offit, Paul. (2005). *The Cutter Incident*. New Haven, CT: Yale University Press.

Sabin, Albert. *Hauck Center for the Albert B. Sabin Archives.* University of Cincinnati. http://sabin.uc.edu/.

"Whatever Happened to Polio?" *Smithsonian Museum of American History.* http://amhistory.si.edu/polio/virusvaccine/.

CAN PATIENTS TRUST MEDICAL RESEARCH?

- **Document:** Henry Beecher, "Ethics in Clinical Research"
- **Date:** 1966
- **Where:** New York, NY
- **Significance:** The 1960s were a tumultuous time in the U.S. and world history. Grassroots activists challenged political and social hierarchies, and consumer and environmental advocates challenged the "What's good for our business is good for America" approach of many corporations. In the medical field, patients' rights groups challenged the traditional "Doctor knows best" attitude of the medical profession. They insisted on the right of all patients to be fully informed about their injuries and illnesses, about the contents of prescription drugs, and about the risks and costs of treatment.

  Some of the most shocking information came from the article below, written, not by a political activist, but by an anesthesiologist, Dr. Henry Beecher (1904–1976). By studying scientific journals, he documented that much of what was done in the name of scientific research completely bypassed any informed consent on the part of the patient.

DOCUMENT

Human experimentation since World War II has created some difficult problems with the increasing employment of patients as experimental subjects when it must be apparent that they would not have been available if they had been truly aware of the uses that would be made of them. Evidence is at hand that many of the patients in the examples to follow never had the risk satisfactorily explained to them, and it seems obvious that further hundreds have not known that they were the subjects of an experiment although grave consequences have been suffered as a direct result of experiments described here. There is a belief prevalent in some sophisticated circles that attention to these matters would "block progress." But, according to Pope Pius XII, "... science is not the highest value to which all other orders of values ... should be subordinated."

I am aware that these are troubling charges. They have grown out of troubling practices. They can be documented, as I propose to do, by examples from leading medical schools, university hospitals, private hospitals, governmental military departments (the Army, the Navy and the Air Force), governmental institutes (the National Institutes of Health), Veterans Administration hospitals and industry. The basis for the charges is broad.

I should like to affirm that American medicine is sound, and most progress in it soundly attained. There is, however, a reason for concern in certain areas, and

I believe the type of activities to be mentioned will do great harm to medicine unless soon corrected. It will certainly be charged that any mention of these matters does a disservice to medicine, but not one so great, I believe, as a continuation of the practices to be cited.

Experimentation in man takes place in several areas: in self-experimentation; in patient volunteers and normal subjects; in therapy; and in the different areas of experimentation on a patient not for his benefit but for that, at least in theory, of patients in general. The present study is limited to this last category . . .

Summary and Conclusions

The ethical approach to experimentation in man has several components; two are more important than the others, the first being informed consent. The difficulty of obtaining this is discussed [in the article] in detail. But it is absolutely essential to strive for it for moral, sociologic and legal reasons. The statement that consent has been obtained has little meaning unless the subject or his guardian is capable of understanding what is to be undertaken and unless all the hazards are made clear. If these are not known this, too, should be stated. In such a situation the subject at least knows that he is to be a participant in an experiment. Secondly, there is the more reliable safeguard provided by the presence of an intelligent, informed, conscientious, compassionate, responsible investigator.

Ordinary patients will not knowingly risk their health or their life for the sake of "science." Every experienced clinician investigator knows this. When such risks are taken and a considerable number of patients are involved, it may be assumed that informed consent has not been obtained in all cases.

The gain anticipated from an experiment must be commensurate with the risk involved.

An experiment is ethical or not at its inception; it does not become ethical post hoc—ends do not justify means. There is no ethical distinction between ends and means.

In the publication of experimental results it must be made unmistakably clear that the proprieties have been observed. It is debatable whether data obtained unethically should be published even with stern editorial comment.

Source: Beecher, Henry. (1966). "Ethics in Clinical Research." *New England Journal of Medicine* 274: 1354–1360. Used by permission of the *New England Journal of Medicine.*

ANALYSIS

Henry Beecher's "Ethics in Clinical Research" is rightly considered to be a foundational work in the ethics and regulation of informed consent and participation in medical research. The reason why it was necessary at all has to do with both the complexity of science and its role in 20th-century history.

Prior to the 20th century, researchers most often tested experimental treatments either on themselves or on patients who were desperately ill and expected to die without them. But the large-scale clinical trials necessary to prove a new treatment both effective and safe meant that researchers had to find a large number of test subjects. During the World War II, many researchers took for granted the value of their research to the war effort and indeed for all humanity. Even the most prominent medical scientists like Jonas Salk carried out clinical trials on residents in what were called caretaker institutions: orphanages, state hospitals, and institutions for those who were mentally or physically incapacitated. Nowadays, those research reports make painful reading, no matter their results. As we read about inmates too incapacitated to accurately report their symptoms and side effects, we have to assume that they were too incapacitated to know they were taking part in a medical experiment.

After the war, money for medical research expanded enormously. Most came in the form of appropriations to the National Institutes of Health (NIH), which then issued grants to medical researchers throughout the United States. In 1945, the NIH had a budget of $700,000. By 1965, the year before Beecher's article was published, the budget was $436 million, and by 1970, it was $1.5 billion. In that year it awarded 11,000 grants, about one-third of which involved human subjects. The project directors were prominent scientists at the major universities and research centers across the United States. Why would anyone think that any additional oversight was required to safeguard the patients under their care?

As Beecher showed, oversight was essential. Research was being carried out on patients too ill or too incapacitated to make informed choices. These included older patients suffering from senility and mentally challenged children placed in residential care. Moreover, medical researchers were clearly not policing their own: as Beecher noted, when he raised these kinds of questions with his colleagues, he was told queries would "block progress" in science.

In response to Beecher, the surgeon general formulated policy requiring that all research involving human subjects be required to undergo independent review, with specific regulations to ensure informed consent. This is the origin of Institutional Review Boards (IRBs) set up to monitor all research involving human subjects. IRB oversight became law and a requirement for federal funding, in 1972. The Hastings Center, an independent bioethics research institute, has established the Henry Knowles Beecher Award, given annually to individuals who have made outstanding contributions to ethics in medicine and science.

FURTHER READING

"Henry Knowles Beecher Award." *The Hastings Center.* http://www.thehastingscenter.org/About/Default.aspx?id=2972.

Katz, Jay. (1993). " 'Ethics and Clinical Research' Revisited: A Tribute to Henry K. Beecher." *The Hastings Center Report* 23: 31–39.

Muraskin, William. (1988). "The Silent Epidemic: The Social, Ethical, and Medical Problems Surrounding the Fight against Hepatitis B." *Journal of Social History* 22: 277–298.

Rothman, David. (2003). *Strangers at the Bedside: A History of How Law and Bioethics Transformed Medical Decision Making.* New Brunswick, Canada: Aldine Transaction.

"Timeline of Laws Relating to the Protection of Human Subjects." *Office of History, National Institutes of Health.* https://history.nih.gov/about/timelines_laws_human.html.

CAN PATIENTS TRUST THE FOOD
AND DRUG ADMINISTRATION?

- **Document:** Frances Kelsey, "Autobiographical Reflections," Food and Drug Administration Oral History Interviews
- **Date:** 1960
- **Where:** Washington, DC
- **Significance:** In the late 1950s, the pharmaceutical company Richardson-Merrell began the Food and Drug Administration (FDA) approval process for a drug, thalidomide, which they hoped to market as a sleeping pill. It was already available in Europe, and Merrell pushed the FDA for a quick approval. The application was handed off to the newest member of the FDA staff, Dr. Frances Kelsey (1914–2015), who required Merrell representatives to answer increasingly tough questions. Her intervention prevented the application from being approved and saved the lives and limbs of many American newborns.

DOCUMENT

I came on the first of August 1960 and I think I got the thalidomide application in early September 1960. I believe it was the second one that was given to me. I was the newest person there and pretty green, so my supervisors decided, "Well, this is a very easy one. There will be no problems with sleeping pills."

So that is how I happened to get the application. I never got another one quite like that one ...

I came to review thalidomide, then, as a new drug application [NDA]. At that time, we had sixty days after receipt of the NDA in which either to reject it, or if we had no objection or if we forgot that the 60 days had elapsed, the drug automatically became approved and the company could put it on the market ...

The thalidomide application was reviewed by three people: a chemist, a pharmacologist for the animal work, and a medical officer, which, of course, was myself ...

All three of us found problems reviewing thalidomide the first time around. The chemist's review showed that there were some matters that had to be cleared up ... Dr. Joseph Murray of Merrell called on ... the chemist who reviewed the application. She had some information on the chemistry, but even at that date— 6 January 1961—the chemistry was not settled completely; there were some problems.

From the pharmacological standpoint, thalidomide looked good, but the pharmacologist did point out that there was a question about absorption. In his review, I think he indicated that how safe it was might be a matter of the absorption of the drug. Thalidomide is relatively non-toxic in animals but it is very poorly absorbed. In animals it could be taken in large doses orally without ill effects.

As regards the clinical area—which was my own area—it was expected that an ideal sleeping pill would meet certain criteria, such as the fact that it would not produce a hangover the next day and so on. The claims made in the NDA for thalidomide were too glowing for the support in the way of clinical back-up. That was the initial thing that perhaps led us to require more substantiation. The claims were just not supported by the type of clinical studies that had been submitted in the application. I cannot remember what the exact number of doctors' reports in the initial submission was, I think about thirty, and many of them were more testimonials than scientific studies. That was the good bulk of them . . .

As I noted, we all three found deficiencies in the thalidomide application, and told Merrell so. Then they brought together more information, but we still found deficiencies so they resubmitted.

In those days, when a drug was under review there would be a great curiosity on the part of the drug companies. It was understandable that the firms would want to know how the review was progressing and, of course, that they would have considerable disappointment when those sixty-day letters came . . . There are more formal meetings set up now, and the firms are discouraged from making continual contacts with FDA reviewers.

I have been asked whether the drug companies had too great an access to me. That is a rather hard question to answer because one has to be fair and see their interests. Many of the drug companies genuinely feel that they have a really good drug (and occasionally they do), and they have spent a lot of time getting these applications ready—lining up the people to do the work, getting the animal studies, etc.—so their hopes are riding high. With thalidomide, because it had been successfully marketed in Europe, I think one of the possible reasons why Merrell's application was so poor was that it seemed like a sort of pushover, that it would have no problem at all being approved . . .

Dr. Joseph Murray was the contact man from Merrell. His background was in bacteriology; he was a bacteriologist, not an M.D. I think he was quite frustrated, to put it mildly, by the problems raised in the review. I suppose he had been given the responsibility of getting the NDA approved as quickly as possible, and to have these roadblocks thrown up must have been quite annoying . . .

Thalidomide had been marketed and very widely distributed in Europe since about 1957. The next step in the story was probably in late January or early February of 1961 when my attention was drawn to a letter to the editor by Dr. Leslie Florence in the *British Medical Journal* of 31 December 1960 in which he reported peripheral neuritis, a very painful tingling of the arms and feet, in patients receiving the drug thalidomide for a fair period of time. This effect was very severe in some cases, and possibly not reversible. I was browsing the journal when I read this in late January or early February 1961. The BMJ was one of the journals we browsed through. Its format is very amenable to that. Although this issue had been published on 31 December 1960, there was a problem with delivery of our journals—I think it was a mail strike—and the journal did not reach us until late January or early February. But the peripheral neuritis did not seem the sort of side effect that should come from a simple sleeping pill. We immediately drafted a letter to the company asking for more information and more proof of safety. It was apparent that this effect might be associated with the use of the drug.

We later learned that this effect had been recognized not only at this time, but earlier in Europe, and it was the main reason why the drug had been removed from over-the-counter status in Germany and made a prescription item. (I do not think it was ever sold over-the-counter in England.) The labeling of the drug by the European companies had carried a warning of the possible side effect of peripheral neuritis, and I believe it was on the labels at the time that the application was submitted to us because these side effects are often realized before they are reported in print in journals. Despite this side effect being known in Europe at the time we received the application, communications were poor in those days, and we were simply not aware of this till we had had the drug for about six to eight months. So there was an awareness of this adverse effect before this publication appeared, but not by us.

We have no way of knowing whether Merrell in general was aware of this problem. They did have representatives overseas, but sometimes the foreign operations of a domestic drug firm are completely separate from those in the United States. Dr. Murray claimed that he had noted the letter in the BMJ at about the same time we did. It seemed to be a surprise to him. But he did not bring it up with us, although we had several phone calls in this period. I asked him about it, I think, on about the third phone call. He had evidently been aware of the report, but had not volunteered the information that thalidomide could cause peripheral neuritis . . .

I cannot recall if I was taken aback by all this, but when I came to the Food and Drug Administration I was unaware of certain things that I learned after I arrived here! For instance, the fact that many of these clinical studies were poorly conducted and poorly reported, and that there was some laxness in attention to details such as this.

It appeared then as though Dr. Murray had not promptly drawn this side effect to our attention. He did go rather promptly overseas to Europe to look into the matter and certainly gave the impression on his return when he reported to us that this side effect was not particularly serious and possibly was tied in with an inadequate diet— perhaps some vitamin deficiencies—because he stated there were regional differences in where it was noted. I never did see this claim written up anywhere in the literature.

It was not until sometime later that we learned that this was apparently a severe side effect, and quite widely distributed; quite a number of people suffered from it. We were not impressed by Dr. Murray's report. We requested documentation and we asked him to contact all the investigators in the United States who had used the drug in patients for a prolonged period of time to find out if they had any cases of peripheral neuritis in their patient population. I believe several were located by this means. Also, of course, we were not aware of the widespread distribution that thalidomide had had in the United States.

I had asked Merrell earlier for a list of investigators who had been given thalidomide, and the list had some thirty or forty investigators on it. We asked that each of these be specifically questioned as regards the peripheral neuritis. Now, the wording in the letter to Merrell was such that it gave an excuse for them to provide the FDA only with a list of those investigators who had had thalidomide long enough to have had patients on it for a period of time; I think we asked for the names of those patients who had been using it for four months or so. We did not get the list of the persons that had received thalidomide in the drive to publicize the drug, that is, the other thousand or so patients. We did not become aware of this widespread distribution of thalidomide until after the drug had been withdrawn. There were the genuine investigators who had worked with it for a long period and whose findings had been submitted to us, and then there were those physicians who were told that the drug was about to come to market and that they need not bother much about keeping records.

The next development was that in April 1961 the company tried a new approach to move its application forward by trying to prove the value of the drug through making comparisons of its safety to the lack of safety of barbiturates. It was continually being said that you could not commit suicide with thalidomide. I did not think that was a sufficient reason unto itself. Marilyn Monroe's death coincided with the time the publicity on thalidomide appeared, and this was, and still is, a favorite quote: "If Marilyn Monroe had taken thalidomide she would still be alive." I should point out that I think there is a grain of truth in the argument that many people make a suicide gesture and will take pills hoping and assuming that somebody will find them in time and pump them out. One could admittedly take many thalidomide tablets in most cases and survive. But this did not outweigh the potential danger, and it did not outweigh what was unknown about thalidomide at that time.

On 25 May 1961, I wrote a letter to Dr. Murray expressing concern that evidence of neurological toxicity apparently was known to Merrell without being forthrightly disclosed in the application. I think Dr. Murray was rather upset at receiving this letter. He thought it was slightly libelous ...

It was the side effect of peripheral neuritis that led us to ask about the use of thalidomide in pregnancy because, at just about that time, there was an interest in the effects of drugs in the fetus. The agency was alerted to a problem about embryos and newborns being unable to handle drugs in the same way that an adult can. They do not have the mature enzyme systems, the mature kidney systems, and so on ... The pediatricians in the FDA were working very closely to develop guidelines about the safety of drugs in infants. These would include, of course, the safety of drugs for fetuses that might be used in pregnancy. Also just about that time steroid hormones were used in threatened miscarriages, and it turned out that a number of the female babies born to mothers who had this treatment had some degree of masculinization because of these progestin type drugs. All of these things were making us think, "When you give a drug to a pregnant woman you are exposing, in fact, two people to the drug, the mother and the child ..."

So when the thalidomide-peripheral neuritis question came up, then we wanted to know what had been the experience with thalidomide in pregnancy. Here was a drug that given for three or four months could cause severe neuropathy. With thalidomide, a growing infant might, perhaps, be exposed to it for five or six or up to nine months. This was the sort of drug that was taken as a mild sedative/hypnotic, and the mother might take it a lot during pregnancy ...

Merrell, the drug company, did not know of any problems with thalidomide in pregnancy, but they had not conducted a study, except for one using it in late pregnancy in order that the mother might be more comfortable, which we did not feel was sufficient. We pointed out that this was a relatively short period of use compared to what might be the effects of nine months of use. Of course we were not thinking in terms of absent arms or legs necessarily. We just thought that if it did something to the adult in this period of time, it might well have an adverse effect on the child. The drug company was unwilling to undertake a study, but they did agree to put a big warning on the labeling, that this drug should not be taken during pregnancy since it was not known what its effects would be. We were really more concerned about the peripheral neuritis, which they were also willing to put on the labeling, but, for one reason or another, they never quite satisfied our demands. Then, quite suddenly, the news came from Europe about the deformities.

In the meantime, Dr. Murray was growing more frustrated. He was particularly disappointed because Christmas is apparently the season for sedatives and hypnotics, and the company had hoped that with the submission in September 1960 the drug would be out in time for that Christmas season. Then it looked like a second Christmas season was coming around with no drug. He indicated in a memo that they wished to get it out because it was a seasonal drug.

Merrell continued to try and convince me and the FDA. In early September 1961, Merrell held a conference in which they called in their clinical investigators. This sort of event is difficult, because the drug company brings in people from the outside, sometimes people associated with universities and so on, who have worked for the firm and are interested in pharmacology and drugs. They think the Food and Drug Administration is obstructionist and so on. Of course, the drug company has selected the people whom they know are going to back them. So such a conference is quite an ordeal, there is no question about it. But when the question "Is thalidomide safe in pregnancy?" arose at Merrell's conference, that ended the criticism of the FDA as people realized that the data were not there. The drug really could not be said to be safe. I think it was at that time the suggestion was advanced that if thalidomide were to be released they would have to put on a disclaimer that its safe use in pregnancy was not known. This type of disclaimer was the sort of thing we had done before, and I think we said, "If you can just give us some case histories of where it has been used throughout pregnancy . . ." The ironic thing was that Dr. Murray said, "Had there been any problems with this they would have been observed since the drug has been so widely used." Thus there was a realization of the increase in this type of birth defect, but it had not been connected to the drug . . . In fact, FDA records show that one of Merrell's clinical investigators had delivered deformed babies . . .

Now the extraordinary thing was that it was quite a long time before a positive connection between thalidomide and the deformities was made. The company claimed it was a false association and that it could not possibly be the drug. It had been so widely used, and it was not possible that this was just coming to public attention. Even the specialists, the teratologists who specialized in birth defects, had difficulty, because this was not a typical drug that caused a typical defect.

The defects occurred in doses that had absolutely no effect in the mother. Even if one looked only at the mother, the drug did not have many adverse effects (perhaps a little drowsiness), so it was unusual in this respect. This, I think, was another reason why it took so long for general acceptance that the drug was at fault.

On 30 November 1961, Dr. Murray of Merrell informed the FDA that the German firm was withdrawing the drug from the market. I remember very well when he called and told us about the information they had received from Germany possibly linking the drug with birth defects. I was—I admit it—very surprised. This was what we had been wanting to make sure would not happen with the drug and it appeared it had. Our objections, as I have pointed out, were really on theoretical grounds, largely based on the fact that there was no evidence that it was safe. Until we had such evidence we had to question the safety . . .

At a certain point the FDA began to suspect that all was not right. My recollection is that when we got the letter in March 1962 indicating the company wished to withdraw the application, it indicated that in December 1961 all active investigators had been notified of the problem and told to discontinue studies until the matter was cleared up. The company then stated that a letter had now been issued on 21 February 1962 to all investigators—all who had received the drug—telling them of this. This led us to think at the FDA that there might have been some people who had not received the earlier letter. My recollection is that this is what led us to request the list of all the physicians who had been supplied with the drug.

This was the letter the FDA sent to Merrell on 11 April 1962. Now, in any drug trial, one expects a certain number of the physicians never to bother to test the drug or just to indicate they are disinterested in it, so one knows that often fewer persons have used the drug than those who have been sent it. Certainly the latter is the bigger number.

We got reinforcement of our belief that it was the drug that caused the deformities from Dr. Helen Taussig, a renowned woman pediatric cardiologist, at the Johns Hopkins University. Dr. Taussig was famous for developing the Blalock-Taussig surgery for blue babies . . . She learned of this problem of deformities from a German physician who had trained with her in Baltimore. Her specialty was pediatric heart defects, and the German physician wrote to her that many of these children had cardiac defects and that she should come to Germany and look them over. She came back with striking photographs after having talked to everyone over there. She talked to drug manufacturers, to parents of deformed children, to scientists, and to epidemiologists. She received support for this trip from the American Heart Association, the Maryland Heart Association, and the NIH, and she spent about six weeks in Germany visiting various centers where they had had experience with these deformities. We always link thalidomide with limb defects, but actually a number of the children had congenital heart disease, too. This, of course, was her primary interest.

Dr. Taussig called Dr. Nestor about the end of March or early April 1962 and told him she was just back from Europe where she had seen some very shocking effects, apparently due to a drug; she wished to discuss them with representatives of the Food and Drug Administration. On 6 April 1962 he and I drove over to her home in Baltimore and she told us what she had learned. She was the first-hand contact who was able to show us the evidence—the pictures, the case histories, and the various bits and pieces of evidence that led to the conclusion that this was definitely drug-related. I remember she was particularly struck by the fact that some of these affected children were children of employees of the drug firms in question. She was not aware at the time that this drug was on clinical trial in this country . . .

She was named president of the American Heart Association, so she was much esteemed. She talked about the drug at that society's meeting, and got people much more concerned than they had been in the past. She informed a meeting of the American College of Physicians on 11 April 1962 ... She even talked before the House Committee that was considering, at that very time, strengthening the United States drug laws. She presented her findings there, and I was in the audience.

Our request for the complete list from Merrell followed our visit with Dr. Taussig and our realization that this was a very definite association and that therefore we would have to take all the measures we could to make sure that none of the drug was remaining in this country where it might be used. The letter was sent on 11 April 1962. In supplying this list, the company also gave us the copies of the form letters they had sent out dated December 1961 and March 1962. In their wording the company stated that all active investigators as well as others who had received the drug were contacted by letter on 20 March 1962. This was what made us realize that not all the investigators had received the letter of December 1961. There might be persons who were unaware of the problem and had supplies of the drug in their possession. So this was the beginning of the inspection of every individual investigator who had gotten the drug and there were over 1,000. Following the receipt from Merrell of the complete list of more than 1,000 physicians who had received the drug, we broke down the list into specialty areas in various states. This was the prelude to going around to each one of the doctors individually, pick up the supplies of the drug they had on hand, find out if they had used the drug, and if it was being used in any pregnant women, and if they had any birth defects as a result.

This recall, of course, caught the eye of the persons who were pressing for drug reform, and there was a very striking newspaper article in the *Washington Post* by a reporter, Morton Mintz, that also got a lot of attention. In next to no time, the fighting over the new drug laws that had been going on for five or six years suddenly melted away, and the 1962 amendments were passed almost immediately, and unanimously.

The 1962 Kefauver-Harris Amendments and the 1963 investigational drug regulations introduced a number of new procedures which led to the strengthening of the control of drugs entering the market in the United States. The greatest change was that before a company could even start testing a drug in man it had to submit to the FDA the information that led it to believe it was safe to do so. This would consist of certain chemistry background material and not necessarily be as complete as would be required for a New Drug Application. Then there would be animal studies, the extent of which, in initial submission, would depend on the type of clinical trials it was proposed to undertake. Third, the company would describe the proposed clinical trials: who they would be done by; the qualifications and facilities of the investigators; and the type of population that would be involved—whether it was volunteers, women, children, sick patients, and so on. Then, as additional investigators were added to the trials, their names would be submitted to the FDA so they were aware of the extent of the investigation. And at least once a year the company was required to send in a report bringing information up-to-date. In the interim, if any severe or alarming side effects developed, the company was required to tell the Food and Drug Administration immediately. When the drug company selected investigators to do their studies, these investigators in turn were required to make certain commitments to the company: that they were qualified; that they would keep good records; that they would advise the company of any adverse effects; that they would get patient consent; that they would supply complete case histories; and so on.

One very dramatic last minute addition to the 1962 amendments was by Senator Jacob Javits of New York. He had raised the question, "Do people know they are getting investigational drugs?" It was very clear from our survey of these 1,000 doctors in the thalidomide case that many of the mothers and patients had not been told this, and the doctors themselves did not quite understand the status of the drug. So a very important amendment to the law, not a regulation, was that patient consent must be obtained before a new drug, an unapproved drug, was given in a clinical trial.

Nowadays we know exactly what is being tested and who is testing it and we get results back as soon as possible. Then if we get reported adverse reactions, we may stop the studies and so on. We have much better exchange of information with other countries. Other countries adopted these particular types of regulations that are the same as ours, and I hope that this will do something at least to prevent another thalidomide or elixir of sulfanilamide tragedy. The trouble is that with these great new developments that come along at intervals—we are now in a very dramatic period where we are getting all these exciting new drugs—the entry of new drugs can outrun, or go faster, than our regulations control. We hope this will not be the case and we keep a very sharp eye on it.

I believe the news about the widespread distribution of thalidomide was the entree to getting the Kefauver-Harris Amendments approved. My endeavors in investigating the safety of thalidomide also led to my receiving the President's Award for Distinguished Federal Civilian Service in August 1962. It is actually documented somewhere that it was Kefauver's group that sent my name forward to the president, because the list of selectees that year had already been announced, and I was very much a last minute addition, just two or three weeks before the event . . .

The event itself was interesting. I thought that I was accepting the medal on behalf of a lot of different federal workers. This was really a team effort. I guess one person had to be singled out. But, anyway, there is no doubt that thalidomide did ensure that there would be some improvements in the law on drug regulation. But, it has to be remembered that I was very new to the agency and pretty naive about how things were done and brought about when I was involved with thalidomide.

Source: Kelsey, Frances. (1960). *Autobiographical Reflections.* Food and Drug Administration Oral History, 49–78. http://www.fda.gov/downloads/AboutFDA/WhatWeDo/History/OralHistories/SelectedOralHistoryTranscripts/UCM406132.pdf.

ANALYSIS

Thalidomide is another medical tragedy: it caused severe birth defects, including deformed or missing limbs in approximately 10,000 children worldwide, and only about 50% survived beyond the first year of life. As Frances Kelsey describes in this document, thalidomide had been given to pregnant women without any testing to ensure its safety for the fetus. The review process revealed another, even more frightening, aspect of the application: Merrell had distributed the drug worldwide to many doctors, who had not informed their patients that they were using an experimental drug.

Yet, the thalidomide story is also a victory for federal regulation of biological materials. It showed that the government could take a tough stand against industry pressure. Indeed it led to still stricter regulations of clinical drug trials, to ensure that new drugs are not distributed prior to FDA approval, and that all patients involved in clinical trials know exactly what they are participating in and what potential risks might be.

There were only 17 cases of birth defects linked to thalidomide in the United States. For her part in making that possible, Frances Kelsey received the President's Award for Distinguished Federal Civilian Service in 1962. She continued to work for the FDA until she retired in 2005 at the age of 90. In 2010, she was the first recipient of the FDA's annual Dr. Frances O. Kelsey Drug Safety Excellence Award.

FURTHER READING

Fleming, John. (1982). "Drug Injury Compensation Plans." *The American Journal of Comparative Law* 30: 297–323.

Hawthorne, Fran. (2005). *Inside the FDA: The Business and Politics behind the Drugs We Take and the Food We Eat*. New York: Wiley.

Hilts, Philip. (2003). *Protecting America's Health: The FDA, Business, and One Hundred Years of Regulation*. New York: Knopf.

Seidman, Lisa and Noreen Warren. (2002). "Frances Kelsey & Thalidomide in the US: A Case Study Relating to Pharmaceutical Regulations." *The American Biology Teacher* 64: 495–500.

Stephens, Trent and Rock Brynner. (2001). *Dark Remedy: The Impact of Thalidomide and Its Revival as a Vital Medicine*. New York: Basic Books.

"VACCINATING ON TIME MEANS HEALTHIER CHILDREN, FAMILIES, AND COMMUNITIES"

- **Document:** Centers for Disease Control and Prevention, "Vaccines for Children Program"
- **Date:** 1994
- **Where:** Atlanta, GA
- **Significance:** By the 1980s, American children were as healthy as they had been in the nation's history. Many people considered vaccine-preventable diseases a thing of the past. The nation was shocked, however, when a series of task forces found there were enormous inequities in childhood health, based on wealth and access to healthcare. As a result, Congress passed the Vaccines for Children Program, making access to vaccines a right guaranteed by law for everyone aged 18 or younger.

DOCUMENT

History of the Vaccines for Children Program

In 1989–1991, a measles epidemic in the United States resulted in tens of thousands of cases of measles and hundreds of deaths. Upon investigation, CDC found that more than half of the children who had measles had not been immunized, even though many of them had seen a health care provider.

In partial response to that epidemic, Congress passed the Omnibus Budget Reconciliation Act (OBRA) on August 10, 1993, creating the Vaccines for Children (VFC) Program. VFC became operational October 1, 1994. Known as section 1928 of the Social Security Act, the Vaccines for Children program is an entitlement program (a right granted by law) for eligible children, age 18 and younger.

Recommended Vaccines Protect against 16 Diseases
Diphtheria
Haemophilus influenzae type b (Hib)
Hepatitis A
Hepatitis B
Human Papillomavirus (HPV)
Influenza (flu)
Measles
Meningococcal disease
Mumps
Pertussis (whooping cough)
Pneumococcal disease
Polio

Rotavirus
Rubella (German measles)
Tetanus (lockjaw)
Varicella (chickenpox)

Source: "Vaccines for Children Program." "CDC Features." *Centers for Disease Control and Prevention.* http://www.cdc.gov/vaccines/programs/vfc/about/index.html.

ANALYSIS

In 1993, President William Clinton (1946–) announced a new initiative: $300 million to support the infrastructure for childhood vaccination for one year, followed by an increase of that budget to $667 million the following year. "It is unacceptable," he stated, "that the United States is the only industrial country that does not guarantee childhood vaccination for all children . . . It is ironic that the country that develops and produces the majority of the world's vaccines does not have an effective or affordable mechanism for distributing them to doctors and clinics who treat children" (Robinson, 1993, 419).

The Vaccination Assistance Act, passed in 1962, was the first in U.S. history to support nationwide immunization efforts. Although it empowered the Centers for Disease Control (CDC) to initiate short-term, intensive vaccination campaigns in case of clear public danger, it was not initially intended to provide ongoing access to routine vaccinations for children. Throughout the 1960s, most public officials assumed children would get their yearly "shots" through their family doctors. In the 1970s and early 1980s, as the number of vaccinations available increased, the funding available for the Vaccination Assistance Act did not. The result was a significant gap in access to vaccines among American families. Middle-class children got all their shots. Poor children got the bare minimum necessary for them to attend school.

Public health leaders had been arguing for increased federal support for childhood vaccination for years, and the measles epidemic of 1989–1991 gave them the ammunition they needed. Though most people thought of measles as a mild disease, there had been 55,467 cases and 132 deaths. The 11,251 hospitalizations and associated medical treatment had led to $150 million in direct medical costs. And that did not take into account the loss of school time for affected children and in work time for parents who had to stay home to take care of them. The measles vaccine only cost $24 per dose when administered by physicians in private practice and $16 per dose when administered at public health locations. Even assuming the higher price, the cost of vaccinating those 55,467 children would only have come to $1.33 million. Why would any sensible government want to pay $150 million rather than $1.3 million?

The reason why the U.S. government was getting hit with the bill for the epidemic was that the children least likely to be vaccinated were those closest to the poverty line. Studies clearly linked "failure to be vaccinated" to the following risk factors: "low educational level, large family size, low socioeconomic status, members of ethnic or minority groups, receiving services through public health clinics, single parent families, starting the immunization series late, and inadequate insurance coverage for immunization services" (Robinson, 1993, 420).

The result was an immunization rate that left the United States, humiliatingly, among the worst in the world and the absolute worst among First World countries. "Of all the nations in this hemisphere," Clinton told a national audience, "only Bolivia and Haiti have worse immunization rates for their children than the United States of America" ("Children at Risk").

By 2013, the Vaccines for Children Program was estimated to have provided coverage against vaccine-preventable illness for over 90% of vulnerable children. It prevented "322 million illnesses (averaging 4.1 illnesses per child) ... 21 million hospitalizations ... and 732,000 premature deaths." (Whitney, 2014, 353). The price tag to the taxpaying public was $107 billion in direct medical costs. But the net savings to that same public was $295 billion in direct medical costs. The dry, bureaucratic cost-accounting language of government programs can best be summed up with the old proverb: an ounce of prevention had clearly been worth a pound of cure.

FURTHER READING

Conis, Elena. (2013). *Vaccine Nation: America's Changing Relationship with Immunization.* Chicago: University of Chicago Press.

Hinman, Alan, Walter Orenstein, and Anne Schuchat. (2011). "Vaccine-Preventable Diseases, Immunizations, and MMWR—1961–2011." *Morbidity and Mortality Weekly Report (MMWR)* 60 (4): 49–57. http://www.cdc.gov/mmwr/preview/mmwrhtml/su6004a9.htm.

Krogh, Peter and Antonia Novello. (1993). "Children at Risk." *The Dean Peter Krogh Foreign Affairs Digital Archives at Georgetown University.* https://repository.library.georgetown.edu/handle/10822/552520.

Robinson, Chester A., Stephen Sepe, and Kimi Lin. (1993). "The President's Child Immunization Initiative—A Summary of the Problem and the Response." *Public Health Reports* 108: 419–425.

Whitney, Cynthia, Fangjun Zhou, James Singleton, and Anne Schuchat. (2014). "Benefits from Immunization during the Vaccines for Children Program Era—United States, 1994–2013." *Morbidity and Mortality Weekly Report (MMWR)* 63 (16): 352–355.

CAN PATIENTS TRUST VACCINES?

- **Document:** Barbara Loe Fisher, "Vaccine Safety Research Priorities: Engaging the Public"
- **Date:** April 11, 2008
- **Where:** Washington, DC
- **Significance:** By the 1980s, middle-class parents expected to have healthy children, and they also expected those children to remain healthy to adulthood and beyond. But alarmingly, the decade also revealed a hidden history of environmental contamination, as national newspapers and scientific studies revealed the impact of air and water pollution on everyday health and well-being. Those same studies and newspapers often pointed to cover-ups, manufacturers, and even state and federal agencies that had known of harmful chemicals but said nothing to the public.

  If there could be pollutants in backyards, school playgrounds, and local streams, why not in vaccines? These three excerpts, from anti-vaccination activist Barbara Loe Fisher, medical scientist Dr. Paul Offit (1951–), and actress Keri Russell (1976–), show the rhetoric of vaccination and its critics in the uncertain environment of the late 20th century.

DOCUMENT

The National Vaccine Information Center is a non-profit educational organization founded in 1982 to prevent vaccine injuries and deaths through public education (www.nvic.org). We represent the vaccine injured as well as families with healthy children and health care professionals united in support of the ethical principle of voluntary, informed consent to vaccination.

I am the mother of three children, including a son who suffered a brain inflammation within hours of his fourth DPT shot in 1980 and was left with multiple learning disabilities. I worked with parents and Congress on the National Childhood Vaccine Injury Act of 1986, which created the federal Vaccine Injury Compensation Program and vaccine safety provisions, including mandatory adverse event reporting and recording, as well as the Vaccine Adverse Events Reporting System and also mandated the Institute of Medicine's 1991 and 1994 reviews of the scientific literature for evidence that vaccines can cause injury and death.

During the past three decades that I have served on committees or forums at the FDA, Institute of Medicine, and CDC, including acting as chair of the subcommittee on vaccine adverse events for the National Vaccine Advisory Committee between 1988 and 1991, the greatest challenge has been to convince public health officials and pediatricians to take seriously the concerns parents have about the quality and quantity of scientific information available to them when making informed vaccination decisions for their children. From the parent's perspective ... the Number One question for many parents raising young children is:

Why are so many of our highly vaccinated children so sick?

Vaccination rates with multiple vaccines in America are at an all-time high, and, with 1 in 6 vaccinated child in America now learning disabled; 1 in 9 suffering with asthma; 1 in 150 developing autism, and 1 in 450 becoming diabetic, this is a legitimate question. America spends more than 75 percent of the $2 trillion price tag for health care to treat the chronically ill and disabled, and it is estimated that, by 2025, 1 in 2 Americans will be chronically ill or disabled.

The scientific, economic, political and moral imperative for addressing the new epidemic of chronic disease and disability, which has developed in the last quarter century and is compromising more children than were ever harmed by any infectious disease epidemic, including polio, makes the vaccine safety research agenda you are developing the most important federal health research funding priority today. It is a funding priority that must not take money from the vaccine injury trust fund created in 1986 to compensate vaccine injured children, but urgently requires independent appropriations by Congress to support a national research program created in collaboration with those most concerned about vaccine safety to generate evidence-based information the people will trust. With more than 2,000 clinical trials worldwide that will bring dozens of new vaccines to market soon, the first step in securing public trust is to add at least two more well informed consumer representatives critical of vaccine safety to this NVAC Working Group and the general National Vaccine Advisory Committee ...

Whether you believe vaccines rarely, if ever, cause injury or death and that government should force everyone to take vaccines without exception, or you believe that vaccines are pharmaceutical products that carry risks which are greater for some than others and that government should allow voluntary, informed consent to taking a vaccine risk that is not equal for all, most reasonable people do agree that individuals genetically or otherwise biologically at high risk should be identified so their lives can be spared.

Parents today are using mass communication and new technology to educate themselves about vaccines. When they evaluate the components of vaccines—from mercury, aluminum and formaldehyde—to animal and human cell substrates that can be contaminated with adventitious agents—they are finding no credible scientific studies proving safety; when they question pediatricians about the safety of giving their babies 8 vaccines on one day, they are being denied medical care instead of being given proof of safety; when they tell their doctor their child regressed after vaccination into autism, they are often told it is all a "coincidence" and so no report is ever made to the Vaccine Adverse Event Reporting System; when their children suffer vaccine reactions and are re-vaccinated again and again, despite deterioration into chronic poor health, they are losing faith in a mass vaccination system that dismisses individual health as unimportant compared to public health when implementing a one-size-fits-all, no exceptions policy.

We have the technology today to investigate and define the pathology involved in vaccine induced brain and immune system dysfunction at the cellular and molecular level. A 20-year study that prospectively enrolls and compares the health outcomes of two groups of children, one group who will be vaccinated with the CDC recommended 48 doses of 14 vaccines by age six and 60 doses of 16 vaccines by age 12 versus another group, who will remain unvaccinated, will give us preliminary answers in six years about measured pathological changes in immune and brain function in both groups, including information about genetic variability and the development of learning disabilities, ADHD, autism, severe allergies, asthma, juvenile diabetes and other chronic disease and disability . . .

What doctors in positions of power in the Department of Health and Human Services need to know at this critical point in time is this:

Young parents today, who trusted doctors to give them good advice about how to keep their children well, do not understand why their children are never well when they have been given twice as many vaccines as children in previous generations received. They want a full-scale, transparent scientific investigation into all potential environmental causes of autism and other chronic immune and brain disorders conducted by extramural researchers who are not connected to vaccine makers and policymakers with a bias toward existing policy. They want a greater separation of the vaccine risk assessment and safety oversight responsibilities from the vaccine policymaking and promotion activities more in the model of the National Transportation Safety Board . . .

If we can agree that individual health and life is to be valued and that the most vulnerable among us should be protected; if we can agree that when one of us is sick or suffering, we are all diminished if we do nothing; if we can agree that the individual biological differences among us must be acknowledged when making vaccine policies because biodiversity is what strengthens the human race and distinguishes our humanity, then there is no reason we cannot find answers to outstanding questions about vaccine risks and develop public health policies that truly protect the biological integrity, the health and well being, of our individual children, our communities, our nation and the world.

Source: Fisher, Barbara Loe. (2008). "Vaccine Safety Research Priorities: Engaging the Public." Testimony to the National Vaccine Advisory Committee Safety Working Group, April 11. Available online at *National Vaccine Information Center.* http://www.nvic.org/injury-compensation/nationalvaccine.aspx.

- **Document:** Paul Offit, Vaccine Schedule
- **Date:** November 4, 2014
- **Where:** Children's Hospital of Philadelphia, Philadelphia, PA

DOCUMENT

Vaccine Schedule—Timetable

The following list provides a suggested timetable. Although vaccine schedules can differ slightly, you can generally expect the following vaccines at the ages indicated below . . .

Hepatitis B

- First dose: at birth
- Second dose: 1 to 2 months
- Third dose: 6 to 18 months

Rotavirus

- First dose: 2 months
- Second dose: 4 months
- Third dose: 3 months. Depending on the type of rotavirus vaccine used, the third dose may be omitted.

Diphtheria/Tetanus/Pertussis (DTaP)

- First dose: 2 months
- Second dose: 4 months
- Third dose: 6 months
- Fourth dose: 15–18 months

Haemophilus influenzae type b (Hib)

- First dose: 2 months
- Second dose: 4 months
- Third dose: 6 months
- Fourth dose: 12–15 months

Pneumococcal

- First dose: 2 months
- Second dose: 4 months
- Third dose: 6 months
- Fourth dose: 12–15 months

Polio

- First dose: 2 months
- Second dose: 4 months
- Third dose: 6 to 18 months

Influenza

Two doses one month apart, then one dose every year starting at 6 months of age

Measles/Mumps/Rubella (MMR)

First dose: 12–15 months
Varicella (Chickenpox)
First dose: 12–15 months

Hepatitis A

Two doses six months apart: 12–23 months
Vaccine Schedule: Altering the Schedule
Deciding whether to alter the immunization schedule

In this age of choices about everything from which songs are on our personal listening devices to which custom drinks we want at the local coffee shop, we are used to deciding what we want and don't want for ourselves and our families. This notion has also started to pervade healthcare. For example, some parents now feel they should approach the childhood immunization schedule in an a la carte manner, giving their children only those vaccines that they feel are appropriate.

While this may seem reasonable on its surface, sometimes these individual decisions are not based on complete information or follow false logic. If you are considering picking and choosing which vaccines to give your child, please consider the following:

- Evaluate each disease fairly. Of course all diseases are not created equal. Some are very scary, some are more deadly, and some are more easily spread. Unfortunately, the ones that are deemed less scary, less deadly or less contagious may seem like good candidates to forego when choosing vaccines. This kind of logic is like deciding only to treat one's cancer if it is more deadly or affecting a certain part of the body. The fact of the matter is that every type of cancer—and every vaccine-preventable disease—can kill. Whether the death rate is 1 in 100 or 1 in 10,000, we can't predict who will be spared and who will not.

- Consider whether vaccine immunity is "good enough." When the disease is considered mundane, some parents would prefer their children experience the infection rather than the vaccine, in part because diseases often create stronger immunity than vaccines. Parents should remember that the disease is not mundane for everyone, vaccine-induced immunity is typically good enough, and immunity from vaccines comes without paying the price of natural infection. For example, although chickenpox is a benign disease in most, every year before the chickenpox vaccine was first used, about 70 children died from the disease, most of whom were previously healthy. Because you never know who is going to be severely affected by chickenpox, all children are recommended to receive the vaccine.

- Realize the full scope of the "wait-and-see" approach. When a new vaccine is developed, some people prefer to delay using it in order to make sure that it works well and is safe. However, each vaccine must be extensively tested before being added to the schedule, and millions of vaccines are given by the approved schedule each year. On the other hand, when people arbitrarily make a schedule based on personal preferences, they are essentially subjecting their children to a vaccine without the benefit of data. In one case, the vaccines are delayed to "wait and see" if they are safe despite the existence of data from tens of thousands of people and years of studies. In the other case, the vaccines are given without the benefit of previous experience or data creating a potentially dangerous "wait- and- see" situation.

- Understand the importance of timing. Many parents focus on the number of vaccines given at a single visit and understandably feel that there are too many given at once, particularly for younger infants. However, three issues should be considered:

  - Vaccines are added to the schedule based on when an infant is likely to be most susceptible to the disease. During the first few months of life, babies are somewhat protected from infectious diseases by maternal antibodies present in their bloodstream at birth or in their mother's milk. However, protection afforded by maternal antibodies wanes during the first year of life and is somewhat variable. For example, studies have shown that maternal antibody levels in infant blood increase right before delivery, so babies who are born prematurely tend to have lower levels than their full-term counterparts. Because the length of protection and robustness of the maternal response cannot be predicted, maturing the infant's own immune response before the maternal response wanes is the most conservative approach.

    Because most vaccines require more than one dose, limiting the number given at one appointment makes getting all of the doses in a timely manner a tremendous feat. A small percentage of parents have willingly scheduled monthly visits to the doctor's office in order to give only one or two vaccines to their child at a time. This is similar to the difference between going to the grocery store every day to get the ingredients for dinner and getting a single order on the weekend; in the long run, you have accomplished the same thing, but you've probably spent less time and money if you used the latter plan. Unfortunately, when it comes to childhood vaccines, the decision goes beyond time and money because children who are given vaccines one or two at a time are vulnerable to some diseases longer and may experience more stress. Specifically, in a study completed a few years ago, children given multiple vaccines at once did not experience more stress than children given only a single shot, so multiple visits to the doctor would cause more stress and more needle phobia over the long term.

  - If a baby is not too young to get the disease, she is not too young to get the vaccine. All vaccines expose recipients to a smaller number of antigens (parts of viruses or bacteria that generate an immune response) than the actual virus or bacteria. Even when multiple vaccines are given together, the number of antigens is limited compared with the number of pathogens to which infants are exposed during a normal day. The difference is we know when our children were exposed to antigens through a vaccine, but we aren't always aware of their exposures to diseases.

  - Consider ingredients in the appropriate context. Many vaccine-related concerns center on the ingredients that are in vaccines. Contemplating giving our children aluminum, mercury, formaldehyde or any of the other oft-mentioned chemicals in vaccines can be scary; however, thinking about what is in a vaccine should be kept in perspective. For example, consider how we have all become adept at reading nutrient labels; ingredients like unsaturated, polyunsaturated, and trans fats are all in many foods; however, we evaluate the foods based on the quantities of these items. The same should be true for vaccines; the quantities of ingredients in vaccines are not sufficient to cause harm even when multiple vaccines are given at the same time. Further, the quantities of vaccine ingredients that at very high levels could do harm (like mercury) is well below the level that is harmful.

Vaccines are arguably the safest, best-tested products we put into our bodies, so the choice not to get them is a choice to take a different and much more potentially serious risk.

Sources: Offit, Paul. (2014). "Vaccine Schedule—Timetable." *The Children's Hospital of Philadelphia.* http://www.chop.edu/centers-programs/vaccine-education-center/vaccine-schedule/timetable#.VcYJpCgg76g; "Vaccine Schedule—Altering the Schedule." *The Children's Hospital of Philadelphia.* http://www.chop.edu/centers-programs/vaccine-education-center/vaccine-schedule/altering-the-schedule#.VcYLrCgg76h. © 2016, The Children's Hospital of Philadelphia. All rights reserved. Used by permission.

- **Document:** Keri Russell, "Protecting Her Newborn from Pertussis"
- **Date:** 2007

DOCUMENT

Preparing for my role as a mom was a little overwhelming. There was a lot to think about.

I learned that pertussis, or whooping cough, has been on the rise in recent years, even though it is a vaccine-preventable disease. Following the birth of our son River, I spoke with my pediatrician about what I could do to protect our young child. She recommended my husband and I both get the pertussis booster. My pediatrician explained that parents actually cause more than half the cases in infants, which is why it is so important for adults and adolescents in close contact with infants to be immunized.

I'm partnering with Parents of Kids with Infectious Diseases (PKIDs) to raise awareness about the importance of booster shots for new parents and people who come in close contact with infants. Like any parent, I would do anything to protect my baby, and that is why I followed my pediatrician's recommendation to get the pertussis vaccine myself.

I'm very excited to be working with PKIDs to spread the word and help other parents learn how to best protect their babies from this deadly but preventable disease.

Source: Russell, Keri. (2007). "Protecting Her Newborn from Pertussis." *PKIDs Online.* http://www.pkids.org/diseases/pertussis/silence_the_sounds_of_pertussis/ keri_russell.html. Used by permission of Parents of Kids with Infectious Diseases.

ANALYSIS

Parents have asked the question, "Why should I put a foreign, potentially harmful substance in my healthy child?" from Lady Mary Wortley Montagu's time to our own. For much of the history of vaccines, doctors and vaccines manufacturers had two common answers. The first was that the disease itself was much worse and much more certain than any harm that could come to children from the vaccination. The second was that the vaccines were perfectly safe, and any statements to the contrary came from ignorant troublemakers. Patients should, therefore, trust in their doctors to know what was right for them.

By the 1970s and 1980s, neither argument was very effective. Few middle-class parents had ever experienced a vaccine-preventable disease, and they could not imagine any circumstance that would put them or their children in any danger from them. And trust in doctors—even family physicians—had been seriously eroded. Indeed, most physicians no longer wanted their patients to trust them blindly. Instead, they wanted them to become informed consumers of medical treatment, partners in their own health care. It seemed, therefore, entirely reasonable on all sides when consumer and patient advocates called for more openness and transparency from family physicians, medical scientists, and pharmaceutical companies about what they were putting in their vaccines and how they knew those vaccines were safe.

As often happens with respect to controversial topics, the debate did not stay reasonable for long. As Barbara Loe Fisher explains in the excerpt above, she became convinced that her son's continued disability had been due to the Diphtheria, Pertussis, Tetanus (DPT) vaccine. The organization she founded was originally called Dissatisfied Parents Together, with reference to DPT, but she later changed the name to the National Vaccine Information Center. She worked with other parents and personal injury lawyers to bring vaccine manufacturers to court and gained millions of dollars in settlements.

The National Childhood Vaccine Injury Act was passed in 1986 in large part to deal with the thousands of potential lawsuits. Parents who believed their children had been injured by vaccines could no longer sue the manufacturer without first bringing their cases to a special court run by the Vaccine Injury Compensation Program (VICP). It was funded by a tax of $ .75 on every dose of vaccine and for the first four years, seems to have taken the settlement of claims as its highest priority. Certainly, later review found that many of the claims settled by the court were not valid; that is, the evidence did not show a clear connection between vaccines and the disabilities claimed by parents.

By the 1990s, the VICP required more rigorous evidence before awarding compensation. Ongoing scientific studies, carried out worldwide as demanded by Fisher and other activists, simply did not show any between vaccines and most of the disabilities claimed in court. There was no evidence that DPT caused Fisher's son's illness, and after 1995, the VICP refused to award compensation for seizures after the DPT vaccine. In 2009, the VICP ruled that there was no evidence linking vaccines to autism and refused compensation based on that claim.

Anti-vaccination activists have been effective consumer advocates even for those who are pro-vaccine. They have acted as industry watchdogs, demanding that both the pharmaceutical industry and federal agencies tell consumers exactly what they are doing and why. The VICP has worked to regulate what could have been a free-for-all of personal injury lawsuits. And by asking questions like "Won't multiple vaccinations make my child sick?" activists have forced scientists to come up with the answers. As Paul Offit notes in the excerpt above, "In a study completed a few years ago, children given multiple vaccines at once did not experience more stress than children given only a single shot." In fact, "children who are given vaccines one or two at a time are vulnerable to some diseases longer."

Indeed, in some ways, the late-20th-century anti-vaccination movement became a victim of its own success. Anti-vaccination rhetoric on television shows in the 1990s was met by its pro-vaccination counterpart. Celebrity support for Fisher's National Vaccine Information Center was countered by celebrities like Keri Russell, spokesperson for PKIDS Online (http://www.pkids.org). And heartrending Internet sites with stories of children damaged by vaccines have been met by equally heartrending stories of children who died because they were not vaccinated.

Sadly, the most important reason for the decline in anti-vaccination activism in the 21st century has been the recurrence of vaccine-preventable diseases. For the first time since the 19th century, it is not poor children but those of the middle class who are most in harm's way during outbreaks of deadly epidemics.

FURTHER READING

Brown, Megan. (2011). "A Shot in the Dark: Vaccinations and Redundant Risks." *Women's Studies Quarterly* 39: 141–160.

Conis, Elena. (2013). "A Mother's Responsibility: Women, Medicine, and the Rise of Contemporary Vaccine Skepticism in the United States." *Bulletin of the History of Medicine* 87: 407–435.

Newton, David. (2013). *Vaccination Controversies: A Reference Handbook.* Santa Barbara, CA: ABC-CLIO.

Offit, Paul. (2011). *Deadly Choices: How the Anti-Vaccine Movement Threatens Us All.* New York: Basic Books.

Rothstein, Aaron. (2015). "Vaccines and Their Critics, Then and Now." *The New Atlantis* 44: 3–27.

MEDICAL FRAUD AND THE AUTISM SCARE

- **Document:** Statement from Henry Waxman on "The Status of Research into Vaccine Safety and Autism," U.S. House of Representatives
- **Date:** June 19, 2002
- **Where:** Washington, DC
- **Significance:** In the late 1990s, many parents believed that there was a link between the frightening increase in autism and the administration of childhood vaccines. Some parents wanted legal compensation, but many more wanted validation of their own experience. They wanted medical scientists to investigate what they believed to be true: that autism was a disease that came from outside their families and attacked its most vulnerable members.

  Research carried out by Andrew Wakefield (1957–), then associated with the University of London Medical School, at first seemed to confirm their fears and beliefs. In a study published in 1998 prestigious London medical journal *The Lancet*, Wakefield claimed to have found a link between the Measles Mumps Rubella (MMR) vaccine and autism. No other scientist could reproduce his research, and it was later exposed as outright fraud. In 2001, he was asked to resign his research affiliation, but he continued to travel throughout Great Britain and America promoting his views. By 2002, when he testified before the U.S. House of Representatives, his unfounded allegations had done considerable harm, as Representative Henry Waxman from California pointed out in the document below.

DOCUMENT

Mr. Waxman. Mr. Chairman, today you have convened a hearing about the safety of vaccines. This is an important topic and also a familiar one to this committee. Over the last several years, you have held a series of hearings raising questions about the safety of vaccines—questions that undoubtedly have caused real concern among some parents and clinicians.

These hearings have had some positive effects. Your interest over the years has led to unprecedented attention to vaccine safety. Since your first hearing on the topic, many respected researchers have chosen to investigate whether vaccines are associated with inflammatory bowel disease, autism, diabetes and other assorted conditions among children. While rare side effects from vaccines are always possible, these studies have not found that vaccines are associated with any of these serious health problems.

Since your first vaccine safety hearing, a blue-ribbon panel of scientists convened by the Institute of Medicine has reviewed many of the most widely disseminated theories alleging harm from vaccines. This esteemed panel evaluated the allegation that the MMR vaccine causes autism. It studied the claim that thimerosal, a vaccine preservative, caused developmental delay. It reviewed whether the hepatitis B vaccine causes neurological injury. It assessed the theory that multiple vaccinations cause allergies and asthma. In each case, the Institute of Medicine panel has found that scientific evidence does not validate the theories. Expert panels in other nations have reached similar conclusions.

Mr. Chairman, you have challenged the public health system to defend itself against numerous allegations that vaccines cause a wide variety of problems. I am not aware of an allegation about the safety of vaccines that you have not pursued. So far, the subsequent investigations and expert reviews have found vaccines to be safe. Because of your efforts in this area, Americans can have more confidence today in the safety of the vaccine supply than ever before.

There has also been a negative consequence to your approach. You have repeatedly provided a forum for unsubstantiated allegations about vaccine safety that have alarmed and confused parents. Although the scientific evidence for vaccine safety has grown stronger, parental concerns about vaccine safety have also increased since you started these hearings. This is a potentially dangerous development because it can lead to lower immunization rates and more disease.

I recently asked CDC to describe what would happen if MMR immunization rates dropped. According to CDC, if immunization rates dropped to the levels they were in 1989 we could see over 26,000 hospitalizations for measles, 8,500 cases of pneumonia, 135 cases of encephalitis, and 224 deaths.

According to CDC, even a drop in immunization rates of 10% could result in an additional 2 million kids being susceptible to measles. It would also significantly increase susceptibility to rubella and Congenital Rubella Syndrome, which can cause serious birth defects such as blindness, deafness, and stillbirths.

Congenital Rubella Syndrome is also a well-known cause of autism, a disease we all want to prevent. How tragic it would be if an unjustified vaccine scare caused some children to die, others to have permanent brain deficits, and still others to suffer from autism ...

While I am strongly opposed to reckless allegations about vaccine risks that scare parents and are not supported by the science, I also recognize that questions about vaccines will always arise. That's why I support efforts to fund additional research on vaccine safety. Some of the theories on the agenda for today do require additional research, and I am pleased the government is supporting such studies.

I also support making sure that the government does not lose the ability to conduct valid vaccine safety studies. We must assure the future of initiatives like the Vaccine Safety Datalink Project. This is a unique collaboration between CDC and several large HMOs that allows for valid and timely research on vaccine safety. Indeed, this research has led to many important policy changes over the years.

Today, we will hear from scientists at CDC who work closely with the Vaccine Safety Datalink project. These scientists are quite concerned about your threats to subpoena the raw data from this data base to pursue a vaccine-related allegation. Because the raw data contain identifiable information from the medical records of more than 6 million Americans, a Congressional subpoena would constitute a serious violation of medical privacy. According to CDC, a subpoena could have the effect of driving HMOs from the program and "destroying CDC's ability to scientifically test hypotheses relating to adverse effects potentially associated with vaccines."

You have an alternative to a subpoena. CDC has worked with the HMOs to create a process for allowing independent researchers access to this data. I continue to urge you to accept this solution and renounce your subpoena threat.

Finally, I would like to address some allegations that Dr. Wakefield makes in his written testimony. Dr. Wakefield implies that a witness who testified here last year, Dr. Michael Gershon, either perjured himself or was guilty of sloppy science by noting problems in the lab that Dr. Wakefield used in his research. Dr. Gershon did not lie to this committee and this portion of his testimony did not involve his scientific expertise and thus was not sloppy. Dr. Gershon related what he was told by Dr. Michael Oldstone of the Scripps Institute, who had performed an evaluation of this lab. Dr. Gershon continues to stand by his testimony. Dr. Wakefield also is planning to make a needless attack on Dr. Gershon's wife, who he alleges may have a financial interest in the chickenpox vaccine. In fact, according to Dr. Gershon, while his wife did conduct research relevant to a chicken pox vaccine patent, neither he nor his wife has any financial interest in the vaccine or its manufacturers. Dr. Wakefield's allegation is therefore groundless as well as gratuitous. Dr. Gershon's testimony last year was quite lengthy and he raised many scientific issues, but Dr. Wakefield has not refuted any of them. Instead, he resorts to name-calling, which does not move these scientific issues along and is unproductive . . .

Source: U.S. Congress House. Committee on Government Reform. (2002, June 19). "The Status of Research into Vaccine Safety and Autism." Statement of Representative Henry A. Waxman. http://democrats.oversight.house.gov/sites/democrats.oversight.house.gov/files/documents/20050124102618-35520.pdf.

ANALYSIS

Andrew Wakefield's 1998 article, "Ileal-lymphoid-nodular Hyperplasia, Non-Specific Colitis, and Pervasive Developmental Disorder in Children," which claimed to show a link between MMR vaccine and the onset of autism, was a classic example of bad science. In the course of four pages, Wakefield and his fellow authors managed to break almost every rule designed to safeguard scientific integrity. First, there were only 12 children in the study, and they were not in any way a random sample. They were, instead, chosen because their symptoms seemed to be most useful for making the case against MMR. Several had been recruited by an attorney who was preparing litigation against MMR manufacturers. Second, Wakefield was hardly an impartial observer. He had received personal fees from the Legal Aid Commission of £435,643 in 1996 for the purpose of assisting in that litigation and an additional £55,000 had come from the Legal Aid Commission to fund the research. Third, the actual data contained in the report was falsified: later comparison of patient records with the published version demonstrated that Wakefield had simply altered facts as it suited him. Fourth, Wakefield did not wait for his own results to be replicated, or even analyzed, by his fellow scientists, before claiming they had shown a clear causal link between MMR vaccines and autism. In what has been called "science by press conference," he announced to the British press that such a link existed and called for an immediate suspension of the vaccine.

These and many other examples of conflict of interest and unprofessional behavior were fully disclosed by 2004. Britain's General Medical Council, which licenses physicians, carried out a full investigation into Wakefield's conduct and removed him from the medical register in 2007. The *Lancet* retracted the article in 2010. Retractions by other medical journals soon followed. Wakefield has refused to admit any wrongdoing. In 2016, as his vindication, he released the film *Vaxxed: From Cover-up to Catastrophe*, which he wrote and directed.

Wakefield was only one of a series of unscrupulous experts who found themselves in a position to earn a great deal of money by claiming a connection between vaccines and autism. As personal injury lawsuits against vaccine manufacturers proliferated, medical testimony played an increasingly important role. But what made Wakefield's article so troubling was that it was published in the *Lancet*, one of the most prominent, peer-reviewed journals in the world. Nor was Wakefield the sole author: he had 11 coauthors, not one of whom, apparently, took the time to analyze the data independently. And his fraud was detected, not by the scientific establishment but by Brian Deer, an investigative journalist, then working for *The Sunday Times*. "Why," as Harvey Marcovitch asked in the *British Medical Journal*, "did it take more than a decade for Andrew Wakefield's paper to be retracted, six years for the General Medical Council to complete its task, and an investigative journalist's detailed investigation to uncover scientific fraud?" (Marcovitch, 2011, 206) Why was the scientific establishment, which is supposed to police its own, asleep at the wheel?

Perhaps the clearest answers are the obvious ones: that any kind of fraud is hard to find and even harder to prove and that many scientists agreed in principle with many parents who felt that if there was even the slightest link between MMR vaccine and negative side effects, research establishing that link should be given a fair hearing. Certainly that was the view of the U.S. Vaccine Injury Compensation Program, which eventually reviewed over 5,000 claims from parents of children with autism in what was called the Omnibus Autism Proceeding. Overwhelmingly, the judges rejected those claims. "Sadly," they wrote, "the petitioners in this litigation have been the victims of bad science, conducted to support litigation rather than to advance medical and scientific understanding of autism spectrum disorder" ("Court Says Vaccine Not to Blame for Autism"). By 2009, the evidence from both scientific studies and legal experts was clear: there was simply no connection between MMR or any other vaccine and autism.

In the 21st century, advocates for the autism spectrum community have shifted their focus from litigation to raising funds for greater awareness, for research, and for support services. Bob Wright (1943–), cofounder of Autism Speaks (http://autismspeaks.org), has posted a statement that "scientific research has not directly connected autism to vaccines. Vaccines are very important. Parents must make the decision whether to vaccinate their children. Efforts must be continually made to educate parents about vaccine safety. If parents decide not to vaccinate they must be aware of the consequences in their community and their local schools."

FURTHER READING

Alaszewski, Andy. (2011). "How Campaigners and the Media Push Bad Science." *BMJ: British Medical Journal* 342: 231.

Colgrove, James. (2006). *State of Immunity: The Politics of Vaccination in Twentieth-Century America.* Berkeley, CA: University of California Press.

"Court Says Vaccine Not to Blame for Autism." (2009). *NBC News.* http://www.nbcnews.com/id/29160138/ns/health-mental_health/t/court-says-vaccine-not-blame-autism/.

Deer, Brian. (2004). "Revealed: MMR Research Scandal." *The Sunday Times,.* http://briandeer.com/mmr/lancet-deer-1.htm.

Marcovitch, Harvey. (2011). "MMR and Scientific Fraud: Is Research Safe in Their Hands?" *British Medical Journal* 342: 206.

Nicol, Caitrin and Cathleen Zafaras. (2007). "Shot in the Dark: Autism and the Vaccines Controversy." *The New Atlantis* 18: 107–115.

Wright, Bob. "Policy Statement." *Autism Speaks.* https://www.autismspeaks.org/science/policy-statements/information-about-vaccines-and-autism.

"YOU'RE PUTTING OTHER CHILDREN AT RISK"

- **Document:** Rich Harris et al., "Watch How the Measles Outbreak Spreads When Kids Get Vaccinated—and When They Don't"
- **Date:** February 2015
- **Where:** Disneyland, Anaheim, CA
- **Significance:** In December 2014, there was a serious outbreak of measles in the United States. The two excerpts below, from the British newspaper *The Guardian* and the American news program *Frontline*, show the status of vaccination debates when potentially fatal diseases are no further away than a trip to Disneyland.

DID YOU KNOW?

"Measles in Virgin Soil"

In April 1951, a sailor returned from mainland Denmark to his native Greenland, a mountainous country with towns and villages clustered around the coast. He celebrated by joining a dancing party, where several thousand people came together before returning to their homes. Unbeknownst to anyone there, the sailor had brought with him a most unwelcome guest: measles, one of the most infectious human diseases. Within the next two months, 4,257 out of the susceptible population of 4,262 individuals contracted the disease, what is technically known as a morbidity of 999 out of 1,000. Seventy-seven people died, a mortality rate of 18 per 1,000.

Epidemiologists call this a "virgin soil" outbreak, because the disease had attacked a previously unexposed population. Measles itself was not a new disease. Prior to the development of the vaccine in 1963, it was endemic in Denmark as in the rest of the world. The reason it had not appeared in Greenland had to do with the difficulty of reaching such a remote place prior to widespread air travel. Measles can only travel if people do, and there were few reasons for outsiders to travel to Greenland until cruise ships in the late 1950s. Measles had been diagnosed in children of Danish parents arriving by ship in the late 1940s, but alert quarantine officials had kept them from carrying the infection ashore. The most likely way for measles to enter the country was in fact the way it happened—a Greenlander returning from abroad—but even

DOCUMENT

Measles is back in the US—and it's spreading. More than 100 cases across 14 states and Washington DC have been confirmed by US health officials since an outbreak began at Disneyland last December. With a majority of those infections in unvaccinated people, widespread blame—from Washington to the rest of the world—has fallen on parents who chose not to vaccinate their children.

Part of the problem, according to Dr Elizabeth Edwards, professor of pediatrics and director of the Vanderbilt Vaccine Research Program, is just that: vaccination is understood by many as an individual choice, when science makes clear that the choice—to vaccinate or not to vaccinate—can affect an entire community.

"When you immunize your child, you're not only immunizing your child. That child's immunization is contributing to the control of the disease in the population," Edwards explained.

That sheltering effect is called herd immunity: a population that is highly immunized makes for a virus that can't spread easily, providing protection to the community—or the herd—as a whole.

Despite the high overall measles vaccination rate in the US, vaccine skeptics—and their unimmunized kids—often congregate in like-minded communities, creating pockets of under-immunization.

California, where the bulk of current measles cases can still be found, is a prime example. It's one of 20 states that allow parents to skip vaccination based on their personal, philosophical beliefs—even though legislators introduced a bill on Wednesday that would ban such an opt-out provision.

In populations where a large enough proportion of children are not immunized, everyone has a greater risk of catching the disease

But California remains home to communities with some of the highest vaccination opt-out rates in the country. Santa Cruz County, for example, has a personal belief exemption rate of 9.35%, nearly three times the state average. Some California school districts see exemption rates higher than 10%. That's enough to put a dent in herd immunity and fuel local outbreaks of measles.

Experts recommend that 92–95% of Americans be vaccinated against measles to protect everyone in the community, especially those who can't get the shot: babies under one year old, people born before the measles vaccine was introduced in 1963 and have never had measles themselves, and immunocompromised kids and adults like Rhett Krawitt, a young boy who recently went through chemotherapy.

That's a high threshold for herd immunity, but it's needed because of measles' extreme spreadability. As James Colgrove, professor of sociomedical sciences at Columbia University's Mailman School of Public Health, explained, "the more quickly a disease spreads, the higher level of herd immunity you need."

that was something of a fluke, since his particular strain of the disease had a longer-than-usual incubation period.

Once the outbreak started, the same difficult travel conditions that had previously hindered the spread of infection made it harder for medical personnel to get to the sick. "Two doctor's boats were available ...," noted a medical report. "The travelling speed of the boats in ice-free water and under favourable weather conditions was five to six nautical miles per hour ... a round trip to all the places" within the medical district "took at least 48 hours in travelling time alone." And that was in good conditions. Since the outbreak took place from April through July, the medical staff faced "difficulties often created by the heavy ice ... Transport might then be paralysed for several days and nights when gales packed the enormous ice blocks together in fjords and sounds and along the shore."

Even a year later, it was clear that Greenland's era of isolation was over with respect to infectious diseases. "The economic and technical developments in recent years," the same report continued, "have caused a great reduction of travelling time from Denmark to Greenland as a consequence of the use of faster ships and aircraft. As a result of this the time that is necessary for travel to South Greenland is now often shorter than the period of incubation of many communicable diseases" (Christensen et al., 1953, 521).

There are fewer places in the world now than in 1951 that could be labeled as "virgin soil." But pockets of vaccine-preventable diseases, like measles, still remain.

Source: Christensen, Povl Elo, Henning Schmidt, H. O. Bang, Vera Andersen, Bjarne Jordal, and Oskar Jensen. (1953). "An Epidemic of Measles in Southern Greenland, 1951. Measles in Virgin Soil." *Acta Medica Seandinavica* 144: 313–322.

Just how infectious is measles? The virus is highly airborne; it can stay on surfaces for up to two hours; and infectivity begins four days before a rash, so you can feel healthy but spread the disease. Measles is so contagious that "if one person has it, 90% of the people close to them who are not immune"—we'll call them susceptibles—"will also become infected," according to the CDC.

Luckily, the measles vaccine—administered in the form of the MMR for measles, mumps and rubella—is very effective. If delivered fully (two doses), it will protect 99% of people against the disease. But, like all vaccines, it's not perfect: 1% of cases are likely to result in vaccine failure, meaning recipients won't develop an immune response to the given disease, leaving them vulnerable. Even with perfect vaccination, one of every 100 people would be susceptible to measles, but that's much better than the alternative.

The bottom line: in populations where a large enough proportion of children are not immunized, everyone has a greater risk of catching the disease—the unprotected, but also those who are vaccinated, Edwards told the Guardian.

"You're putting other children at risk by deciding not to immunize your own," she added.

Source: Harris, Rich, Nadja Popvich, and Kenton Powell. (2015, February 5). "Watch How the Measles Outbreak Spreads When Kids Get Vaccinated—and When They Don't." *The Guardian.* http://www.theguardian.com/society/ng -interactive/2015/feb/05/-sp-watch-how-measles-outbreak-spreads-when-kids-get -vaccinated. Copyright Guardian News & Media Ltd 2016. Used by permission.

- **Document:** Seth Mnookin, Interview by Sarah Moughty, *Frontline*
- **Date:** March 24, 2015
- **Where:** Boston, MA

DOCUMENT

Why did you write *The Panic Virus?*

I started work on *The Panic Virus* not long after my wife and I had got married. We moved from Manhattan to Brooklyn and started doing adult things like go to dinner parties and socialize with other couples, and we both noticed that this subject of vaccine safety and efficacy kept coming up in conversations. We were not parents or expectant parents at the time.

But what struck both of us was that when we asked our friends how they were making these decisions, a lot of them said that essentially they were going on their intuition. They weren't deciding based on a doctor's recommendations or based on scientific literature. And that really surprised me. . . .

At the time, I actually didn't know which side in this debate was right. As someone who's been a journalist for a long time, the idea that there was some big conspiracy was kind of appealing to me in terms of the story. So when I started looking into it, I was essentially coming at it with no background and no preconceptions. And what I thought would be maybe a yearlong project I guess now is seven years and counting. . . .

So characterize your Brooklyn friends. Would they have fit into any category of types who would not vaccinate?

The friends that I was spending time with and that were having these conversations about vaccines tended to look a lot like me. They might not have been

journalists; they might have been lawyers or computer programmers, people in advertising, people in tech, you know, usually in their 30s, maybe early 40s, tended to be well educated, some graduate school, some of the college graduates, but were essentially my peer group, not only in age but in occupation and a lot of other things. . .
.

I knew obviously that there were scientific debates in which people said, "Well, I don't care what the evidence is; I don't believe that humans are contributing to climate change," or, "I don't believe in evolution." But I also I guess had some biases about that and assumed that people who thought that way were not people that I knew. It was some other group of people that lived somewhere else. . . .

So one of the questions I wanted to get into when I started work on the book was really just, what is the nature of truth? How do we decide, as individuals, as a society, what qualifies as truth? Is it what experts tell us? Is it what the government tells us? Is it what our friends tell us? Or is it what we feel in our gut? . . .

Why is that essential question about what is the truth, why does that translate so hard into the vaccine debate?

I think one of the reasons that the issue of vaccines has been such a difficult question for parents and for people is because it gets to some of the most primal and basic decisions that we need to make, and that's, how are we going to care for our children? . . .

I think that, combined with the fact that we also are living in a time in which there are a lot of factors that make us feel powerless, have sort of combined to make the vaccine debate this one area where people have the illusion of control. . . .

[That's] combined with the fact that vaccines really have been a victim of their own success. Parents in my generation don't know kids who grew up in iron lungs. You don't know kids that were blinded by rubella, haven't had experience with kids spending weeks in intensive care because of measles. . . .

Yet here we are seeing outbreaks. Talk about what has changed about the vaccine war in the last five years.

Right. There have been a couple of big developments surrounding the debates and the vaccine wars, essentially, over the last four or five years.

Probably the biggest is that this paper by Andrew Wakefield that was really kind of the foundational paper of a lot of the anti-vaccine sentiment that still is going on today, that purported to link the measles, mumps, and rubella (MMR) vaccine to a gut disorder, and then that gut disorder to something like autism—that paper has been retracted. It was found to be partially fraudulent. Andrew Wakefield has lost his medical license.

So one would think—and I actually did think when all this was happening—that that was going to kind of close the door on this. . . . That has obviously not turned out to be the case at all. People are still concerned about the MMR. Sometimes they express that in different ways than specifically talking about autism.

But I think what we've seen and what we've learned in the last five years is that once you scare someone, you can't just unscare them. You can't just say, "OK, actually, never mind; wipe that from your from your memory," because as humans, once you've introduced the idea that something bad could happen, we are naturally going to think about that possible bad thing that could happen. So I think that's been a big shift.

Another big shift in the vaccine wars over the past five years is that I think the media coverage today is much more responsible than it was five years ago, definitely 10 years ago. Even then there was an enormous amount of scientific evidence on the side of vaccines being safe, having absolutely no connection with autism and really no evidence to the contrary. You had a lot of stories that express this as an on-the-one-hand/on-the-other-hand debate. I think those stories did a huge, huge disservice to public health, and you really don't see that anymore.

That is what I'm interested in. It seems the climate has really changed both for the anti-vaccine camp and pro-vaccine camp. Five years ago there was a greater sense of pro-vaccine sentiment acknowledging the other side as a reasonable, other way of looking at. Now that's different.

When I started working on this in 2008, what I encountered was parents who were skeptical of vaccines, were oftentimes very vocal about that. And the vast majority—the 90-plus percent of parents who do vaccinate—were not vocal about that. They sort of felt like it wasn't their place to tell other parents what they thought they should be doing. . . .

That's something that has definitely changed over the past couple of years, I think in large part because of the outbreaks that we've been seeing, the measles outbreaks, not just in 2015. For the last several years we've had many, many more measles cases than we had been having. Those numbers are so striking to people in public health because measles had been eliminated in the United States. We've had pertussis [whooping cough] outbreaks that have swept across the country. We've had deaths from pertussis.

So I think parents now who are vaccinating their children also understand that parents who don't vaccinate are having an impact on the rest of society. Even if your own child is vaccinated, there are public health costs associated with these outbreaks, pretty significant public health costs. . . .

Years ago, doctors were predicting that outbreaks of disease would happen. Now we are seeing whooping cough and measles. What do you think is the trajectory? Where do we stand now?

I think we're in a very critical time in all of this. There have been hundreds of measles infections this year, really a striking number, a vast majority of them coming out of this Disneyland outbreak. But still, in a nation of 300 and something million, that's a very small number of people.

What makes the public health community so nervous is that you do have these communities where enough people are not vaccinated so that tomorrow you could have 30, 40, 50 new infections. Even if none of those 30, 40, 50 kids ends up hospitalized for an extended amount of time, the most recent study that I've seen indicated that it costs more than $10,000 per case of measles to contain it . . . The efforts to contain it, the efforts to track down everyone that the infected person has come in contact with, are just incredibly, incredibly expensive. So even though we're only seeing hundreds of cases, that can have a pretty significant impact on public health.

But I do think we are at this point where it's possible that education and awareness, stemming partially from what's happened, could mean that the 90-plus percent of parents that are vaccinating now rises up to 93 percent. . . . That, I think, is sort of a best-case scenario.

A worst case scenario is we look overseas at what happened in France, where they had several dozens of cases a couple of years ago and now have tens of thousands of cases. And that's tens of thousands of cases in a country essentially the size of Texas. So you extrapolate that out to the U.S., and you start to get pretty big numbers.

That's an absolute worst case scenario. I don't see that happening in the United States because of school-age vaccination requirements and other factors, but it's certainly not out of the realm of possibility.

So that brings me to exemption laws. . . . Can you describe how these laws work around the country and what you know about how they've changed or been used in ways that amount to lowering immunities?

So in the country as a whole, you have several different types of exemptions. You have medical exemptions, which every state has, which no one, I think, is arguing that you should not have. Doctors think there should be medical exemptions. The public health community thinks there should be medical exemptions.

Who would get a medical exemption?

Medical exemptions could be applicable for someone with a not fully developed immune system, someone who's immune-compromised. . . .

You also could have situations where the medical recommendation is to delay a vaccine, ranging from something as simple as a child is sick at that time and they don't want to give them a shot right then to there's some larger issue that will resolve over time and they're going to wait until that issue does resolve. So I think medical exemptions are not going away; no one thinks they should go away. . . .

There are essentially two types of non-medical exemptions in this country: religious exemptions and personal-belief exemptions. They're sometimes also called philosophical exemptions.

The way those two types of exemptions are administered around the country vary widely. In some places, you essentially just need to say, "It is my personal belief that I should not vaccinate my child," and sign a piece of paper, and that's that. In some states, you need to have a conversation with a medical professional and sign a piece of paper saying that you understand the risks of not vaccinating and those risks include X, Y and Z. . . .

Some states are looking at tightening up the mandates and wiping personal-belief exemptions from the list at all.

I think another illustration of how the vaccine debate has kind of ebbed and flowed over the past couple of years is that right now, you're seeing a lot of legislation being introduced that would tighten up exemptions or get rid of personal-belief exemptions. And again, I think that's because you have a larger portion of the public understanding what the risks are of having a large number of non-vaccinating people in their community.

What you saw a couple of years ago were when there were new laws introduced about exemptions, oftentimes it was because you had anti-vaccine forces who were kind of rallying their troops and sending a lot of letters.

Right now, you're seeing the opposite. You're seeing legislators who are aware of the risks. You are seeing constituents who are saying: "I don't want to live in a school district where there's an incredible likelihood of a measles outbreak. I don't want to be in a place where, if there's a child with leukemia, he or she needs to fear for his life because we have 30 percent of kids who aren't vaccinated in this community." . . .

[Some parents have said] this is a First Amendment issue; this is parental choice; this is freedom of religion or expression. Just in terms of voters, how will politicians process this issue to win votes? . . .

There are parents who try and frame the vaccine question as a First Amendment issue, as a right to express themselves the way that they want. That's a ridiculous argument. There are all sorts of behaviors that impact public health that we do not have a First Amendment right to. I do not have a First Amendment right to drive drunk, even though I may want to express myself that way. I do not have a First Amendment right to take my infant child and put him in a car without a car seat and without a seat belt, even though I may want to express myself that way.

So this is not some infringement on First Amendment rights by any stretch of the imagination. Protecting its citizens is one of the most fundamental jobs that a government has, and we have all sorts of laws and regulations aimed to do exactly that. . . .

At the end of your book, you get quite sympathetic for the parents of autistic children . . .

I think one of the big tragedies, and a tragedy that doesn't get as much attention as it should [have] in the last 10 or 15 years of the vaccine wars, is the extent to which the autism community has just been done a horrible disservice. We don't know nearly as much as we should about autism, and there have been just untold amounts of research dollars essentially poured down the drain because of this insistence of again and again going after this illusion that there was some connection between vaccines and autism. All of that was research money that could have been spent on projects that actually needed to be done.

Another huge tragedy is that in this country in 2015, families with autism very often don't get the support that they need or deserve, and unfortunately now there's this incredibly charged situation where you have researchers who are afraid to look into questions having to do with autism because they don't want to all of a sudden be in the crosshairs of the most fervent anti-vaccine camps. . . .

Does the vaccine story seem fated to wax and wane forever?

If you look throughout history, there have been anti-vaccine movements and anti-vaccine sentiment for all sorts of different reasons.

One thing that you see pretty consistently is that when a disease is endemic in a society, there's not a lot of anti-vaccine sentiment. And when a disease kind of disappears from both people's consciousness and from that society, that's when you start to get these anti-vaccine concerns. . . .

When the polio vaccine was introduced in this country, there was actually a batch of tainted vaccines that paralyzed some people and killed some people. That did not completely sidetrack the polio vaccination efforts because everyone in the country knew what a concern polio was. Kids knew that they weren't allowed to go swimming. They saw their neighbors in iron lungs. So even when there was real cause to be concerned, the public health organization and the doctors were able to get that effort back on track. . . .

[Can you give us an overview of the Disneyland measles outbreak? What does it say about where we are today in the vaccine debate?]

. . . You had one case at Disneyland that has now spread to over 100 infections, not just in California, to different states around the country, and because of that, it's something that's gotten a lot of attention.

I think that this is another one of those examples of how the national conversation is shifting, because I think what that has done is really highlight and bring awareness to the fact that a single person infected with this disease can have implications that are going to go on for months for hundreds of people, and, as a result, are going to cost millions of dollars.

Measles is the single most infectious microbe known to humankind. If you have one person with measles in a room, that person can leave the room; two hours later someone else can come in and still get infected. So when you have someone in a public place like Disneyland or on a plane or in a shopping mall, the ripple effects of that can be almost impossible to quantify. . . .

Source: Mnookin, Seth. (2015, March 24). "How the Vaccine War Has Changed." Interview by Sarah Moughty. *FRONTLINE, The Vaccine War.* http:// www.pbs.org/wgbh/pages/frontline/health-science-technology/the-vaccine-war/ seth-mnookin-how-the-vaccine-war-has-changed/. © 1995–2016 WGBH Educational Foundation. Used by permission.

ANALYSIS

The outbreak of measles at Disneyland in 2015 dramatized the shift in public acceptance of vaccines, from fear of vaccines to renewed fear of infectious diseases. The basic dynamic should be familiar. Throughout the history of vaccination, fears about disease and even death lead to an upswing in vaccinations and a downswing in fears about vaccine safety. The clear and present danger of the disease and its cost to individuals, families, and communities are much more frightening than the vaccine.

As vaccinations successfully reduce the spread of infectious disease, the danger appears more remote. Individuals, families, and communities invoke other costs—fears about vaccine safety, about civil liberties, about uncertain environmental outcomes—as higher priorities than protection against a disease they believe they will never experience. As Eula Biss has put it, "The belief that public-health measures are not intended for people like us is widely held by people like me" (Biss, 2013).

But from the point of view of bacteria or viruses, all people look the same whatever we believe, and what all unvaccinated people look like are potential host organisms. Vaccines are the only sure way we can block microbes from using us for their purposes. That is the main lesson of the vaccine wars for the 21st century.

FURTHER READING

Biss, Eula. (2013). "Sentimental Medicine: Why We Still Fear Vaccines." *Harper's Magazine*. https://harpers.org/archive/2013/01/sentimental-medicine/.

Hensley, Scott. (2015). "Vaccination Gaps Helped Fuel Disneyland Measles Spread." *SHOTS: Health News from NPR*. http://www.npr.org/sections/health-shots/2015/03/16/393336901/vaccination-gaps-helped-fuel-disneyland-measles-spread.

Kirkland, Anna. (2012). "Credibility Battles in the Autism Litigation." *Social Studies of Science* 42: 237–261.

"Measles Cases and Outbreaks." (2015). *Centers for Disease Control and Prevention*. http://www.cdc.gov/measles/cases-outbreaks.html.

Mnookin, Seth. (2011). *The Panic Virus: A True Story of Medicine, Science, and Fear*. New York: Simon and Schuster.

8

GLOBAL VACCINATION IDEALS AND REALITY (2000–PRESENT)

ESSENTIAL VACCINATIONS FOR CHILDREN

- **Document:** World Health Organization, Model List of Essential Medicines for Children
- **Date:** August 2015
- **Where:** Geneva, Switzerland
- **Significance:** The greatest challenge for vaccination in the 21st century is not development of new vaccines but the global distribution of the vaccines we already have. Families within industrialized countries have the benefits of an established health-care infrastructure: they can simply make doctor's appointments to have their children receive the recommended vaccines. But what happens to children in countries without that infrastructure and without the funding to create it? Since its inception in 1948, the World Health Organization (WHO) has had the responsibility of answering the hard questions about global vaccination efforts.

DOCUMENT

19.3 Vaccines

WHO immunization policy recommendations are published in vaccine position papers on the basis of recommendations made by the Strategic Advisory Group of Experts on Immunization (SAGE).

WHO vaccine position papers are updated three to four times per year. The list below details the vaccines for which there is a recommendation from SAGE and a corresponding WHO position paper as at 27 February 2015. The most recent versions of the WHO position papers, reflecting the current evidence related to a specific vaccine and the related recommendations, can be accessed at any time on the WHO website at:

http://www.who.int/immunization/documents/positionpapers/en/index.html.

Vaccine recommendations may be universal or conditional (e.g., in certain regions, in some high-risk populations or as part of immunization programmes with certain characteristics). Details are available in the relevant position papers, and in the Summary Tables of WHO Routine Immunization Recommendations available on the WHO website at:

http://www.who.int/immunization/policy/immunization_tables/en/index.html.

Selection of vaccines from the Model List will need to be determined by each country after

---

DID YOU KNOW?

Timeline of Human Vaccine Development, 2000–2014

Disease	Year
Cold-adapted influenza	2003
Human papillomavirus	2006
Zoster	2006
Meningococcal B	2014

Source: Plotkin, Stanley, Walter Orenstein, and Paul Offit, eds. (2013). *Vaccines.* Philadelphia, PA: Elsevier Saunders; Centers for Disease Control and Prevention (CDC). Meningococcal Vaccination. http://www.cdc.gov/meningococcal/vaccine-info.html.

consideration of international recommendations, epidemiology and national priorities. All vaccines should comply with the WHO requirements for biological substances. WHO noted the need for vaccines used in children to be polyvalent.

Recommendations for all

- BCG vaccine
- diphtheria vaccine
- Haemophilus influenzae type b vaccine
- hepatitis B vaccine
- HPV vaccine
- measles vaccine
- pertussis vaccine
- pneumococcal vaccine
- poliomyelitis vaccine
- rotavirus vaccine
- rubella vaccine
- tetanus vaccine

Recommendations for certain regions

- Japanese encephalitis vaccine
- yellow fever vaccine
- tick-borne encephalitis vaccine

Recommendations for some high-risk populations

- cholera vaccine
- hepatitis A vaccine
- meningococcal meningitis vaccine
- rabies vaccine
- typhoid vaccine

Recommendations for immunization programmes with certain characteristics

- influenza vaccine (seasonal)
- mumps vaccine
- varicella vaccine

Source: World Health Organization. (2015). "WHO Model Lists of Essential Medicines." http://www.who.int/medicines/publications/essentialmedicines/en/. Used by permission of the World Health Organization.

ANALYSIS

When WHO was founded after World War II, its immediate tasks were to deal with the tremendous dislocation and public health crises produced by the war. Over the next 30 years, WHO increased funding, staff, and public health initiatives. But like other UN agencies, WHO was caught up in Cold War geopolitical conflicts, and the enormous disparities in wealth across the world meant that the poorest, most war-torn countries—where health care was most needed—were the least likely to get it. By 1974, only 5% of the world's children were receiving any vaccines at all. And of those 5%, most lived in wealthy industrialized nations.

To solve this problem, WHO created the Expanded Program on Immunization (EPI) and partnered with another UN agency, the United Nations International Children's Emergency Fund (UNICEF), to increase access to childhood vaccines. This effort was enormously successful. By 1990, 80% of children worldwide had access to the six recommended vaccines, against tuberculosis, diphtheria, tetanus, pertussis, measles, and polio.

But enormous disparities still remained between wealthy and developing countries and among urban, suburban, and rural populations worldwide. During the 1990s, WHO's vaccination efforts slowed down. This was partly for internal reasons, such as funding cuts and competition with other UN agencies. But many public health officials in developing countries also questioned the value of vaccination in regions so poor that children did not have access to primary care basics: clean water, nutritious food, or proper sanitation. Why promote a high-cost, high-tech vaccination program when so many poor children had no access to any other kind of medical care? Why spend billions of dollars developing a vaccine against malaria, when pennies per day could provide mosquito nets to keep mosquitoes against sleeping children? What was the point of sending public health officials into slums to vaccinate children against tuberculosis, without providing the clean water supply that would protect them against cholera?

Between 2000 and the present, public and private donors launched the Global Alliance for Vaccines and Immunization (GAVI), an unprecedented collaboration among WHO, the World Bank, UNICEF, and the Bill and Melinda Gates Foundation. The Bill and Melinda Gates Foundation provided $750 million for the first five years, from 2000 to 2005; WHO provides the technical expertise and establishes the list of recommended vaccines; UNICEF, through EPI, ensures that they get to children in developing countries; the World Bank has responsibility for continued funding and accountability. The effort has been enormously successful in supporting worldwide vaccination efforts. As Dr. Margaret Chan, director-general of WHO, reported in 2012, "The Decade of Vaccines was launched in 2010. The following year, leading drug companies announced significant slashes in vaccine prices for the developing world, including a 95% price reduction for the new rotavirus vaccines. Also in 2011, donors pledged more than $4 billion to support the work of GAVI, an amount that exceeded expectations" (Chan, 2012, 2).

According to 2012 statistics, access to vaccination saves the lives of 2–3 million children every year from diphtheria, tetanus, pertussis, and measles (Global Immunization Data).

FURTHER READING

Brimnes, Niels. (2007). "Vikings against Tuberculosis: The International Tuberculosis Campaign in India, 1948–1951." *Bulletin of the History of Medicine* 81: 407–430.

Chan, Margaret. (2012). "Keeping Promises: Accountability of Dr Margaret Chan during Her First Term as WHO Director-General." *World Health Organization.* http://www .who.int/dg/Report_card_cover_28_06.pdf?ua=1.

Global Alliance for Vaccines and Immunization (GAVI). *The Vaccine Alliance.* http://www .gavi.org/.

Global Immunization Data. (2013, July). http://apps.who.int/immunization_monitoring/ Global_Immunization_Data_v2.pdf?ua=1.

Vargha, Dora. (2014). "Between East and West: Polio Vaccination across the Iron Curtain in Cold War Hungary." *Bulletin of the History of Medicine* 88: 319–342.

THE END OF SMALLPOX

- **Document:** Kathy Nellis and Jason Weisfeld, "Smallpox Eradication: Memories and Milestones"
- **Date:** 2007
- **Where:** Washington, DC
- **Significance:** Smallpox, the first disease to have a vaccine, was also the first to be eradicated. Rinderpest, a cattle disease, was declared eradicated in 2011. Guinea worm, with only 23 cases worldwide in 2015, may be the next to be completely eliminated from the catalog of human diseases.

DID YOU KNOW?

The Bifurcated Needle

Sometimes a simple change in technology can make all the difference. In 1965, Benjamin Rubin (1917–2010), working for Wyeth Pharmaceuticals, developed the bifurcated needle as a smallpox vaccination device, and his invention is credited with saving the lives of millions of people.

Up to that point, the standard way to deliver the vaccine was with the rotary lancet. As Rubin explained in his patent application, there were a number of problems with it.

The conventional technique of vaccination is to put a drop of vaccine on the skin either from a capillary tube or a syringe. An ordinary single-pointed straight needle from a sterile capillary is then applied. For proper vaccination, the needle should be pressed against the skin parallel to the plane of the skin. The tip of the needle should rest in the drop of vaccine and this tip has to be pressed firmly against the skin approximately twenty times. The excess vaccine is then uneconomically wiped off. The skin should show a small red area, preferably approximately one-eighth inch in diameter, but no blood. Unfortunately, the very nature of the prior art single-pointed needles is conducive to various errors in technique. The usual error is that the needle is not pressed against the skin firmly enough, or else it is actually jabbed into the skin point forward.

DOCUMENT

Thirty years ago, on October 26, 1977, a Somali man, Ali Maow Maalin, was diagnosed with a case of smallpox. A World Health Organization (WHO) team led by Jason S. Weisfeld, MD, MPH, from the Centers for Disease Control (CDC), and Karl Markvart from Czechoslovakia, conducted a surveillance and containment program that confirmed this to be the last case of endemic smallpox in the world. This historic achievement was possible only through the persistent efforts of thousands of local health workers who identified people with smallpox and vaccinated around them to prevent the spread. International leadership was vital, but without the dedication of local and national governments, eradication would not have been possible . . .

[Interview with Jason Weisfeld]

Who were you and why were you in Somalia?

At the time of my assignment in Somalia, I was a Career Development officer with CDC having completed two years of EIS, more than a year seconded to WHO for Smallpox Eradication Programmes in India and Bangladesh, a Preventive Medicine residency and an MPH at Harvard. I felt very privileged to be selected for the first group of Westerners invited to work in Somalia and had begun work in various endemic areas of central Somalia in May 1977.

What was the smallpox situation in Somalia?

Although national authorities had attempted to conceal active transmission prior to our arrival, intense surveillance and active public participation soon revealed that smallpox was being transmitted in many areas of southern and central Somalia. By the time of the last case in October 1977, we had interrupted all of the known chains of transmission and there was heightened anticipation that we would soon identify any last remaining cases.

How did the last case become infected? How was his case identified?

Ali Maow Maalin was a 23-year-old cook at the Merca Hospital along the coast of southern Somalia when he became infected. He had volunteered for the local Smallpox Eradication Programme staff and had been immunized, but no one checked his vaccination site and his subsequent illness revealed that he must not have had a successful immunization and was not protected.

One evening, after office hours, two cases of smallpox were brought to the hospital and Ali was selected to drive with them in a closed Land Cruiser with the windows closed and the air conditioning running to the local team leader's house. We estimated that Ali was probably exposed to these cases for a maximum of five minutes—but that was sufficient. When Ali became symptomatic with fever and rash, his history of being immunized against smallpox led the local hospital staff to assume that he had chickenpox. He was hospitalized briefly but then discharged to the small room he rented near the hospital. When being visited by one of the male nurses from the hospital, it was suspected that he might have smallpox and the team leader reported the suspect case to the Ministry of Health in Mogadishu.

What action did finding Ali precipitate?

Upon confirming the diagnosis, the National Smallpox Eradication Programme initiated a major response. Dr. Karl Markvart, a Czech colleague, and I were requested to transfer immediately to Merca and assume responsibility for the management of the outbreak. We had the full support of additional international and national staff as well as the local police and Party authorities.

Our first priority was to organize surveillance within Merca Town and to establish working relationships with local authorities and community groups to immunize the

Either of these methods will yield a poor vaccination. (Rubin, 1965)

Rubin had the idea of taking a sturdy sewing machine needle and grinding of the end, thus creating a tiny, precise, two-pronged fork. Between the two prongs was exactly the right amount of space to hold exactly the right amount of vaccine. To get it into the patient, all the vaccinator had to do was hold it at right angles to the patient's skin and push. The vaccine then entered the patient's bloodstream through the two punctures. "The field trials showed that the technique was easy to teach," remembered William Foege, an important consideration with a worldwide effort. Success rates were 98%, and vaccinators used only about 20% of the vaccine needed with other technologies. "The needles were also inexpensive, costing about a half-cent each . . . Supplies were lightweight and could be taken easily from door to door, and vaccinators could, under good conditions, do up to five hundred vaccinations in a day" (Foege, 2011, 101–102).

Though made of steel, Rubin's bifurcated needle became the gold standard for global vaccination efforts.

Sources:

Foege, William. (2011). *House on Fire: The Fight to Eradicate Smallpox.* Berkeley, CA: University of California Press.

Rubin, Benjamin. (1965). "Pronged Vaccinating and Testing Needle US 3194237 A." U.S. Patent Office. https://docs.google.com/viewer?url=patentimages.storage.googleapis.com/pdfs/US3194237.pdf.

entire population of the town and surrounding areas. We established check-points at all entrances to the town and local staff kept log books of who arrived, and departed, and their immunization status. Vaccinators were stationed at these check-points and immunized anyone who had not been recently immunized.

What was your role?

I was requested to identify all contacts and then to immunize them and their families as well as to maintain rash-and-fever surveillance on all of them every two days for six weeks. By establishing a close, personal relationship with Ali in his containment camp, I was eventually able to identify 161 contacts and their close family members. With the assistance of a local team of dedicated health workers and a fleet of motorcycles, we were able to maintain close surveillance for the required six-week period.

What were your thoughts when it was realized that this was the last case of smallpox?

As mentioned, even prior to the identification of Ali's case, most of the Programme staff were quite aware that we had interrupted almost all of the remaining chains of transmission within Somalia. Special attention was being given to ensuring that an outbreak among a nomadic group near Merca was prevented from spreading to non-protected populations. So, when I was asked to shift to Merca to assist with Ali's case, I had the premonition that I was being given a major responsibility and would need to be especially rigorous in whatever ways I could assist. In addition to coordinating the immunization and surveillance of contacts, I also helped Karl supervising night-time immunizations of the town population.

Of course, some of us were not very confident that this WAS the very last endemic case until sometime after Ali's recovery. We still feared ongoing transmission in inaccessible areas of Ethiopia. But this never came to pass . . .

What has become of Ali? Did he become involved with EPI?

When I visited Somalia in the mid-1990s for UNICEF, I tracked down Ali in a small roadside town near Merca. He was working as an untrained drug seller in a local shop and we had a wonderful reunion over a proverbial cup of sweet tea. Subsequently, I understand that he joined the national Polio Eradication Programme . . . fulfilling his earlier dream of helping out with Smallpox Eradication.

Source: Nellis, Kathy. (2007). "Smallpox Eradication: Memories and Milestones." *CDC Connects, Global Health Chronicles.* http://www.globalhealthchronicles .org/archive/files/869774faa96420dc6f1a1628e3fa7127.pdf.

ANALYSIS

The distinctive biology that made smallpox such a good candidate for Edward Jenner's cowpox vaccine also contributed to its eradication efforts. Smallpox is highly visible: it produces a very distinctive rash, and smallpox patients become very sick. There is really no such thing as smallpox without symptoms. Its transmission through a region is easy to monitor: it only passes from person to person, and there is no animal or insect vector. If public health officials can establish an effective cordon preventing infected persons from coming into contact with a vulnerable population, there is no other way for the disease to spread. Though the disease has a 10–12-day incubation period, during which the patient may not know s/he is sick, s/he is also not contagious until the first pox appears. And since smallpox patients are so sick, they cannot continue to move through their communities spreading the disease.

The first commitment to large-scale eradication of smallpox came from the Pan American Sanitary Organization in 1950, which pledged to eliminate smallpox in the Western Hemisphere. The WHO made a similar commitment a few years later. These early efforts were successful in cutting down on smallpox incidence in many countries, but overall, the results were disappointing. Smallpox, which had had a successful vaccine for 160 years, was still endemic: in 1966, there were around 10–15 million cases worldwide. It is a measure of the challenge that WHO could not provide a more precise number for the incidence of the disease.

In 1966, then, WHO launched a global smallpox eradication campaign, with funding of $2.4 million annually for what was expected to be a 10-year effort. The money went to support two programs, each of which would contribute to the overall effort. The first involved distributing high-quality vaccine to countries through established public health authorities. This was expected to reach at least 80% of the population and also to further strengthen each country's public health infrastructure. Through this part of the vaccination program, public health officials would be able to provide resources and educate parents about the value of primary health care for children.

The second program became known as "surveillance and containment." Special teams were recruited to serve in regions with especially high incidence of smallpox, especially those with few doctors or clinics in remote areas. The first step was to quickly identify cases of smallpox as soon as they appeared. That is the "surveillance" part. The next step was to vaccinate every single person that the original patient had been in contact with, for even the briefest period. This is sometimes called the "ring method," since the idea was to create a ring of vaccinated people around the original patient. This "ring" was not necessarily based on location: if a person who later developed smallpox had taken a bus to work, public health officials would vaccinate not only his/her family, neighbors, and coworkers but also try to track down everyone who had been on that bus. Jason Weisfeld describes the mechanics of this in the excerpt above.

WHO succeeded in its goal of eradicating smallpox worldwide within 10 years: Ali Maow Maalin, diagnosed in 1977, was indeed the last victim. He volunteered for the polio eradication campaign in Somalia and was interviewed when it succeeded in 2008. "Somalia was the last country with smallpox," he told reporters, "I wanted to help ensure that we would not be the last place with polio too." He was still vaccinating children in 2013, when he caught malaria and died.

FURTHER READING

"Disease Eradication." *History of Vaccines.* http://www.historyofvaccines.org/content/articles/disease-eradication.

Henderson, Donald. (2009). *Smallpox—The Death of a Disease: The Inside Story of Eradicating a Worldwide Killer.* Amherst, NY: Prometheus Books.

Neelakantan, Vivek. (2010). "Eradicating Smallpox in Indonesia: The Archipelagic Challenge." *Health and History* 12: 61–87.

"The Smallpox Eradication Programme—SEP (1966–1980)." (2010). *World Health Organization.* http://www.who.int/features/2010/smallpox/en/.

Stepan, Nancy. (2011). *Eradication: Ridding the World of Diseases Forever?* Ithaca, NY: Cornell University Press.

"I'M GOING TO GIVE YOU AN ELEPHANT"

- **Document:** Mary Guinan and Melissa McSwigan, "Mary Guinan Oral History—India"
- **Date:** 2008
- **Where:** Washington, DC
- **Significance:** Dr. Mary Guinan, now a distinguished dean of the University of Nevada, Las Vegas, School of Community Health Sciences, and professor of epidemiology and community health, was one of many women who turned to public health as a pathway into medicine. Though she faced many obstacles due to negative stereotypes about women, her gender could also be an advantage in connecting with her patients and their communities, as she described in the interview below.

DOCUMENT

Melissa McSwigan: This is an interview with Mary Guinan on July 10, 2008 at the Centers for Disease Control and Prevention in Atlanta, Georgia, about her involvement with the Smallpox Eradication Program. The interview is being conducted as part of our reunion, marking the 40th anniversary of the program in Asia and East Africa . . .

Mary Guinan: Well-I'm not sure how my education and upbringing brought me into Public Health, but I'll tell you how I decided that I wanted to be part of the Smallpox Eradication Program. I was born in New York City, a child of immigrants. My parents were immigrants from Ireland. They were farmers. They had maybe three years of education, 3rd Grade education level and they came to follow the American dream . . . they believed in education. They believed that that was the way to move ahead and they loved this country because of its freedom and lack of persecution for your political views and they were very, very . . . very loyal Americans and felt that this was really an important place to be and that we should be grateful . . . for being born in this country and for exactly what we had available to us . . .

So when I was a young teenager my dad died very suddenly and my mother had no means of support and we all got jobs to work our way through school; and I worked my way through school and graduated from high school. I worked my way through college. I wanted to be a physician, but women weren't being admitted to medical school then; and also, one of the criteria for medical school was that you had to have money to pay for it; and there weren't scholarships available or other things available to students like me who really didn't have the means to do that. So I decided then that I would pursue other things. I majored in Chemistry in college and when I graduated, I couldn't get a job because they didn't hire woman Chemists . . .

I got a job in a Chewing Gum Factory . . . the American Chicle Company and they made Chiclets and all sorts of chewing gum. . . . It was not terribly rewarding kind of existence, but there wasn't really much available for women then and I try to look for fellowships and I applied to many schools, to graduate school, and I was rejected mostly because I was a woman; and if I was accepted, I couldn't get a fellowship program because they didn't give them to women at that time. But at the time the Space Program was in full bloom and with Sputnik, President Kennedy had said we wanted to be on the moon; that we were going to the moon; and there were lots of . . . fellowships for scientists. So I found out that . . . the University of Texas Medical Branch in Texas had a program for scientist in Aerospace Medicine and that the Director of the Medical Program, Chuck Berry—Dr. Chuck Berry, had an appointment at the University of Texas there. So I applied there to get my PhD in Physiology and Space Medicine and I wanted to be an astronaut. Of course I didn't tell anybody then that I wanted to be an astronaut because women didn't do those sorts of things.

So I went to Texas and people in New York said: You won't last there-about six months. You know you're a New York person born and brought up in New York. But I did, I lasted four years and I went to NASA. I applied—all of my class in physiology and space medicine there at the University took a test for the Astronaut Program and I was the only woman who took it and I was the only one who passed the test. The reason I passed the test was I had 20/20 vision; and all the other people wore glasses . . . I got to see all the astronauts, I took classes at NASA. The astronauts, you know like John Glenn and Neil Armstrong gave classes and talked about their experiences in space.

It was really exciting; I was really excited as a scientist; and I did a post doctoral fellowship; I got a Post Doctoral Fellowship at the National Institutes of Health in Bethesda, Maryland; and it was during the Vietnam War and I actually had gotten a place that was for a man who had been drafted. So I filled in and I knew that I wouldn't really be there very long because they saved the places for men who had been drafted and had gone to war; and it was very difficult for me to get a job at NIH because I didn't have an MD degree, and my mentor there at NIH said to me, "It would be so easy to get you a job if you had an MD."

. . . So I applied to two medical schools. Since I was living in Maryland, I applied to the University of Maryland to Johns Hopkins; and I got rejected from the University of Maryland and accepted at Johns Hopkins which tells you something about the crazy system we have about being accepted into medical school . . . So I went to medical school and I graduated from Johns Hopkins in 1972 and during that time period, I was continuing my career, I had done my PhD, my doctorate in physiology in the area of blood coagulation and I was wanting to continue my career and be a hematologist, oncologist, and go in academic medicine. That's what I thought I would want to do. Never thought about public health, didn't really know about public health. I went to medical school at Johns Hopkins where one of the premiere Public Health Schools in the nation is, and took courses but really had no interest in public health at that time.

But I was interested in tropical medicine and I did a tropical medicine fellowship in Mexico during my senior year at Hopkins . . . Then, as I was graduating, this was the end of the 60's and beginning of the 70's and what happened during my last year of medical school really changed my life, in that what happened was Kent State … People were killed for demonstrating. This is a free country, our Government. The United States Government, which I was very proud of being an American and was very, very upset about what happened in the anti-war demonstrations that went on; and then these students in Kent State were killed, unarmed students, by the National Guards that had been even called out. People killed and I thought: What has happed to this country that I live in? How can this be-that we're living in this country where they're killing unarmed demonstrators? Our whole history of our country was revolution and fighting for freedom and doing what we thought was right.

… I decided I wasn't sure what I was going to do and so in my senior year I read in this magazine, sort of like a magazine at Hopkins about the Smallpox Eradication Program. That there was this idea to eradicate smallpox in the world and I thought, "Isn't that wonderful? What a great idea that we could eliminate a scourge. It would be the first time in history that by the design of man or woman, there would be a human disease eliminated from the world and smallpox, a very frightening disease." … Then I found out that the people who were going were being assigned from CDC [Centers for Disease Control], so you had to come to CDC and somehow get a job at CDC and then you could be assigned to the Smallpox Eradication Program.

… I applied to the EIS [Epidemic Intelligence Service] Program and in 1973 I guess, I was accepted; and I came to interview and I was the only woman physician in my class that was accepted … we used to have a Tuesday morning seminar in Auditorium-B every week for all the EIS Officers and we'd attend this meeting and there'd be announcements at the beginning and every time somebody from the smallpox program would go up and say, "We are looking for volunteers for the Smallpox Eradication Program." You know it was a three or four-month assignment in India …; and I applied to go and they told me, they were not taking women. Now, Indira Gandhi was the Prime Minister of India so it's like to say, "Well, how is it possible?" That was the first round and then each week, you know, they'd have somebody and finally … I said [to the head of the program], "You know, I keep volunteering and I keep getting turned down, but I don't know why. Can you tell me what the criteria are?" So I think they thought I might make a fuss …

When I applied to the EIS, I was accepted, but we had to get three references from physicians who knew us, and they sent me the reference sheets that had to be completed and it was: "Will you please rate this candidate on his background on his—whatever he does and is he a leader? Is he going to …" You know, there wasn't a parenthesis with "she" and so I sent back the forms, I said, "I'm sorry. I'm a woman. Do you have forms for women?" and apparently that caused some issues here at CDC before I arrived, so they figured, "Oh, oh-this is trouble coming." They wrote back and said, "We do not discriminate, but we don't have any female forms." So, they crossed out the "he" and put "her" and "she" in the appropriate spots. So … finally, they said, "You're going. You're going to India." So I went in December of '74 through early May of '75.

Melissa McSwigan: And what was your exact role while you were in India?

Mary Guinan: What our roles were was that we would be assigned to a district . . . and you did surveillance for smallpox, looked for smallpox cases and then if you found one, you quarantine the case and then surrounded it with a ring of immunity in a five or 10-mile radius around because smallpox spread locally.

So . . . we were sent to Uttar Pradesh and there were still smallpox in Uttar Pradesh. There were two provinces in India, Uttar Pradesh and Bihar that still had smallpox. So it was like a competition between Bihar and Uttar Pradesh; who would come first down to smallpox zero? What we'd do is, we would go out into the field; we would go and do surveillance. You were assigned a driver and a paramedical assistant and then you were given all these traveler's checks like in Rupees because you had to hire people, and you had to pay them. Then I would go to the bank and cash these checks so I'd have lots of money to pay people to immunize. You had to get vaccinators. You had to get people to work for you. I didn't realize what the whole system was in India, but since my driver and paramedical assistant had been working, and my paramedical assistant was Shaffy Mohamed, he was a Muslim, and my driver was a Hindu, and they spoke different languages actually. Shaffy spoke English perfectly, but his native language is Urdu not Hindi, so that we had this three way thing going on trying to communicate with Urdu, Hindi and English. I didn't speak any of either, but I learned to read the Hindi symbols so I could read the road signs and they were very small—rarely was there a road sign, but if there were, the driver couldn't read, so I would phonetically sound the symbols so I could tell which way the direction was pointing. . . .

The paramedical assistant acted as your interpreter, your cook. To find a place to stay, we were issued . . . sleeping bags and these mattresses. You know, thinking about India, I thought it would be very hot and didn't bring any warm clothes, but Uttar Pradesh is up North near Nepal and it got very cold. It was three degrees (3°) centigrade when I arrived at the Delhi airport and it was cold. So I had made a quilt, so I would wrap it around me because I didn't have any warm clothes. We would go out and we would offer a reward; we'd go . . . to a village and the paramedical assistant would get up and say to the villagers, they had never seen a foreigner before so I was a great source of interest to people like: look at me, this is incredible..

We would go to the village and we had these picture postcards that showed cases of smallpox and we would say, "Ten Rupees to anyone who can show me a case of smallpox" and . . . 10 Rupees was a lot of money then for the average person. So if there was smallpox in the village they would bring you to the person. Very often it was chickenpox, not smallpox; or something else. It wasn't smallpox; and you were supposed to be the expert, not having ever seen a case of smallpox, it was like strange to think that you were going to be the expert and tell whether this was smallpox or chickenpox. Of course we were taught at all of these training sessions how to do it.

So we heard about a report of smallpox in a village that was supposed to be free of smallpox . . . So I went there and I looked at the case and it sure looked like smallpox to me; and at that time we took a culture of the lesions and put them in a little vial and a mailing case. Then I mailed it off to Delhi and they would either confirm, because they wanted to culture every case to see if it was really a case; but it would take weeks and weeks before the results came back. I declared it as smallpox and so we started our immunization. There were vaccinators who actually worked in all the villages. There's this infrastructure in India where they have these people who are vaccinators; and they could be hired. So my paramedical assistant would just let out the word and people would come and want to work for you because we paid very well. So what we would do, we would pay the people's family to be guards at the door. This is a mud hut in these villages and then we would pay a family member to be the guard at the door and the only people—they'd have to vaccinate them. Anybody who went in or out of the house had to be vaccinated . . .

So we went about, and I found out that when we go to the villages surrounding it, we didn't have maps, it wasn't like you'd say, "Okay let's draw a five-mile radius around this and try and find some maps to figure out what the radius was or how you could do this." So, we got these rather rudimentary maps and we started going to the villages to try to vaccinate. We found out when people would come—we had a jeep . . . and they were provided by the Indian Government, the jeeps; and when the jeeps came and the only time the villagers ever saw a jeep come in was when the Family Planning person came and there was a big initiative in India at that time to reduce the population and to introduce birth control, and they used to pay the men to have a vasectomy, gave them a portable radio was one of the gifts that the men would get . . .

[T]he Family Planning people had told us that they had to meet every month. They had to have so many vasectomies and so many tubal ligations and they were not terribly receptive people so they saw this jeep coming and they thought it was the Family Planning people and they all ran away. So nobody would be there. So we said, "We couldn't find anybody to vaccinate, everybody disappeared." . . .

The whole idea of us being Family Planning people caused problems for us to be able to do the immunization. So what we decided to do was to do a survey of the town, to get all the names, and this was something that we understood what the people used to do that gave—what the politicians used to do to give resources to a town or village. They would take a census of the village . . . and then take the census of everybody who lived in each house in the village and maybe there were 50 or 60 or 70 houses in the village or less, and there usually would be sometimes 10 or 15 people living in that one room mud hut. So we would just go in and say we're doing a census; and we'd go to the village Elder and talk to him and tell him first that we were going to do the census; and then we would tell him after we did the census when we had all of the—then we would ask the Elder if we could vaccinate the village and why. If the elder agreed then, we could go and start the vaccination.

So we would go, but we knew how many people were there. They would all sort of list all these children and you always knew that there was a child every year, so if you had a one-year-old that look like one, you would look for the baby somewhere underneath, hidden in blanket somewhere there was always a baby. So we would find a baby. So we would come back regularly to check every two or three days. Sometimes there wouldn't be the guard at the door and we say, "Okay, where is the guard?" and we had the guard and the vaccinator had a book in which he listed all the people he vaccinated so we'd know who were vaccinated . . .

As we went from village to village, I'd find another one and declare it then, I would culture the lesion and send it off to the post office and this is a big thing to do, to find a post office that would take this and send it off to Delhi. You'd never know if it would arrive there or not, because sometimes they didn't have stamps at the post office so you couldn't buy stamps and it was a complicated system that you had to try and figure out how to ensure that your specimen got sent.

So I kept sending them off and then we kept moving around from village to village; and the person who was in-charge of Uttar Pradesh at the time of the Smallpox Eradication Program was Don Francis and he would come to visit . . . to see what we were doing because they wanted to make sure, you know I was new, of what you were really doing and actually, I was a woman and they weren't sure women could do those things at that time. So Don came down and he said, "Listen, this place was declared free of smallpox and you are sending off all these sample saying there's smallpox. Are you sure these are smallpox?" I said, "As sure as I can be . . . All I can say is, to the best of my ability I call them smallpox." "Sure they weren't chickenpox?" "I think they were smallpox, it's a possibility that they were." He said, "Are you sure because you're causing a big sensation here." The leader, the Indian Public Health leader in the area was very upset because he had declared his districts free of smallpox and I was saying it wasn't. So that caused a little political problem . . .

Melissa McSwigan: Let me interrupt you for a second. How would you say that this experience that you had, the six months that you had in India, how would you say that affected your career after that?

Mary Guinan: Well, I became a believer. I believed that this was the way to go. I decided that I was going to have a career in public health because it was so successful. I mean, I couldn't believe it, what you were doing and all the things you were doing and all the problems you were having . . . and it's working. It's actually working, so you were reinvigorated to go out in the field and keep doing what you were doing because you can't really see the results and you often see the errors that are made and sometimes things slipped through the cracks, somebody didn't guard the patient, and did they possibly infect someone else and you had a whole trail of small-pox moving about. You're always worried about that, but it worked. So I decided to work in public health-that changed my life . . .

Melissa McSwigan: It sounds like you faced a lot of challenges before you went for the Smallpox Eradication Campaign. Particularly, you've talked a lot about being a woman and how that presented some obstacles as far as getting into school and so on. Did you find that in this particular campaign that being a woman affected the work that you were doing? You talked a little bit about when Don Francis, I think you said, came to visit you, how they kind of doubted maybe your effectiveness?

Mary Guinan: Well, they were worried. You know, as I would've been in Don's place. It turned out they were all smallpox. But I think it did affect the people—I think it helped me a lot. People were much more trusting of a woman than a man in that situation when I'd go into a village.

Melissa McSwigan: That was as far as the Indians were concerned?

Mary Guinan: Yeah, as far as the Indians were concerned. Because I was such a curiosity to them; and also, people helped me a lot . . . We had problems traversing the rivers and the only way to get across was a boat, a camel or an elephant. So there were always camel drivers and we would just wait until a camel came along then I would rent the camel and then we'd get across; and how I got back from over the other side: we'd hope another camel would come or somebody would show up with a rowboat and would row us across. We'd pay them to take us across.

So one day, while we're working in the village, this local Raja Saab they call him came, and he said, "What are you doing?" And I told him what we were doing and he said, "That's wonderful." He said, "Well, since you're having this difficulty, I have an elephant and I'm going to give you an elephant so you can have this elephant to go across the river." So I got this elephant. I mean elephants swim and they're wonderful. Camels are nasty and they want to bite you. It's really difficult getting on a camel . . . [The] elephant [was] very sweet and there was a Mahout, an elephant driver, and he said to me, "When the elephant swims over this river, he will take you up in his trunk, so you won't get wet." I said, "No. No. I'm not doing that. I'll get wet-it's okay if I get wet." So when we would go across . . . [the elephant was female] she would take the Mahout in her trunk and carry him over, and swim to the other side and then I'd go; and then we'd come back and then somehow somebody would call an elephant. The elephant would come and then take me back to the other side. Of course Don Francis heard about this naturally, and he came saying he wants an elephant ride. He came down, he says, "I want my first ride." So he got an elephant ride.

I think this man, because I was a woman, he thought I needed help in getting across and so, he gave me an elephant. I gave it back to him. I didn't take it home.

Source: Guinan, Mary. (2008). "Mary Guinan Oral History—India." Interview by Melissa McSwigan. *The Global Health Chronicles.* http://www.globalhealth chronicles.org/items/show/3539.

ANALYSIS

For many idealistic health workers from the world's wealthiest countries, their experiences shaped their own identities and their futures. As William Foege said of his time with the smallpox eradication campaign in Nigeria, "To practice community health in another culture requires an understanding and appreciation of that culture. But it's also arrogant to assume you can truly understand it . . . As much as we learned, the differences between the villagers' experience and ours always remained starkly evident. For one thing, we could leave any time we wanted. For another, we had access to basic health knowledge and the money to be able to apply it, while the villagers did not. To cite just one example, we arrived in the village at the end of a whooping cough epidemic. The characteristic coughs, or whoops, which often go on for weeks, persisted throughout the village at night during our early weeks in the village, making clear the price paid for not having routine childhood immunizations. We were able to provide our child not only with immunizations but also with prophylaxis against malaria, screened windows to protect against mosquitoes, bed nets, and safe water. The villagers could not do this for their children. They did not have access to such basic health practices. They had to spend the little money they had, the equivalent of $1 per day, on food and shelter" (Foege, 2011, 33–34).

Both Mary Guinan and her supervisor, Don Francis, returned to the United States in time to become key figures in the CDC's effort to control HIV and AIDS. They found themselves practicing community medicine in the United States, using techniques of surveillance as the first incidents of lethal disease spiraled into an epidemic. They appear as characters in the 1993 movie *And the Band Played On*, with Glenne Headly as Guinan and Matthew Modine as Francis.

FURTHER READING

Bhattacharya, Sanjoy. (2006). *Expunging Variola—The Control and Eradication of Smallpox in India, 1947–1977*. New Delhi: Orient Longman.

Bhattacharya, Sanjoy, Mark Harrison, and Michael Warboys. (2005). *Fractured States: Smallpox, Public Health, and Vaccination Policy in British India 1800–1947*. New Delhi: Orient Longman.

Foege, William. (2011). *House on Fire: The Fight to Eradicate Smallpox*. Berkeley, CA: University of California Press.

The Global Health Chronicles. A Collection of Materials on Public Health Efforts to Prevent, Control, and Eradicate Global Disease. http://globalhealthchronicles.org/.

Guinan, Mary. (2016). *Adventures of a Female Medical Detective: In Pursuit of Smallpox and AIDS*. Baltimore, MD: Johns Hopkins University Press.

THE END OF POLIO

- **Document:** "Ending an Outbreak: The Importance of Strong Surveillance"
- **Date:** 2015
- **Where:** Ethiopia, Kenya, Somalia
- **Significance:** Smallpox eradication in 1977 was heralded as a major public health triumph, and many public health officials looked forward to future eradication efforts in order to save the lives of still more millions of children. For many groups, polio seemed the ideal target: its biology seemed well-understood, there was an existing vaccine for it, and philanthropies like the Rotary Club had been raising money for it for years. In 1988, the polio eradication campaign was launched, with the stated goal of eliminating polio by the start of the 21st century. By the year 2000, there was a 99% worldwide decrease in cases of polio.

  That last 1%, however, has proven much harder to achieve. The efforts of local community health leaders have been crucial, as the documents in this section show.

DOCUMENT

No "polio-free" without surveillance

In June, an outbreak response assessment team in the Horn of Africa declared that transmission of poliovirus has been interrupted in Ethiopia and Kenya. The site of an outbreak of polio two years ago that led to the paralysis of 223 children across Ethiopia, Kenya and Somalia, the Horn of Africa has seen an outbreak response that has increased population immunity, strengthened community engagement and extended surveillance systems.

The assessment sought to determine whether or not polio transmission has been stopped, to outline the work still be done to achieve and maintain polio-free status, and to provide recommendations for strengthening acute flaccid paralysis (AFP) surveillance across the region. AFP is the symptom that indicates the possible presence of poliovirus, yet it can also have other causes. Surveillance systems must be strong enough to pick up on every case of AFP and ensure it is tested for polio in order to be 100 % sure that it is caused by something other than polio, that polio is not present in the country. This is why strengthening surveillance plays such an important role in closing polio outbreaks.

In all three outbreak countries, efforts were taken to strengthen contact with at-risk populations, particularly pastoral and nomadic communities as a way to involve them in surveillance. By identifying water points and markets, engaging with nutrition and water, sanitation and hygiene programmes, and veterinarian services, plans were strengthened to ensure children from these communities didn't slip through the net. In Somalia, joint human and animal vaccinations were held in Puntland, which reached 26,400 children with the oral polio vaccine (OPV), measles vaccines and vitamin A tablets, 36% of whom had never received the polio vaccine before. In Ethiopia, social mobilisers succeeded in informing parents of the risks of polio and upcoming campaigns in 80 % of the Somali region. Making these connections and raising awareness helps communities understand the importance of looking for and reporting AFP cases.

Further to go

In Somalia, while immunity in urban areas and amongst mobile population has improved, there remain significant concerns about rural communities. Only 68 of 115 districts are fully accessible, leaving around 350,000 under 5s unreached by polio vaccines. The assessment team determined that it was premature to close the outbreak in Somalia and recommended a minimum of 12 months without detection of poliovirus and with good and validated surveillance before a decision can be made.

While surveillance was considered sufficient in Ethiopia and Kenya to declare confidently that transmission has stopped, the assessment team emphasised that there was much further to go to expand and strengthen surveillance in all three countries in order to keep children in the region safe from polio.

While Somalia saw an improvement in surveillance following the outbreak, the assessment team found enough gaps not to be confident that transmission has stopped.

The people at the heart of surveillance

For every 100,000 children under the age of 15, a strong surveillance system would expect to pick up on one to two cases of AFP. Every district that does not identify and report this one case per 100,000 is therefore labelled a 'silent' district, as those AFP cases are not reaching the ears of those in the surveillance system. In all countries, being able to test that one case for polio in a laboratory is the one thing that enables the system to reliably vouch for the presence or absence of polio. And ultimately, it is that knowledge that will enable us to corner and eliminate the threat of the virus for ever.

'Active' surveillance is the most useful tool in tackling silent districts, and is being expanded in Ethiopia, Kenya and Somalia. Amina Ismail is a surveillance officer in Kenya who works to improve the sensitivity of surveillance by visiting health centres, schools, traditional healers and any other sites that could pick up on AFP cases, strengthening the knowledge of the people who form the heart of the system.

"Through my work, I ensure that every health worker knows about the polio eradication initiative and they know the case definition of AFP. This means it is not likely that they can miss a case," explains Amina. "We have community health workers especially in hard to reach areas that are helping in active case searches. Our confidence in the strength of the surveillance system lies in the knowledge of health workers.

"As we approach the end of polio across Africa I am getting more energy, because once we have eradicated polio I will have achieved something that I will be able to tell my grandchildren: that I was key in eradicating a very serious disease in this world. So that is what is pushing me; surveillance is part of polio eradication history."

Source: "Ending an Outbreak: The Importance of Strong Surveillance." (2015, June 26). *Polio Global Eradication Initiative.* http://www.polioeradication .org/mediaroom/newsstories/Ending-an-Outbreak—The-Importance-of-Strong -Surveillance/tabid/526/news/1251/Default.aspx. Used by permission of the Global Polio Eradication Initiative, World Health Organization.

- **Document:** "The People at the Heart of Polio Eradication in Afghanistan"
- **Date:** 2015
- **Where:** Afghanistan

DOCUMENT

... Meet religious leaders, health care workers, volunteer vaccinators, programme monitors and parents as they play their unique roles in protecting children across the country from polio.

Ensuring that no child is missed during polio vaccination campaigns in Afghanistan is essential to securing a polio-free future for its children, and children around the world. More than 65,000 people across the country are volunteering and working towards this goal ... [including] supervisors who are transporting polio vaccines for an upcoming campaign to the remote districts and villages of Kunar province.

Living with polio

Ashoqullah is just three years old, and his right arm and leg have been paralysed by polio. He never received a dose of the oral polio vaccine because vaccinators had not visited his village, Dama Kohistanat, in the Behsood district of Nangarhar province. Campaigns in 2015 need to reach every single child with multiple rounds of polio vaccines in Afghanistan, so that children ... are protected against polio which is incurable, meaning that those affected are crippled for life.

Paediatricians

Mirwais Hospital in Kandahar city is a very busy place, and Doctor Mohammad Sidiq is a very busy man. As a Senior Pediatrican and acute flaccid paralysis (AFP) focal point for the hospital, he sees many children every day. He checks to see whether they have been vaccinated and, in case of a child presenting with floppiness or weakness in their arms or legs, he informs his WHO colleague who collects a stool sample for laboratory testing. AFP surveillance is one of the core pillars of global polio eradication efforts. According to Dr. Sidiq, '. . . polio vaccination campaigns are the key solution to eradicate poliovirus from all places in the country.'

Pharmacists

'As a pharmacist, I am often in touch with people more than a doctor is, especially with the villagers', says Shah Mahmmod Qurishi, a pharmacist in downtown Kandahar city. When parents come to him, he asks them if the vaccination team reached their home or not. There are still some parents who do not see the need for their children to be vaccinated every round, thinking that one time is enough. So the pharmacist explains to them that all children, including new-borns, need to receive two drops, every single time the vaccinators come to call. As a volunteer working in AFP surveillance, he also refers children with weak or floppy limbs to the AFP focal point, who then informs WHO so that a stool sample can be taken to the laboratory to be tested for polio.

Vaccinators

Hamid Ullah works as a volunteer vaccinator within Spinboldak city in Kandahar province. On campaign days, he eagerly sets to work with his team, going house-to-house to vaccinate every child under 5 years in the area. While his team mate vaccinates children and marks their finger as evidence for the monitors that they have received the vaccine, his role is to fill in the tally sheet, to record when children weren't able to be vaccinated in each household so that they can be reached another time, and to mark every door. The door-marking indicates how many children were vaccinated in every home, enabling the monitors to check that no child is missed.

Campaign monitors

Nargis is a 22 year old Post Campaign Monitor in Jalalabad city, Nangarhar province. She trains vaccinators on how to carry out and monitor campaigns properly. After each polio campaign, Nargis checks doors and finger markings through household visits to assess the performance of the campaigns. Post campaign assessment helps the polio programme to estimate the number of children vaccinated, and to track the number of and reason for missed children. 'There are many problems that we have to handle through different methods and techniques in order to obtain reliable information,' says Nargis.

Campaign monitors

At Asadabad Central Hospital in the capital of Kunar province, an Afghan mobile vaccinator marks the finger of a little girl who has been given the oral polio vaccine as part of a polio campaign. These dots of ink on the finger make it possible for monitors to check which children have received protection, and which still need the crucial dose of the vaccine that each campaign seeks to provide.

Religious leaders

Masoom Jan is a preacher at Etifaq Mina Mosque in Paktia province of Eastern region. 'Islam has not forbidden vaccination drives, which are to benefit members of a society and to keep them healthy and strong,' he explains to parents. 'One of my happiest moment in the mosque is when I inform the residents during Friday prayers that a polio vaccination campaign is about to start in the province.'

Female volunteer vaccinators

Like their male colleagues, female volunteer vaccinators leave the Team Support Centre in the mornings with a supply of vaccines, ready to go house-to-house during polio campaign days. They vaccinate all children below 5 years, ask in each household for any child with floppiness/weakness, mark fingers and doors, and record on their tally sheet. 'As female volunteers, we are serving our community and at the same time we do have access to ladies in the houses,' says one vaccinator. While women working during a campaign is accepted in Jalalabad, and can make it easier for vaccinators to enter a home, it can be challenging in other provinces depending on cultural norms, where it may not be acceptable for women to work outside the home.

Families

Families have a crucial role to play in the eradication of polio. Most families are made aware of the threat of polio and the importance of vaccines by media campaigns, preachers, village elders and teachers. Mohammad Nasir is 61 years old and has three children under the age of 5, and grandchildren from his older children in Gardez City of Paktia province. He knows all about the dangers of polio, and has always vaccinated his family. 'They are my life and my only hope for the future is to have healthy children. I cannot see innocent children being paralyzed.'

The end goal

[Vaccinated children have dots on] their fingers which show that they were reached with polio vaccines during a polio vaccine campaign on the outskirts of Kandahar city. The hard work of every single person involved in polio campaigns and the love of the parents of children like these results in their being protected against polio for life. These hard working individuals are just some of thousands going house-to-house during each and every day of campaigns to reaching children with the polio vaccine. Afghanistan and neighbouring Pakistan will be the countries to take the world over the finishing line of polio eradication—thanks to the people from all walks of life who commit their time and passion to seeing the job done.

Source: "The People at the Heart of Polio Eradication in Afghanistan." (2015, August 6). Photo Essay. Polio Global Eradication Campaign. http://www.polioe radication.org/Mediaroom/Photos/Photoessays.aspx#prettyPhoto[Afghanistan]/0/. Used by permission of the Global Polio Eradication Initiative, World Health Organization.

ANALYSIS

The polio eradication campaign has proven much more controversial than the campaign to eradicate smallpox. A lot of the reason lies in the word *eradication.* No one would question a campaign to eliminate polio or any other disease as an ongoing threat to the world's children, if it could be done quickly, easily, and cheaply. That was the original premise of the WHO in 1988. Unfortunately, the campaign proved to be neither quick and easy nor cheap. *Eradication* means "eliminating every single incidence of the disease," and polio is much harder to get rid of than smallpox. It spreads more easily, patients can infect other people before showing any symptoms, and it is endemic in some of the most dangerous, war-torn areas of the world, with the fewest opportunities for primary health care of any kind.

Some of the problems of polio had to do with limits of vaccine technology. The original eradication efforts were based on use of the Sabin oral vaccine, which had proved so effective in industrialized countries. But the Sabin vaccine used an attenuated but still live virus, and there were outbreaks of polio that could be directly linked to that vaccine. Naturally, that hampered polio immunization efforts in those communities. An updated version of the Salk vaccine, which completely inactivated the virus, was improved and introduced very successfully. But communities who had participated in the early polio vaccination efforts were unhappy at being told they needed still more vaccines. If this medicine was supposed to be so valuable, why had scientists not gotten it right the first time around?

But at the heart of the polio eradication controversy was the question of opportunity costs: why were all those billions of dollars being spent on polio, when they could have been better spent on building up primary health-care systems? If the world's poorest families had basic health care available to them, clinics and regular checkups and school screenings—all the infrastructure available in industrialized nations at the start of the 20th century—then there would be no need for a polio eradication campaign. Millions of children's lives would be saved by regular immunizations, according to the schedule set by WHO itself. Not to mention the benefits that would come from ongoing doctor's visits and community health education.

William Muraskin, author of *Polio Eradication and Its Discontents*, has stated, "Polio was not a disease that was eradicated because of a massive demand from the countries that suffered from polio. It wasn't a disease that was being eradicated because polio experts wanted it to be eradicated . . . In the 1980s . . . most of the world's health community said, No more of these vertical, come in, eradicate, and leave programs. We want primary health care, we want to build routine immunization systems, we want systems that will last for ever, and will produce and deliver health goods to children into the future." Muraskin argues that a small but determined group of world health leaders, backed by an equally determined cluster of philanthropies like the Rotary Club and the Bill and Melinda Gates Foundation, called for polio eradication as a public health tool. Their goal was to show that smallpox eradication had not been a one-shot deal. Instead, eradication as an ongoing public health strategy could work on a global level.

Muraskin is not convinced that it has. "The opportunity costs" of the eradication efforts to the developing world, he noted, "are very high." That high-cost, top-down effort was bought at the price of primary health care. "The attraction of eradication," he explained, "is that it appeals to politicians and philanthropists because they feel they're going to get something for it. I give my money and I get eradication: there's a beginning, a middle, and an end." In contrast, "building long-term structures is not glamorous." It takes ongoing maintenance, and its outcomes are harder to measure.

Health-care experts on the ground with the polio campaign disagree with Muraskin. As of 2014, there were fewer than 200 polio cases worldwide; in 2015, there were 73 cases of what is called "wild poliovirus"—that is, from the disease occurring naturally in the population—and 28 induced by the Sabin vaccine. "The countries where polio eradication has not happened," explained Philippe Duclos from the WHO, ". . . are areas where health systems are weak, access is a problem, security may be a problem as well, so everything comes together . . ." As he noted, "There are big debates, what is the legacy of the polio program . . . But this infrastructure" created for the polio eradication campaign "in many places, it's the only infrastructure that exists. Polio has more than 10,000 people in the field," while primary health care has very few people in hard-pressed areas. That means that whatever happens with primary health care for the world's most vulnerable children, according to Duclos, "it's already dependent on polio infrastructure" (Finnegan, 2014).

These debates will continue. Eradication advocates are already thinking about the next disease to target. Some of the candidates for eradication via immunization include measles, mumps, and rubella. But for other diseases with more complex causes, other kinds of interventions may be more effective. Malaria, for example, can be eliminated more easily by eradicating the parasite that spreads it than by vaccine. And guinea worm disease, which affected an estimated 3.5 million people worldwide, had been reduced to 22 cases in 2015, largely as a result of community education efforts.

FURTHER READING

Finnegan, Gary. (2014). "Is Polio Eradication Worth It? *Vaccines Today.* http://www .vaccinestoday.eu/vaccines-for-me/is-polio-eradication-worth-it/.

"How the Focus on Polio Eradication in Nigeria Undermines Itself." *Humanosphere.* http:// www.humanosphere.org/global-health/2014/11/how-the-focus-on-polio-eradication -in-nigeria-undermines-itself/.

Muraskin, William. (2012). *Polio Eradication and Its Discontents: A Historian's Journey Through an International Public Health (Un)Civil War.* Telangana, India: Orient Blackswan.

"War-Torn Somalia Eradicates Polio." (2008). *BBC News.* http://news.bbc.co.uk/2/hi/africa/ 7312603.stm.

Yahya, Maryam. (2007). "Polio Vaccines: 'No Thank You!' Barriers to Polio Eradication in Northern Nigeria." *African Affairs* 106: 185–204.

NEW EPIDEMICS, NEW VACCINES?

- **Document:** Brant Goode, "Stories from the Field"
- **Date:** January 2015
- **Where:** Liberia
- **Significance:** As the CDC reminds us, viruses and bacteria are only a plane ride away. As global communication and transportation networks expand, so too do the opportunities for serious infectious diseases. Outbreaks of Ebola virus disease in 2014 and of Zika virus in 2015–2016 raise most basic health-care questions for the 21st century: do we rely on quarantine, or do we seek new vaccines?

DOCUMENT

As the world is witnessing, Liberia is experiencing severe impact from Ebola among both the general population and healthcare workers. Around the time of my deployment, 18 of 24 infected healthcare workers at the C.H. Rennie Hospital in Kakata died from Ebola, including the lead infection preventionist. To be sure, this scenario heightened the world's urgency to slow and stop the spread of Ebola. I knew that I could help.

After undergoing training at CDC headquarters in Atlanta, I traveled to Liberia to aid infection prevention and control (IPC) efforts. My work included training healthcare workers and community members, providing expert technical assistance to Government of Liberia personnel, and consulting with partners including the World Health Organization (WHO), UNICEF, and Save the Children.

One of the things that surprised me most as I traveled from clinic to clinic in Liberia was the emphasis on the use of personal protective equipment (PPE) for infection control. With over 25 years of experience, I knew that while PPE is important, there are other important IPC measures, and these other measures were not being as actively embraced. IPC efforts should include safe practices that remove hazards to begin with, and I was concerned that if facilities didn't implement these IPC measures in addition to PPE, case counts would increase and the facilities' already limited resources would be stretched even further.

DID YOU KNOW?

Zika: "Carried Widely by International Travel"

Zika virus, transmitted by *aedes* mosquitos, is everything we do not want to have in an epidemic disorder. It was first identified in Uganda in 1947 and subsequently spread across Africa and Asia, causing a mild illness. By 2007, though, it had created a larger-scale outbreak on the island of Yap in the Federated States of Micronesia. By 2013, it had spread further across the South Pacific, and researchers reported more serious effects. In 2015, Zika was reported in Brazil and other areas of South and Central America, and infants whose mothers had contracted Zika while pregnant were found to have a higher incidence of microcephaly, smaller than usual heads. Outbreaks of Zika were also associated with Guillain-Barré syndrome, an autoimmune disorder. In the past, the geographical spread of Zika would have been linked to the mosquitos that transmitted it. But since the 19th century, the *aedes* mosquitos, which also transmit yellow fever, have demonstrated they can travel around the world. As the WHO Zika timeline puts it, "The future transmission of Zika infection is likely to coincide mainly with the distribution of Aedes mosquito vectors, although there may be rare instances of person-to-person transmission (other than mother to child, e.g. through semen). Beyond the range of mosquitos, infection has been, and will continue to be, carried widely by international travel" (Kindhauser et al., 2016).

Researchers have said that a vaccine might be available by early 2018. New scientific methods involve using only part of the virus's DNA to create the vaccine in order to avoid serious adverse effects that might be generated by the use of a whole virus, whether live or killed. Preliminary results have been promising, and clinical trials began in August 2016.

Of the many unknowns involved in new vaccine development, the major one for the Zika virus is its connection to Guillain-Barré syndrome. If the virus can produce an upswing in cases, would the vaccine do the same? "There will be a risk . . .," according to the director of the National Institute of Allergy and Infectious Diseases. Yet, with scientists predicting a global pandemic, "the risk of not having a vaccine overwhelms the risk" of Guillain-Barré syndrome. (cited in Maron, 2016).

Should a vaccine be developed and licensed by the FDA, its use will follow the recommendations of the ACIP, based on scientific evaluation of its efficacy and safety, burden of illness, values, and preferences.

Sources:

Kindhauser, Mary Kay, Tomas Allen, Veronika Frank, Ravi Shankar Santhana, and Christopher Dye. (2016). "Zika: The Origin and Spread of a Mosquito-Borne Virus." *Bulletin of the World Health Organization.* http://www. who.int/bulletin/online_first/16-171082/en/.

Maron, Dina Fine. (2016). "Zika Vaccine Could Solve One Problem while Stoking Another." *Scientific American.* http://www.scientificamerican.com/article/zika-vaccine-could-solve-one-problem-while-stoking-another/.

There are many things that should be emphasized in training personnel. When visiting outlying clinics, I taught personnel how to apply some of these IPC measures effectively. At the Weala Clinic, I used a role-playing exercise to teach the clinic's Officer in Charge (OIC) how to assess patients for Ebola before they entered the clinic's waiting area:

"My son is sick and needs medicine!" said the father of a patient.

The OIC stopped him at a distance from the clinic. "Wait there a moment. What's wrong with your son?"

The OIC stepped forward to triage the patient while maintaining a distance of at least two meters from him. From this, he was able to conclude that the patient met the probable case definition for Ebola. The OIC then directed both the patient and father to a different clinic entrance area specifically for Ebola patients. This protected other patients in the waiting area from potential exposure, as well as clinic staff.

One of the easiest and most important things facility managers can do is to strictly control access to clinics and hospitals (an engineering control) using fences where needed and choosing triage points that are located outside of the facility itself. This is especially important in areas where PPE is limited. I found that the C.H. Rennie Hospital had already instituted this kind of system by using chain-link fences with security and a single triage point. I urged another hospital to similarly triage patients at a separate location and they agreed it made sense to do so.

These are just some examples of how successfully prioritizing IPC efforts can lead to reduced transmission risk and better work flow. Measures such as identifying and training IPC leaders within healthcare facilities, implementing engineering controls such as fences to control access, determining appropriate locations to provide care to Ebola patients, and training other personnel to implement appropriate work practices should receive high priority if we are to save lives.

Source: Goode, Brant. (2015). "Stories from the Field: Brant Goode, RN/BSN, MPH, CDC Career Epidemiology Field Officer." http://www.cdc.gov/vhf/ebola/hcp/stories-brant-goode.html.

ANALYSIS

Whenever there are reports of new, frightening diseases, there is public outcry for vaccines to prevent their spread. We are all aware that people and the diseases they spread are hard to control. We can all see that, throughout history, devastating epidemics can be traced to population movements, large and small, through unprotected communities. Through Internet and television, we can see images of Ebola and Zika victims, and we can imagine all too readily what outbreaks might do to our own families, schools, cities, and countries.

As this excerpt shows, there are international organizations like the WHO, UNICEF, and the CDC that monitor outbreaks and take steps to control them. Brant Goode's description of his role in "IPC," infection prevention and control, shows what can be done even in epidemics for which there are no vaccines and no cures. As the WHO website explains, "Community engagement is key to successfully controlling outbreaks. Good outbreak control relies on applying a package of interventions, namely case management, surveillance and contact tracing, a good laboratory service, safe burials and social mobilisation" ("Ebola Virus Disease Fact Sheet." WHO. http://www.who.int/mediacentre/factsheets/fs103/en/).

These interventions are necessary, because vaccines take a long time to develop, typically 10–15 years. In the United States, all vaccines must be licensed by the federal government, and the entire development process is closely monitored. The first exploratory stage consists of basic research on microbe biology, which usually takes two to four years. The next, preclinical stage generally involves testing on animal subjects and can last from one to two years. The next stage is a formal application to the Food and Drug Administration (FDA) for an Investigational New Drug (IND), providing full details of both the previous research and the proposed new scientific study. All clinical details must be reviewed by a clinical review board to ensure that they comply with federal regulations.

If the IND application is approved, the proposed new vaccine undergoes three phases of testing. The first phase tests the vaccine on 20–80 healthy adults. Even if the vaccine is intended for children, it is first tested on adults. This takes about a year. The second phase tests several hundred adults at a time and includes randomized and double-blind studies. It takes about a year to complete. The third phase may test from 1,000–3,000 adults and is specifically designed to look for quality control problems in large-scale production and distribution. This can take about three years. All three phases must follow federal guidelines on informed consent so that all patients involved in the trials are aware of the risks involved.

If the phase three trials are successful, the manufacturer submits a biologics license application to the FDA. After a new vaccine is approved, the FDA may require additional clinical trials to monitor its long-term safety.

Candidates for an Ebola vaccine are currently in clinical trials, and results from phase one have been published. Clinical trials of vaccines for lethal microbes like Ebola virus cannot be ethically carried out on people, so the process has to be modified to allow more weight to be given to animal studies. It is an extremely complicated process, because there are five strains of the Ebola virus, and researchers must study the virology of each one. Since it is so deadly, the studies must be carried out with careful attention to all potential biohazards. Scientists believe it will be many years before a safe, effective Ebola vaccine is available.

It is a truism of virology that the more complicated the epidemiology of a disease, the harder it will be to develop effective vaccines against it. Scientists have been searching for a vaccine for malaria, one of the oldest of human diseases, for more than 40 years. There is one in phase three development, but even if proven effective, global health-care experts believe it will be used in conjunction with existing public health measures like mosquito control and anti-malarial pills. We can expect the CDC's efforts in IPC as well as community health partnerships to be key components of global health care for the 21st century.

FURTHER READING

"How the Ebola Outbreak and WHO's Response Unfolded." *World Health Organization*. http://www.who.int/csr/en/.

McNeil, Donald, Catherine St. Louis, and Nicholas St. Fleur. "Short Answers to Hard Questions About Zika Virus." *New York Times*, February 3, 2016. http://www.nytimes.com/interactive/2016/health/what-is-zika-virus.html?_r=0.

"Vaccine Development, Testing, and Regulation." *History of Vaccines*. http://www.historyofvaccines.org/content/articles/vaccine-development-testing-and-regulation.

Waters, A. P., M. M. Moa, M. R. van Dijk, and C. J. Janse. (2005). "Malaria Vaccines: Back to the Future?" *Science* New Series 307: 528–530.

"Zika Virus." *World Health Organization*. http://www.who.int/topics/zika/en/.

CHRONOLOGY

ca. 900 CE	Abu Bakr Muḥammad Ibn Zakariya al-Razi first distinguishes between smallpox and measles.
ca. 1000 CE	Smallpox inoculation recorded in China
1578	Epidemic of pertussis (whooping cough) recorded in Paris
1713	Emanuel Timonius writes an account of smallpox inoculation in Turkey to the Royal Society of London.
1717	Lady Mary Wortley Montagu writes a letter to a friend about her family's experiences with smallpox inoculation in Turkey. She becomes an advocate for the technique when she returns to Great Britain, sparking the first European dispute between inoculation advocates and adversaries.
1721	Smallpox outbreak in Boston, leading to the first inoculation in America and the first American dispute between advocates and adversaries
1769	Smallpox inoculation made illegal in Virginia
1777	Smallpox inoculation implemented in Continental Army during the U.S. War of Independence
1793–1795	Yellow fever epidemic in cities across the eastern seaboard
1798	Edward Jenner publishes *An Inquiry into the Causes and Effects of the Variolae Vaccinae, or Cowpox*, ushering in the modern era of vaccination.
1800	Benjamin Moseley publishes *A Treatise on Sugar with Miscellaneous Medical Observations*, a sensationalist work opposing Jenner's vaccination.
1802–1807	Vaccination techniques spread throughout Europe, Asia, and the Americas
1826	Pierre Bretonneau provides first clinical description of diphtheria.
1840s	Yellow fever spreads across Atlantic Ocean as global trade increases.

1853	The United Kingdom passes Vaccination Act requiring every child to be vaccinated by the age of four months.
1855	John Snow demonstrated the spread of cholera through contaminated water.
1861	Start of U.S. Civil War; vaccination against smallpox considered an essential military precaution
1865	Claude Bernard writes *An Introduction to the Study of Experimental Medicine*, which promotes scientific research standards in medicine.
1874	Germany passes Vaccination Law.
1876	Robert Koch demonstrates that the anthrax bacillus causes the disease. He develops Koch's Postulates, criteria used to determine whether a particular microorganism causes a particular disease.
1881	Louis Pasteur develops vaccine for anthrax.
1883	Robert Koch identifies cholera bacillus.
1885	Louis Pasteur develops vaccine for rabies.
1896	Development of vaccines for typhoid and cholera
1897	Development of the vaccine for bubonic plague
1901	Walter Reed and his team determine that yellow fever is transmitted by the *Aedes* mosquito.
1901–1903	Smallpox epidemic in the United States
	Death of nine children in Camden, New Jersey, from tetanus after being vaccinated for smallpox
	Tetanus outbreak in St. Louis after contaminated diphtheria antitoxin is administered
1902	U.S. Biologics Control Act
1905	U.S. Supreme Court case *Jacobson v. Massachusetts*, 197 U.S. 11, upheld the authority of states to enforce compulsory vaccination laws; last yellow fever epidemic in North America.
1914–1918	During World War I, fewer soldiers died from communicable diseases than in any previous war, due to vaccination.
1922	Carl Sandburg publishes *Rootabaga Stories*.
1923	Development of vaccine for diphtheria
1925	Great Race of Mercy in Alaska; statue of Balto erected in Central Park, New York City
1926	Development of vaccine for tetanus and pertussis (whooping cough)
1927	Development of vaccine for tuberculosis
1935	Development of vaccine for yellow fever
1936	Development of a vaccine for influenza
	Release of *The Story of Louis Pasteur*, directed by William Dieterle and starring Paul Muni

1938	Development of a vaccine for typhus
	Creation of the National Foundation for Infantile Paralysis, often called the March of Dimes
1955	U.S. Polio Vaccination Assistance Act; the "Cutter Incident"; development of an injected vaccine for polio
1963	Development of an oral vaccine for polio, and a vaccine for measles
1966	Henry Beecher publishes "Ethics in Clinical Research," leading to increased regulation of research on human subjects.
1967	Development of a vaccine for mumps
1969	Development of a vaccine for rubella
1974	Development of a vaccine for meningococcus
1977	Development of a vaccine for pneumococcus
1980	Smallpox eradicated worldwide; development of a vaccine for adenovirus
1981	Development of a vaccine for hepatitis B
1985	Development of a vaccine for H influenzae type b
1988	Launch of Global Polio Eradication Initiative
1989	Development of the modern vaccine for typhoid; poor vaccination rates among low-income children in the United States lead to measles outbreak
1992	Development of a vaccine for Japanese encephalitis
1994	U.S. Vaccines for Children program, providing funding to ensure that all children up to age 18 had access to recommended vaccines
1995	Development of a vaccine for varicella (chicken pox)
1996	Development of a vaccine for hepatitis A
1999	Development of a vaccine for rotavirus
2003	Development of a vaccine for cold-adapted influenza
2006	Development of vaccines for human papillomavirus (HPV) and zoster
2008	Measles outbreaks in the United States due to low vaccination rates
2010	U.S. Affordable Care Act, providing funding for all recommended vaccinations without co-pay
2013–2014	Outbreak of meningococcal B in the United States
2014	Development of meningococcal B vaccine

BIBLIOGRAPHY

Ackerknecht, Erwin. (1953). *Rudolf Virchow. Doctor, Statesman, Anthropologist.* Madison, WI: University of Wisconsin Press.

"An Act to Regulate the Inoculation of the Small-Pox within This Colony." (1821). In *The Statutes at Large: Being a Collection of All the Laws of Virginia,* edited by William Waller Hening. Richmond, VA: George Cochran, 371–374.

Advisory Committee on Immunization Practices (ACIP). (2010, October 27–28). *Summary Report.* Atlanta, GA. http://www.cdc.gov/vaccines/acip/meetings/downloads/min-archive/min-oct10.pdf.

Advisory Committee on Immunization Practices (ACIP). (2015a, June 24–25). *Summary Report.* Atlanta, GA. http://www.cdc.gov/vaccines/acip/meetings/downloads/min-archive/min-2015-06.pdf.

Advisory Committee on Immunization Practices (ACIP). (2015b, October 21). *Summary Report.* Atlanta, GA. http://www.cdc.gov/vaccines/acip/meetings/downloads/min-archive/min-2015-10.pdf.

Alaszewski, Andy. (2011). "How Campaigners and the Media Push Bad Science." *BMJ: British Medical Journal* 342: 231.

Alcott, Louisa May. (1863). *Hospital Sketches.* Boston, MA: James Redpath.

Alden, Dauril and Joseph Miller. (1987). "Out of Africa: The Slave Trade and the Transmission of Smallpox to Brazil, 1560–1831." *The Journal of Interdisciplinary History* 18: 195–224.

Allen, Arthur. (2007). *Vaccine: The Controversial Story of Medicine's Greatest Lifesaver.* New York: W. W. Norton & Company.

Allen, Arthur. (2014). *The Fantastic Laboratory of Dr. Weigl.* New York: W. W. Norton & Company.

al-Razi [Rhazes], Abu Bakr Muhammad Ibn Zakariya. (1848). *A Treatise on the Smallpox and Measles,* trans. William Greenhill. London: Sydenham Society.

America's Second Revolution. Civil War Philadelphia and Its Countryside. http://www.civilwarphilly.net/.

Anderson, Warwick. (2007). "Immunization and Hygiene in the Colonial Philippines." *Journal of the History of Medicine and Allied Sciences* 62: 1–20.

"Another Attack on Polio Workers in Pakistan Leaves 4 dead." (2014). Global Health. *Humanosphere*. http://www.humanosphere.org/global-health/2014/11/another-attack-polio-workers-pakistan-leaves-four-dead/.

"Anti Typhoid Vaccination for Vacationists." (1921, July 2). *Weekly Report of the Department of Health of the City of New York* 10 (27): 209.

Barnes, David. (2006). *The Great Stink of Paris and the Nineteenth-Century Struggle against Filth and Germs*. Baltimore, MD: Johns Hopkins University Press.

Baxby, Derrick. (1981). *Jenner's Smallpox Vaccine: The Riddle of Vaccinia Virus and Its Origin*. London: Heinemann Educational Books.

Bazin, Hervé. (2011). *Vaccination: A History from Lady Montagu to Genetic Engineering*. Esher, England: John Libbey Eurotext.

Becker, Ann. (2004). "Smallpox in Washington's Army: Strategic Implications of the Disease during the American Revolutionary War." *The Journal of Military History* 68: 381–430.

Beecher, Henry. (1966). "Ethics in Clinical Research." *New England Journal of Medicine* 274: 1354–1360. Reprinted in Jon Harkness, Susan Lederer, Daniel Winkler. (2001). "Laying Ethical Foundations for Clinical Research." *Bulletin of the World Health Organization* 79: 365–372. http://www.who.int/docstore/bulletin/pdf/2001/issue4/vol79.no.4.365-372.pdf.

Bellows, Henry. (1866). Sanitary Commission No. 26. Notes of a Preliminary Sanitary Survey of the Forces of the United States, in the Ohio and Mississippi Valleys, near Midsummer, 1861. Reprinted in Documents of the U.S. Sanitary Commission. New York.

Berish, Amy. "FDR and Polio." *Franklin D. Roosevelt Presidential Library and Museum*. https://fdrlibrary.org/polio.

Bernard, Claude. (1927). *Introduction to the Study of Experimental Medicine*, trans. Henry Copley Greene. New York: Henry Schuman, Inc.

Bhattacharya, Sanjoy. (2006). *Expunging Variola—The Control and Eradication of Smallpox in India, 1947–1977*. New Delhi: Orient Longman.

Bhattacharya, Sanjoy, Mark Harrison, and Michael Warboys. (2005). *Fractured States: Smallpox, Public Health, and Vaccination Policy in British India 1800–1947*. New Delhi: Orient Longman.

Biologics Control Act, Public Law 57-244, 57th Congress, 1st session, July 1, 1902. *Office of History, National Institutes of Health*. http://history.nih.gov/research/downloads/PL57-244.pdf.

Birch, John. (1817). *An Appeal to the Public on the Peril and Hazard of Vaccination, Otherwise Cow Pox*. London: J. Harris.

Biss, Eula. (2013). "Sentimental Medicine: Why We Still Fear Vaccines." *Harper's Magazine*. https://harpers.org/archive/2013/01/sentimental-medicine/.

Biss, Eula. (2014). *On Immunity: An Inoculation*. Minneapolis, MN: Graywolf Press.

Black, Francis. (1994). "An Explanation of High Death Rates among New World Peoples When in Contact with Old World Diseases." *Perspectives in Biology and Medicine* 37: 292–307.

Blake, John. (1952). "The Inoculation Controversy in Boston: 1721–1722." *New England Quarterly* 25: 489–506.

Blanplain, Jan. (1978). *National Health Insurance and Health Resources: The European Experience*. Cambridge, MA: Harvard University Press.

Bliss, Michael. (1999). *William Osler: A Life in Medicine*. New York: Oxford University Press.

Booker, John. (2008). *Maritime Quarantine: The British Experience 1650–1900*. Farnham, England: Ashgate Publishing.

Boylston, Zabdiel and Cotton Mather. (1721). *Some Account of What Is Said of Inoculating or Transplanting the Small Pox*. Boston, MA: S. Gerrish.

Bren, Linda. (2002). "The Road to the Biotech Revolution—Highlights of 100 Years of Biologics Regulation." *About FDA*. http://www.fda.gov/AboutFDA/WhatWeDo/History/FOrgsHistory/CBER/ucm135758.htm.

Brimnes, Niels. (2007). "Vikings against Tuberculosis: The International Tuberculosis Campaign in India, 1948–1951." *Bulletin of the History of Medicine* 81: 407–430.

Brock, Thomas. (1988). *Robert Koch, a Life in Medicine and Bacteriology*. Berlin: Springer-Verlag.

Brown, Megan. (2011). "A Shot in the Dark: Vaccinations and Redundant Risks." *Women's Studies Quarterly* 39: 141–160.

Brunton, Deborah. (2004). "Birch, John." "Moseley, Benjamin." *Oxford Dictionary of National Biography*. http://www.oxforddnb.com/.

Brunton, Deborah. (2008). *The Politics of Vaccination: Practice and Policy in England, Wales, Ireland, and Scotland, 1800–1874*. Rochester, NY: University of Rochester Press.

Bucchi, Massimiano. (1997). "The Public Science of Louis Pasteur: The Experiment on Anthrax Vaccine in the Popular Press of the Time." *History and Philosophy of the Life Sciences* 19: 181–209.

Buerki, Robert. (1971). "Reception of the Germ Theory of Disease in The American Journal of Pharmacy." *Pharmacy in History* 13: 158–168.

Burton, John. (2001). " 'The Awful Judgments of God Upon the Land': Smallpox in Colonial Cambridge, Massachusetts." *New England Quarterly* 74: 495–506.

Bynum, William. (1994). *Science and the Practice of Medicine in the Nineteenth Century*. New York: Cambridge University Press.

Caplow, Theodore, Louis Hicks, and Ben Wattenberg. (2001). *The First Measured Century: An Illustrated Guide to Trends in America, 1900–2000*. Washington, DC: AEI Press.

Carmichael, Ann and Arthur Silverstein. (1987). "Smallpox in Europe before the Seventeenth Century: Virulent Killer or Benign Disease?" *Journal of the History of Medicine* 42: 147–168.

Carrell, Jennifer. (2004). *The Speckled Monster: A Historical Tale of Battling Smallpox*. New York: Penguin Group.

Centers for Disease Control and Prevention. (2016a). "ACIP Charter." http://www.cdc.gov/vaccines/acip/committee/charter.html.

Centers for Disease Control and Prevention. (2016b). "ACIP Meeting Information." http://www.cdc.gov/vaccines/acip/meetings/meetings-info.html.

Centers for Disease Control and Prevention. (2016c). "Immunization Schedules for Preteens and Teens." http://www.cdc.gov/vaccines/schedules/easy-to-read/preteen-teen.html.

Chan, Margaret. (2012). "Keeping Promises: Accountability of Dr Margaret Chan during Her First Term as WHO Director-General." *World Health Organization*. http://www.who.int/dg/Report_card_cover_28_06.pdf?ua=1.

Chan, Margaret. (2015). "WHO Director-General Assesses Polio Situation in Pakistan." *World Health Organization*. http://www.who.int/dg/speeches/2015/pakistan-polio/en/.

Chatterjee, Archana, ed. (2013). *Vaccinophobia and Vaccine Controversies of the 21st Century*. New York: Springer.

Christensen, Povl Elo, Henning Schmidt, H. O. Bang, Vera Andersen, Bjarne Jordal, and Oskar Jensen. (1953). "An Epidemic of Measles in Southern Greenland, 1951. Measles in Virgin Soil." *Acta Medica Scandinavica* 144: 313–322.

"CIA Organised Fake Vaccination Drive to Get Osama bin Laden's Family DNA." (2011). *The Guardian*. http://www.theguardian.com/world/2011/jul/11/cia-fake-vaccinations -osama-bin-ladens-dna.

Clausen, Christopher. (2005). "The President and the Wheelchair." *The Wilson Quarterly* 29: 24–29.

Clendening, Logan, ed. (1942). *Source Book of Medical History*. New York: Dover Publications.

Clot, Antoine Barthelemy [Clot Bey]. (1838). "On the Medical Institutions of Cairo." *British and Foreign Medical Review* 11: 592–594.

Code of Federal Regulations of the United States of America. (1939). Title 35: Panama Canal.

Coleman, William. (1987). "Koch's Comma Bacillus: The First Year." *Bulletin of the History of Medicine* 61: 315–342.

Colgove, James. (2004). "Between Persuasion and Compulsion: Smallpox Control in Brooklyn and New York, 1894–1902." *Bulletin of the History of Medicine* 78: 349–378.

Colgrove, James. (2005). " 'Science in a Democracy': The Contested Status of Vaccination in the Progressive Era and the 1920s." *Isis* 96: 167–191.

Colgrove, James. (2006). *State of Immunity: The Politics of Vaccination in Twentieth-Century America*. Berkeley, CA: University of California Press.

Conis, Elena. (2013a). "A Mother's Responsibility: Women, Medicine, and the Rise of Contemporary Vaccine Skepticism in the United States." *Bulletin of the History of Medicine* 87: 407–435.

Conis, Elena. (2013b). *Vaccine Nation: America's Changing Relationship with Immunization*. Chicago: University of Chicago Press.

Cook, Harold. (1994). "Good Advice and Little Medicine: The Professional Authority of Early Modern English Physicians." *Journal of British Studies* 33: 1–31.

"Court Says Vaccine Not to Blame for Autism." (2009). *NBC News*. http://www.nbcnews .com/id/29160138/ns/health-mental_health/t/court-says-vaccine-not-blame-autism/.

Cowing, Hugh. (1895). "Notes on the Epidemic of Smallpox in Muncie." *The Cincinnati Lancet-Clinic* 74: 9–12.

Crosby, Alfred. (2004). *Ecological Imperialism: The Biological Expansion of Europe 900–1900*. New York: Cambridge University Press.

Cross, Gary and John Walton. (2005). *The Playful Crowd: Pleasure Places in the Twentieth Century*. New York: Columbia University Press.

Cunningham, Andrew and Roger French, eds. (1990). *The Medical Enlightenment of the Eighteen Century*. New York: Cambridge University Press.

Curtin, Philip. (1973). *The Image of Africa: British Ideas and Action, 1780–1850*. 2 vols. Madison, WI: University of Wisconsin Press.

Daemmrich, Arthur and Mary Ellen Bowden. (2005). "A Rising Drug Industry." *Chemical and Engineering News* Special Issue 83. http://pubs.acs.org/cen/coverstory/83/8325/ 8325intro.html.

Dammann, Gordon and Alfred Jay Bollet. (2008). *Images of Civil War Medicine*. New York: Demos.

"Data and Statistics." (2016). National Vaccine Injury Compensation Program. *Health Resources and Services Administration*. http://www.hrsa.gov/vaccinecompensation/data/ statisticsreport.pdf.

Davies, Hugh. (2007). "Ethical Reflections on Edward Jenner's Experimental Treatment." *Journal of Medical Ethics* 33: 174–176.

Day, Alison. (2013). " 'The Magical Formula': Reactions and Responses to Diphtheria Immunisation in New Zealand 1920–1960." *Health and History* 15: 53–71.

De Kruif, Paul. (1926). *The Microbe Hunters*. New York: Harcourt Brace and Company.

Dear, Peter. (2001). *Revolutionizing the Sciences: European Knowledge and Its Ambitions, 1500–1700*. Princeton, NJ: Princeton University Press.

Debru, Claude. (1997). "On the Usefulness of the History of Science for Scientific Education." *Notes and Records of the Royal Society of London* 51: 291–307.

Deer, Brian. (2004, February 22). "Revealed: MMR Research Scandal." *The Sunday Times*. http://briandeer.com/mmr/lancet-deer-1.htm.

DeLancey, Dayle. (2010). "Vaccinating Freedom: Smallpox Prevention and the Discourses of African American Citizenship in Antebellum Philadelphia." *Journal of African American History* 95: 296–321.

DePauw, Linda Grant. (1981). "Women in Combat: The Revolutionary War Experience." *Armed Forces and Society* 7: 209–226.

Devine, Shauna. (2014). *Learning from the Wounded: The Civil War and the Rise of American Medical Science*. Chapel Hill: The University of North Carolina Press.

Dewey, Frank. (1983). "Thomas Jefferson's Law Practice: The Norfolk Anti-Inoculation Riots." *Virginia Magazine of History and Biography* 91: 39–53.

"The Diphtheria Antitoxin and Tetanus Outbreak in St. Louis." (1902). *The Sanitarian* 48: 32–34.

"Disease Eradication." *History of Vaccines*. http://www.historyofvaccines.org/content/articles/disease-eradication.

Dobson, Mary. (1997). *Contours of Death and Disease in Early Modern England*. Cambridge, England: Cambridge University Press.

Douglass, William. (1722). *Inoculation of the Small Pox as Practised in Boston, Consider'd in a Letter to A—S—M.D. & F.R.S. in London*. Boston, MA: J. Franklin.

Dr. Ehrlich's Magic Bullet. (1940). Directed by William Dieterle. Warner Brothers.

Dr. Jenner's House and Garden. http://www.jennermuseum.com/.

Dubos, René. (1960). *Pasteur and Modern Science*. Garden City, NY: Anchor Books.

Duffy, John. (1978). "School Vaccination: The Precursor to School Medical Inspection." *Journal of the History of Medicine and Allied Sciences* 33: 344–355.

Duncan, S. R., Susan Scott, and C. J. Duncan. (1994). "Smallpox Epidemics in Cities in Britain." *Journal of Interdisciplinary History* 25: 255–271.

Durbach, Nadja. (2002). "Class, Gender, and the Conscientious Objector to Vaccination, 1898–1907." *Journal of British Studies* 41: 58–83.

Durbach, Nadja. (2005). *Bodily Matters: The Anti-Vaccination Movement in England, 1853–1907*. Durham, England: Duke University Press.

Dyer, R. E. (1944). "The Role of Immunization in Wartime Advances in Medicine." *Proceedings of the American Philosophical Society* 88: 182–188.

Echenberg, Myron. (2011). *Africa in the Time of Cholera: A History of Pandemics from 1817 to the Present*. New York: Cambridge University Press.

"Ending an Outbreak: The Importance of Strong Surveillance." (2015, June 26). Polio Global Eradication Initiative. http://www.polioeradication.org/mediaroom/newsstories/Ending-an-Outbreak—The-Importance-of-Strong-Surveillance/tabid/526/news/1251/Default.aspx.

Fahmy, Khaled. (1997). *All the Pasha's Men: Mehmed Ali, His Army, and the Making of Modern Egypt*. Cairo: American University in Cairo Press.

Fairchild, Amy, Ronald Bayer, James Colgrove, and Daniel Wolfe. (2007). *Searching Eyes: Privacy, the State, and Disease Surveillance in America*. Berkeley, CA: University of California Press.

"FDR Timeline." *Franklin D. Roosevelt Presidential Library and Museum.* http://www.fdrlibrary.marist.edu/archives/resources/timeline.html.

"Federal Control of Vaccine Virus." (1905). *Western Druggist* 27: 433–434.

Fenn, Elizabeth. (2001). *Pox Americana: The Great Smallpox Epidemic of 1775–1782.* New York: Hill and Wang.

Few, Martha. (2010). "Circulating Smallpox Knowledge: Guatemalan Doctors, Maya Indians and Designing Spain's Smallpox Vaccination Expedition, 1780–1803." *British Journal for the History of Science* 43: 519–537.

Finger, Simon. (2010). "An Indissoluble Union: How the American War for Independence Transformed Philadelphia's Medical Community and Created a Public Health Establishment." *Pennsylvania History* 77: 37–72.

Finger, Simon. (2012). *The Contagious City: The Politics of Public Health in Early Philadelphia.* Ithaca, NY: Cornell University Press.

Finnegan, Gary. (2014). "Is Polio Eradication Worth It?" *Vaccines Today.* http://www.vaccinestoday.eu/vaccines-for-me/is-polio-eradication-worth-it/.

Fisher, Barbara Loe. (2008). "Vaccine Safety Research Priorities: Engaging the Public." *National Vaccine Information Center.* http://www.nvic.org/injury-compensation/nationalvaccine.aspx.

Fisher, Richard. (1991). *Edward Jenner 1749–1823.* London: André Deutsch.

Fleming, John. (1982). "Drug Injury Compensation Plans." *The American Journal of Comparative Law* 30: 297–323.

Foege, William. (2011). *House on Fire: The Fight to Eradicate Smallpox.* Berkeley, CA: University of California Press.

Ford, William. (1911). "The Life and Work of Robert Koch." *Bulletin of the Johns Hopkins Hospital* 22: 415–425.

Fortune, Robert. (1989). *Chills and Fever: Health and Disease in the Early History of Alaska.* Fairbanks, AK: University of Alaska Press.

Fuess, Harald. (2014). "Informal Imperialism and the 1879 'Hesperia' Incident: Containing Cholera and Challenging Extraterritoriality in Japan." *Japan Review* 27: 103–140.

Fulford, Tim and Debbie Lee. (2000). "The Jenneration of Disease: Vaccination, Romanticism, and Revolution." *Studies in Romanticism* 39: 139–163.

Galambos, Louis, with Jane Eliott Sewell. (1995). *Networks of Innovation: Vaccine Development at Merck, Sharp & Dohme, and Mulford, 1895–1995.* New York: Cambridge University Press.

Gates, Henry Louis Jr. " '12 Years a Slave': Trek from Slave to Screen." *The African Americans: Many Rivers to Cross.* http://www.pbs.org/wnet/african-americans-many-rivers-to-cross/history/12-years-a-slave-trek-from-slave-to-screen/.

Geison, Gerald. (1978). "Pasteur's Work on Rabies: Reexamining the Ethical Issues." *The Hastings Center Report* 8: 26–33.

Geison, Gerald. (1995). *The Private Science of Louis Pasteur.* Princeton, NJ: Princeton University Press.

Geist, Edward. (2012). "When Ice Cream Was Poisonous: Adulteration, Ptomaines, and Bacteriology in the United States, 1850–1910." *Bulletin of the History of Medicine* 86: 333–360.

German Empire. (1904). *Vaccination Law of April 8, 1874.* Berlin: B. Paul.

Gilje, Paul. (1996). *Rioting in America.* Bloomington, IN: Indiana University Press.

Gillette, Mary. (1981). *The Army Medical Department 1775–1818.* Washington, DC: Government Printing Office. http://history.amedd.army.mil/booksdocs/rev/gillett1/default.html.

Global Alliance for Vaccines and Immunization (GAVI). *The Vaccine Alliance.* http://www
.gavi.org/.

*The Global Health Chronicles. A Collection of Materials on Public Health Efforts to Prevent,
Control, and Eradicate Global Disease.* http://globalhealthchronicles.org/.

Global Immunization Data. (2013, July). http://apps.who.int/immunization_monitoring/
Global_Immunization_Data_v2.pdf?ua=1.

Glynn, Ian and Jenifer Glynn. (2004). *The Life and Death of Smallpox.* New York: Cambridge
University Press.

Goode, Brant. "Stories from the Field: Brant Goode, RN/BSN, MPH, CDC Career Epidemiology Field Officer." http://www.cdc.gov/vhf/ebola/hcp/stories-brant-goode.html.

Gorgas, William. (1911). "Report of Maj. W. C. Gorgas, Medical Corps, United States
Army." In *Yellow Fever, A Compilation of Various Publications,* James Carroll, William
Crawford Gorgas, Robert Latham Owen, and Walter Drew McCaw. Washington,
DC: Government Printing Office, 234–238.

Gould, Tony. (1997). *A Summer Plague: Polio and Its Survivors.* New Haven, CT: Yale
University Press.

Gradmann, Christophe. (2009). *Laboratory Disease: Robert Koch's Medical Bacteriology.*
Baltimore, MD: Johns Hopkins University Press.

Grainger, Samuel. (1721). *The Imposition of Inoculation as a Duty Religiously Considered.*
Boston, MA: Nicholas Boone, *National Library of Medicine.* http://collections.nlm
.nih.gov/bookviewer?PID=nlm:nlmuid-2555032R-bk.

The Great Fever. The American Experience. PBS.org. http://www.pbs.org/wgbh/amex/fever/
index.html.

Grundy, Isobel. (2001). *Lady Mary Wortley Montagu, Comet of the Enlightenment.* Oxford,
England: Oxford University Press.

Guerrini, Anita. (2003). *Experimenting with Humans and Animals: From Galen to Animal
Rights.* Baltimore, MD: The Johns Hopkins University Press.

Guinan, Mary. (2008). "Mary Guinan Oral History—India." Interview by Melissa
McSwigan. *The Global Health Chronicles.* http://www.globalhealthchronicles.org/
items/show/3539.

Guinan, Mary. (2016). *Adventures of a Female Medical Detective: In Pursuit of Smallpox and
AIDS.* Baltimore, MD: Johns Hopkins University Press.

H. K. Mulford Company. (1902). "How Mulford's Vaccine Is Made" and "How Mulford's
Antitoxin Is Made." *Detroit Medical Journal* 2: xxiv–xxvi.

Halsband, Robert. (1953). "New Light on Lady Mary Wortley Montagu's Contribution to
Inoculation." *Journal of the History of Medicine and Allied Sciences* 8: 390–405.

Hamlin, Christopher. (2009). *Cholera: The Biography.* New York: Oxford University Press.

Hammersten, J. F., W. Tattersall, and J. E. Hammersten. (1979). "Who Discovered Smallpox Vaccination? Edward Jenner or Benjamin Jesty?" *Transactions of the American
Clinical and Climatological Association* 90: 44–55.

Hancock, Cornelia. (1937). *South after Gettysburg: Letters of Cornelia Hancock from the
Army of the Potomac, 1863–1865.* Philadelphia, PA: University of Pennsylvania Press.
HathiTrust Digital Library. http://babel.hathitrust.org/cgi/pt?id=mdp.39015027744807.

Hansen, Bert. (2004). "Medical History for the Masses: How American Comic Books Celebrated Heroes of Medicine in the 1940s." *Bulletin of the History of Medicine* 78: 148–191.

Harmaneh, Sami. (1974). "Ecology and Therapeutics in Medieval Arabic Medicine." *Sudhoffs Archiv* 58: 165–185.

Harris, Rich, Nadja Popvich, and Kenton Powell. (2015, February 5). "Watch How the
Measles Outbreak Spreads When Kids Get Vaccinated—and When They Don't."

The Guardian. http://www.theguardian.com/society/ng-interactive/2015/feb/05/-sp-watch-how-measles-outbreak-spreads-when-kids-get-vaccinated.

Harrison, Mark. (2012). *Contagion: How Commerce Has Spread Disease*. New Haven, CT: Yale University Press.

Hau, Michael. (2000). "The Holistic Gaze in German Medicine, 1890–1930." *Bulletin of the History of Medicine* 74: 495–524.

Hawthorne, Fran. (2005). *Inside the FDA: The Business and Politics behind the Drugs We Take and the Food We Eat*. New York: Wiley.

Henderson, Donald. (2009). *Smallpox—The Death of a Disease: The Inside Story of Eradicating a Worldwide Killer*. Amherst, NY: Prometheus Books.

Henderson, Patrick. (1965). "Smallpox and Patriotism: The Norfolk Riots, 1768–1769." *Virginia Magazine of History and Biography* 73: 413–424.

Hennock, Ernest. (1987). *British Social Reform and German Precedents: The Case of Social Insurance, 1880–1914*. Oxford, England: Clarendon Press.

"Henry Knowles Beecher Award." *The Hastings Center*. http://www.thehastingscenter.org/About/Default.aspx?id=2972.

Hensley, Scott. (2015). "Vaccination Gaps Helped Fuel Disneyland Measles Spread." *SHOTS: Health News from NPR*. http://www.npr.org/sections/health-shots/2015/03/16/393336901/vaccination-gaps-helped-fuel-disneyland-measles-spread.

Herbert, Eugenia. (1975). "Smallpox Inoculation in Africa." *Journal of African History* 16: 539–559.

Hilts, Philip. (2003). *Protecting America's Health: The FDA, Business, and One Hundred Years of Regulation*. New York: Knopf.

Hinman, Alan, Walter Orenstein, and Anne Schuchat. (2011). "Vaccine-Preventable Diseases, Immunizations, and MMWR—1961–2011." *Morbidity and Mortality Weekly Report (MMWR)* 60 (4): 49–57. http://www.cdc.gov/mmwr/preview/mmwrhtml/su6004a9.htm.

Historical Collections at the Claude Moore Health Sciences Library, University of Virginia. *The U.S. Army Yellow Fever Commission*. http://exhibits.hsl.virginia.edu/yellowfever/.

"History of Anti-Vaccination Movements." *History of Vaccines. An Educational Resource by the College of Physicians of Philadelphia*. http://www.historyofvaccines.org/content/articles/history-anti-vaccination-movements.

History of Vaccines. An Educational Resource by the College of Physicians of Philadelphia. http://www.historyofvaccines.org/.

Holmes, Frederic. (1974). *Claude Bernard and Animal Chemistry*. Cambridge, MA: Harvard University Press.

Hooker, Claire. (2000). "Diphtheria, Immunisation and the Bundaberg Tragedy: A Study of Public Health in Australia." *Health and History* 2: 52–78.

Houdek, Jennifer. "The Serum Run of 1925." *LitSite Alaska*, University of Anchorage. http://www.litsite.org/index.cfm?section=Digital-Archives&page=Land-Sea-Air&cat=Dog-Mushing&viewpost=2&ContentId=2559.

"How the Ebola Outbreak and WHO's Response Unfolded." *World Health Organization*. http://www.who.int/csr/en/.

"How the Focus on Polio Eradication in Nigeria Undermines Itself." *Humanosphere*. http://www.humanosphere.org/global-health/2014/11/how-the-focus-on-polio-eradication-in-nigeria-undermines-itself/.

"How Vaccines Work." *The History of Vaccines. An Educational Resource by the College of Physicians of Philadelphia*. http://www.historyofvaccines.org/content/how-vaccines-work.

Huerkamp, Claudia. (1985). "The History of Smallpox Vaccination in Germany: A First Step in the Medicalization of the General Public." *Journal of Contemporary History* 20: 617–635.

"The Human Immune System and Infectious Disease." *The History of Vaccines. An Educational Resource by the College of Physicians of Philadelphia.* http://www.history ofvaccines.org/content/articles/human-immune-system-and-infectious-disease.

Humphreys, Margaret. (2013). *Marrow of Tragedy: The Health Crisis of the American Civil War.* Baltimore, MD: Johns Hopkins Press.

"Influenza 1918." *The American Experience.* http://www.pbs.org/wgbh/americanexperience/ films/influenza/.

"Inoculation." *Thomas Jefferson's Montecello.* https://www.monticello.org/site/research-and -collections/inoculation.

Ireland's Great Hunger Museum. http://ighm.org.

Jacobi, Abraham. (1881). "Rudolf Virchow. An Address, Introductory to the Course of Lectures of the Term, 1881–2." Reprinted from *The Medical Record.* New York: Trow's Printing, 11–12.

Jacobs, Charlotte. (2015). *Jonas Salk: A Life.* New York: Oxford University Press.

Jarvis, Eric. (2011). " 'Secrecy Has No Excuse': The Florida Land Boom, Tourism, and the 1926 Smallpox Epidemic in Tampa and Miami." *The Florida Historical Quarterly* 89: 320–346.

Jenner, Edward. (1909). "An Inquiry into the Causes and Effects of the Variolae Vaccinae, or Cowpox. 1798." *The Three Original Publications on Vaccination against Smallpox. The Harvard Classics, 1909–1914.* New York: P.F. Collier and Son Company.

Jenner, Edward. (1983). *Letters of Edward Jenner, and Other Documents Concerning the Early History of Vaccination.* Edited by Genevieve Miller. Baltimore, MD: Johns Hopkins University Press.

"Jenner, Edward." *Science Museum Brought to Life.* http://www.sciencemuseum.org.uk/ broughttolife/people/edwardjenner.aspx.

Jenner, George C. (1805). *Evidence at Large, as Laid before the Committee of the House of Commons, Respecting Dr. Jenner's Discovery of Vaccine Inoculation.* London: J. Murray.

Jesty, Robert, and Gareth Williams. (2011). "Who Invented Vaccination?" *Malta Medical Journal* 23: 29–32.

Johnson, Steven. (2006). *The Ghost Map: The Story of London's Most Terrifying Epidemic— and How It Changed Science, Cities, and the Modern World.* New York: Riverhead Books.

Katz, Jay. (1993). " 'Ethics and Clinical Research' Revisited: A Tribute to Henry K. Beecher." *The Hastings Center Report* 23: 31–39.

Kaufman, Martin. (1971). *Homeopathy in America: The Rise and Fall of a Medical Heresy.* Baltimore, MD: Johns Hopkins University Press.

"Keeping the Army Fit." (1920). In *The Inventive and Industrial Triumphs of the War. Harper's Pictorial Library of the World War,* edited by Austin Lescaboura and J. Bird, eds. 12 vols. New York and London: Harper & Brother's Publishers, 8: 392–393.

Kellogg, Wilfrid. (1923, November 10). "Immunization against Diphtheria." *California State Board of Health Weekly Bulletin* 2 (39).

Kelly, Howard. (1923). *Walter Reed and Yellow Fever.* Baltimore, MD: Norman Remington Co.

Kelly, Joanne. (2007). "Interview, March of Dimes Poster Girl Who Kissed Elvis." http:// www.elvisinfonet.com/interview_joannekelly.html.

Kelsey, Frances. (1960). *Autobiographical Reflections*. Food and Drug Administration Oral History. http://www.fda.gov/downloads/AboutFDA/WhatWeDo/History/Oral Histories/SelectedOralHistoryTranscripts/UCM406132.pdf.

Kindhauser, Mary Kay, Tomas Allen, Veronika Frank, Ravi Shankar Santhana, and Christopher Dye. (2016). "Zika: The Origin and Spread of a Mosquito-Borne Virus." *Bulletin of the World Health Organization*. http://www.who.int/bulletin/online_first/16 -171082/en/.

Kirkland, Anna. (2012). "Credibility Battles in the Autism Litigation." *Social Studies of Science* 42: 237–261.

Klepp, Susan. (1991). "The Swift Progress of Population: A Documentary and Bibliographic Study of Philadelphia's Growth." Philadelphia, PA: American Philosophical Society.

"Koch's Postulates." *History of Vaccines*. http://www.historyofvaccines.org/content/koch's -postulates.

Kondratas, Ramunas. (1982). "The Biologics Control Act of 1902." In *The Early Years of Federal Food and Drug Control*, edited by James Harvey Young. Madison, WI: University of Wisconsin Press, 6–12.

Krogh, Peter and Antonia Novello. (1993). "Children at Risk." *The Dean Peter Krogh Foreign Affairs Digital Archives at Georgetown University*. https://repository.library.georgetown .edu/handle/10822/552520.

Latour, Bruno. (1988). *The Pasteurization of France*. Cambridge, MA: Harvard University Press.

Leahy, Ellen. (2003). " 'Montana Fever': Smallpox and the Montana State Board of Health." *Montana: The Magazine of Western History* 53: 32–45.

Leavitt, Judith Walzer. (1996). *The Healthiest City: Milwaukee and the Politics of Health Reform*. Madison, WI: University of Wisconsin Press.

Lee, Debbie. (2002). *Slavery and the Romantic Imagination*. Philadelphia, PA: University of Pennsylvania Press.

Letterman, Jonathan. (1866). *Medical Recollections of the Army of the Potomac*. New York: Appleton and Company.

Lewis, George W. (1885). *Ten Days in the Laboratory with Dr. Robert Koch*. Buffalo, NY: Times Print.

Lewis, Jane. (1986). "The Prevention of Diphtheria in Canada and Britain 1914–1945." *Journal of Social History* 20: 163–176.

Liebenau, Jonathan. (1987). *Medical Science and Medical Industry: The Formation of the American Pharmaceutical Industry*. London: Macmillan.

Lindenmann, Jean. (2002). "Typhus Vaccine Developments from the First to the Second World War (On Paul Weindling's 'Between Bacteriology and Virology . . .')." *History and Philosophy of the Life Sciences* 24: 467–485.

Linton, Derek. (2010). " 'War Dysentery' and the Limitations of German Military Hygiene during World War I." *Bulletin of the History of Medicine* 84: 607–639.

Lloyd, Christopher. (1968). *The Navy and the Slave Trade: The Suppression of the African Slave Trade in the Nineteenth Century*. London: Frank Cass & Co. Ltd.

Loetz, Francisca. (2010). "Why Change Habits? Early Modern Medical Innovation between Medicalisation and Medical Culture." *History and Philosophy of the Life Sciences* 32: 453–473.

Magowska, Anita. (2014). "The Unwanted Heroes: War Invalids in Poland after World War I." *Journal of the History of Medicine and Allied Sciences* 69: 185–220.

Maitland, Charles. (1722). *Mr. Maitland's Account of Inoculating the Small Pox Vindicated, from Dr. Wagstaffe's Misrepresentations of that Practice*. London: J. Peele.

Marcovitch, Harvey. (2011). "MMR and Scientific Fraud: Is Research Safe in Their Hands?" *British Medical Journal* 342: 206.

Margadent, Jo Burr. (1990). *Madame Le Professeur: Women Educators in the Third Republic.* Princeton, NJ: Princeton University Press.

Maron, Dina Fine. (2016). "Zika Vaccine Could Solve One Problem While Stoking Another." *Scientific American.* http://www.scientificamerican.com/article/zika -vaccine-could-solve-one-problem-while-stoking-another/.

Martin, Emily. (1994). *Flexible Bodies: Tracking Immunity in American Culture from the Days of Polio to the Age of AIDS.* Boston, MA: Beacon Press.

McGaugh, Scott. (2015). *Surgeon in Blue: Jonathan Letterman, the Civil War Doctor Who Pioneered Battlefield Care.* New York: Arcade Publishing.

McGirk, Tim. (2015). "Taliban Assassins Target Pakistan's Polio Vaccinators." *National Geographic.* http://news.nationalgeographic.com/2015/03/150303-polio-pakistan -islamic-state-refugees-vaccination-health/.

Mckiernan-González, John. (2012). *Fevered Measures: Public Health and Race at the Texas-Mexico Border, 1848–1942.* Durham, England: Duke University Press.

McNeely, Ian. (2002). *"Medicine on a Grand Scale": Rudolf Virchow, Liberalism, and the Public Health.* London: Wellcome Trust.

McNeil, Donald. (2012, July 9). "CIA Vaccine Ruse May Have Hurt the War on Polio." *New York Times.* http://www.nytimes.com/2012/07/10/health/cia-vaccine-ruse-in -pakistan-may-have-harmed-polio-fight.html?_r=1&adxnnl=1&pagewanted=all&adxnnlx =1428419574-Aabw93F8haEhgbPvIqVSkg.

McNeil, Donald, Catherine St. Louis, and Nicholas St. Fleur. (2016, February 3). "Short Answers to Hard Questions about Zika Virus." *New York Times.* http://www.nytimes .com/interactive/2016/health/what-is-zika-virus.html?_r=0.

McNeill, J. R. (1999). "Ecology, Epidemics and Empires: Environmental Change and the Geopolitics of Tropical America, 1600–1825." *Environment and History* 5: 175–184.

McWilliam, James Ormiston. (1851). "Some Account of the Yellow Fever Epidemy by Which Brazil Was Invaded in the Latter Part of the Year 1849." *Medical Times* 23: 424–426.

"Measles Cases and Outbreaks." (2015). *Centers for Disease Control and Prevention.* http:// www.cdc.gov/measles/cases-outbreaks.html

Meldrum, Marcia. (1998). "'A Calculated Risk': The Salk Polio Vaccine Field Trials of 1954." *BMJ: British Medical Journal* 317: 1233–1236.

Metropolitan Life Insurance Company. (191–). *The ABC Book of Health for Children.* New York: The Company. HathiTrust Digital Archives. https://babel.hathitrust.org/cgi/pt? id=mdp.39015080463816.

Metropolitan Life Insurance Company. (1929, November). "Lucky Babies." *Boys Own Life*: 32.

Miller, Genevieve. (1957). *The Adoption of Inoculation for Smallpox in England and France.* Philadelphia, PA: University of Pennsylvania Press.

Milroy, Gavin. (1847). *The Cholera Not to be Arrested by Quarantine.* London: J. Churchill.

Milstien, Julie. (2004). "Regulation of Vaccines: Strengthening the Science Base." *Journal of Public Health Policy* 25: 173–189.

Milwaukee Common Council Proceedings, 1894–1895.

Minardi, Margot. (2004). "The Boston Inoculation Controversy of 1721–1722: An Incident in the History of Race." *William and Mary Quarterly* 61: 47–76.

Minchew, Kaye. (1999). "Shaping a Presidential Image: FDR in Georgia." *The Georgia Historical Quarterly* 83: 741–757.

Mnookin, Seth. (2011). *The Panic Virus: A True Story of Medicine, Science, and Fear.* New York: Simon and Schuster.

Mnookin, Seth. (2015, March 24). "How the Vaccine War Has Changed." Interview by Sarah Moughty. *FRONTLINE, The Vaccine War.* http://www.pbs.org/wgbh/pages/frontline/health-science-technology/the-vaccine-war/seth-mnookin-how-the-vaccine-war-has-changed/.

Mondale, Sara, ed. (2002). *School: The Story of American Public Education.* Boston, MA: Beacon Press.

Montagu, Lady Mary Wortley. (1722). "Plain Account of the Inoculating of the Small Pox by a Turkey Merchant." *Oxford Scholarly Editions Online.* http://www.oxfordscholarlyeditions.com/view/10.1093/actrade/9780198124443.book.1/actrade-9780198124443-div1-8.

Montagu, Lady Mary Wortley. (1822). *Letters of Lady Mary Wortley Montague, Written during Her Travels in Europe, Asia, and Africa.* Paris: Firman Didot.

Morman, Edward. (1984). "Guarding against Alien Impurities: The Philadelphia Lazaretto 1854–1893." *The Pennsylvania Magazine of History and Biography* 108: 131–151.

Moseley, Benjamin. (1800). "Cow-Pox." *A Treatise on Sugar with Miscellaneous Medical Observations.* London: John Nichols.

Muraskin, William. (1988). "The Silent Epidemic: The Social, Ethical, and Medical Problems Surrounding the Fight against Hepatitis B." *Journal of Social History* 22: 277–298.

Muraskin, William. (2012). *Polio Eradication and Its Discontents: A Historian's Journey through an International Public Health (Un)Civil War.* Telangana, India: Orient Blackswan.

Mustakeem, Sowande'. (2008). " 'I Never Have Such a Sickly Ship Before': Diet, Disease, and Mortality in 18th-Century Atlantic Slaving Voyages." *The Journal of African American History* 93: 474–496.

Nancrede, Joseph. (1828). "Memorial of Joseph G. Nancrede, Vaccine Physician, Philadelphia." Washington, DC: Gales & Seaton.

"National Health Service." *The National Archives.* http://www.nationalarchives.gov.uk/cabinetpapers/themes/national-health-insurance.htm.

Neelakantan, Vivek. (2010). "Eradicating Smallpox in Indonesia: The Archipelagic Challenge." *Health and History* 12: 61–87.

Nellis, Kathy. (2007). "Smallpox Eradication: Memories and Milestones." *CDC Connects, Global Health Chronicles.* http://www.globalhealthchronicles.org/archive/files/869774faa96420dc6f1a1628e3fa7127.pdf.

Newton, David. (2013). *Vaccination Controversies: A Reference Handbook.* Santa Barbara, CA: ABC-CLIO.

Ngalamulume, Kalala. (2004). "Keeping the City Totally Clean: Yellow Fever and the Politics of Prevention in Colonial Saint-Louis-du-Sénégal, 1850–1914." *The Journal of African History* 45: 183–202.

Nguyen, Thuy Linh. (2010). "French-Educated Midwives and the Medicalization of Childbirth in Colonial Vietnam." *Journal of Vietnamese Studies* 5: 133–182.

Nicol, Caitrin and Cathleen Zafaras. (2007). "Shot in the Dark: Autism and the Vaccines Controversy." *The New Atlantis* 18: 107–115.

Nixon, J. A. (1939). "British Prisoners Released by Napoleon at Jenner's Request." *Proceedings of the Royal Society of Medicine* 32: 877–883.

Northrup, Solomon. (1855). *Twelve Years A Slave.* New York: Miller, Orton, and Mulligan.

Nugent, Frank. (1936, February 10). "Review of *The Story of Louis Pasteur.*" *New York Times.*

Offit, Paul. (2005). *The Cutter Incident.* New Haven, CT: Yale University Press.

Offit, Paul. (2011). *Deadly Choices: How the Anti-Vaccine Movement Threatens Us All*. New York: Basic Books.

Offit, Paul. (2014). "Vaccine Schedule—Altering the Schedule." *Children's Hospital of Philadelphia*. http://www.chop.edu/centers-programs/vaccine-education-center/vaccine-schedule/altering-the-schedule#.VcYLrCgg76h.

Offit, Paul. (2014). "Vaccine Schedule—Timetable." *Children's Hospital of Philadelphia*. http://www.chop.edu/centers-programs/vaccine-education-center/vaccine-schedule/timetable#.VcYJpCgg76g.

Oldstone, Michael. (1998). *Viruses, Plagues, & History*. New York: Oxford University Press.

Olsen, Louis. (1923, November 10). "Palo Alto Enlisting Parents' Cooperation." *California State Board of Health Weekly Bulletin* 2 (39).

O'Malley, Charles and Allen Debus, eds. (1974). *Medicine in Seventeenth Century England*. Berkeley, CA: University of California Press.

Oshinsky, David. (2006). *Polio: An American Story*. New York: Oxford University Press.

Osler, William. (1913). *Man's Redemption of Man*. London: Constable & Co, Ltd.

Outbreak. (1995). Directed by Wolfgang Petersen. Warner Brothers.

Pasteur, Louis. (1942). "Prevention of Rabies." In *Source Book of Medical History*, edited by Logan Clendening. New York: Dover Publications, 388–392.

"Peace." *Commemorative Medals Relating to Napoleon*. http://fortiter.napoleonicmedals.org/medals/history/peace.htm.

Peet, Amanda. "Are They Safe? A Mother's Choice." *Vaccinate Your Baby*. http://www.vaccinateyourbaby.org/safe/choice.cfm.

"The People at the Heart of Polio Eradication in Afghanistan." (2015, August 6). Photo Essay. Polio Global Eradication Campaign. http://www.polioeradication.org/Mediaroom/Photos/Photoessays.aspx#prettyPhoto[Afghanistan]/0/.

Phebus, George. (1995). *Alaskan Eskimo Life in the 1890s: As Sketched by Native Artists*. Fairbanks, AK: University of Alaska Press.

Philadelphia Dispensary. (1803). *A Comparative View of the Natural Small-Pox, Inoculated Small-Pox, and Vaccination in Their Effects on Individuals and Society*. Philadelphia, PA: Jane Aikin. Medical Heritage Library. https://archive.org/details/8206600.nlm.nih.gov.

Philadelphia Medical Museum. (1805–1809). *Medical Heritage Library*. http://www.medicalheritage.org/journal-titles-o-r/.

Pierce, John and Jim Writer. (2005). *Yellow Jack*. Hoboken, NJ: John Wiley and Sons.

Plotkin, Stanley Walter Orenstein and Paul Offit, eds. (2013). *Vaccines*. Philadelphia, PA: Elsevier Saunders.

"Poliomyelitis Fact Sheet." (2014). *World Health Organization*. http://www.who.int/mediacentre/factsheets/fs114/en/.

Pormann, Peter and Emilie Savage-Smith. (2007). *Medieval Islamic Medicine*. Washington, DC: Georgetown University Press.

Porter, Dorothy. (1989). *Health for Sale: Doctors and Doctoring in Eighteenth-Century England*. Stanford, CA: Stanford University Press.

Pratt, Joan Klobe. (2002). "The Free Economic Society and the Battle against Smallpox: A 'Public Sphere' in Action." *The Russian Review* 61: 560 578.

"Prevent Tetanus by Using Tetanus Antitoxin." (1921, July 2). *Weekly Report of the Department of Health of the City of New York* 10 (27): 210.

"Profile: Shakil Afridi." (2012). *BBC News*. http://www.bbc.com/news/world-asia-18182990.

Pryor, Elizabeth. (1987). *Clara Barton: Professional Angel*. Philadelphia, PA: University of Pennsylvania Press.

Pūyān, Nāsir. (2014). "Al-Razi (Rhazes), an Independent Medical Thinker Who Gave the First Description of Measles and Smallpox and Distinguished between Them." *Journal of Microbiology Research* 4: 183–186.

Reed, Walter. (1911). "The Prevention of Yellow Fever." In *Yellow Fever, A Compilation of Various Publications*, James Carroll, William Crawford Gorgas, Robert Latham Owen, and Walter Drew McCaw. Washington, DC: Government Printing Office, 131–148.

"Regulations for the Sale of Viruses, Serums, Toxins, and Analogous Products." (1909). *Public Health Reports* (1896–1970) 24: 629–633.

Report of the Governor of Alaska to the Secretary of the Interior. (1925). Washington, DC: Government Printing Office.

"Review of a Treatise on the Lues Bovilla; or Cow Pox." (1805). *The Critical Review* 5: 329–330.

Rhoads, William. (1983). "Franklin D. Roosevelt and the Architecture of Warm Springs." *The Georgia Historical Quarterly* 67: 70–87.

Richardson, Alan. (1993). "Romantic Voodoo: Obeah and British Culture, 1997–1807." *Studies in Romanticism* 32: 3–28.

Rigau-Perez, Jose. (1989). "The Introduction of Smallpox Vaccine in 1803 and the Adoption of Immunization as a Government Function in Puerto Rico." *The Hispanic-American Historical Review* 69: 393–423.

Roberts, Edward. (1994). Oral History Interview. *State Government Oral History Program. California State Archives.* http://archives.cdn.sos.ca.gov/oral-history/pdf/roberts.pdf.

Robinson, Chester A., Stephen Sepe, and Kimi Lin. (1993). "The President's Child Immunization Initiative—A Summary of the Problem and the Response." *Public Health Reports* 108: 419–425.

Rogers, Naomi. (1992). *Dirt and Disease: Polio before FDR.* New Brunswick, Canada: Rutgers University Press.

Rogers, Naomi. (2013). *Polio Wars: Sister Kenny and the Golden Age of American Medicine.* New York: Oxford University Press.

Roosevelt, Franklin Delano. (1938). *The President's Birthday Magazine.* National Foundation for Infantile Paralysis. http://www.disabilitymuseum.org/dhm/lib/detail.html?id=2155&&page=all.

Ropes, Hannah Anderson. (1980). *Civil War Nurse: The Diary and Letters of Hannah Ropes*, edited by John Brumgardt. Knoxville, TN: University of Tennessee Press.

Rose, David. (2003). *March of Dimes (NY): Images of America.* Charleston, SC: Arcadia Publishing.

Rosenberg, Charles. (1987a). *The Care of Strangers: The Rise of America's Hospital System.* New York: Basic Books.

Rosenberg, Charles. (1987b). *The Cholera Years: The United States in 1832, 1849, and 1866.* Chicago: University of Chicago Press.

Rosner, Lisa. (2012). "What's in a Name? Or, Will Vaccination Turn Your Children into Cows?" *History of Vaccines.* http://www.historyofvaccines.org/content/blog/what's-name-or-will-vaccination-turn-your-children-cows.

Rothman, David. (2003). *Strangers at the Bedside: A History of How Law and Bioethics Transformed Medical Decision Making.* New Brunswick, Canada: Aldine Transaction.

Rothstein, Aaron. (2015). "Vaccines and Their Critics, Then and Now." *The New Atlantis* 44: 3–27.

Rothstein, William. (2012). "The Decrease in Socioeconomic Differences in Mortality from 1920 to 2000 in the United States and England." *Journal of the History of Medicine and Allied Sciences* 67: 515–552.

Rousch, Sandra, Trudy Murphy, and the Vaccine-Preventative Table Working Group. (2007). "Historical Comparisons of Morbidity and Mortality for Vaccine-Preventable Disease in the United States." *Journal of the American Medical Association* 298: 2155–2163.

Rubin, Benjamin. (1965). "Pronged Vaccinating and Testing Needle US 3194237 A." U.S. Patent Office. https://docs.google.com/viewer?url=patentimages.storage.googleapis.com/pdfs/US3194237.pdf.

Rudacille, Deborah. (2000). *The Scalpel and the Butterfly: The Conflict between Animal Research and Animal Protection.* Berkeley, CA: University of California Press.

Rusnock, Andrea. (2002). *Vital Accounts: Quantifying Health and Population in Eighteenth-Century England and France.* Cambridge, England: Cambridge University Press.

Rutkow, Ira. (2005). *Bleeding Blue and Gray: Civil War Surgery and the Evolution of American Medicine.* New York: Random House.

Sabin, Albert. *Hauck Center for the Albert B. Sabin Archives.* University of Cincinnati. http://sabin.uc.edu/.

Salisbury, Gay and Laney Salisbury. (2005). *The Cruelest Miles: The Heroic Story of Dogs and Men in a Race against an Epidemic.* New York: W. W. Norton & Company.

Sandburg, Carl. (1922). "How Bimbo the Snip's Thumb Stuck to His Nose When the Wind Changed." *Rootabaga Stories.* New York: Harcourt, Brace and Company, Inc., 123–124.

Sanitary Commission No. 40. (1866). A Report to the Secretary of War on the Operations of the Sanitary Commission, and upon the Sanitary Condition of the Volunteer Army, Its Medical Staff, Hospitals, and Hospital Supplies. Washington, DC: McGill and Witmerow, Printers, 1861. Reprinted in Documents of the U.S. Sanitary Commission. New York.

Schell, Marc. (2005). *Polio and Its Aftermath: The Paralysis of Culture.* Cambridge, MA: Harvard University Press.

Schiebinger, Londa. (2004). *Plants and Empire: Colonial Bioprospecting in the Atlantic World.* Cambridge, MA: Harvard University Press.

Schlicht, Thomas. (2000). "Linking Cause and Disease in the Laboratory: Robert Koch's Method of Superimposing Visual and 'Functional' Representations of Bacteria." *History and Philosophy of the Life Sciences* 22: 43–58.

Schroeder-Lein, Glenna R. (2008). *Encyclopedia of Civil War Medicine.* New York: ME Sharpe.

Schultz, Jane. (1992). "The Inhospitable Hospital: Gender and Professionalism in Civil War Medicine." *Signs* 17: 363–392.

Seidman, Lisa and Noreen Warren. (2002). "Frances Kelsey & Thalidomide in the US: A Case Study Relating to Pharmaceutical Regulations." *The American Biology Teacher* 64: 495–500.

Semple, Robert, ed. (1859). *Memoirs on Diphtheria from the Writings of Bretonneau, Guersant, Trousseau, Bouchut, Empis, and Daviot.* London: The New Sydenham Society.

Senate Bill S. 2501 authorizing grants to the states to assist in providing children and expectant mothers with the vaccination against poliomyelitis. Report no. 839. 84th Congress, 1st Session, July 13, 1955.

Shapin, Steven. (1994). *A Social History of Truth: Civility and Science in 17th Century England.* Chicago, IL: University of Chicago Press.

A Short History of the National Institutes of Health. https://history.nih.gov/exhibits/history/index.html.

Silver, Julie and Daniel Wilson. (2007). *Polio Voices: An Oral History from the American Polio Epidemics and Worldwide Eradication Efforts.* Westport, CT: Praeger.

Simmons, Duane. (1880). *Cholera Epidemics in Japan*. Shanghai: Statistical Department of the Inspectorate General of Customs, 4–10.

Simon, John. (1857). *Papers Relating to the History and Practice of Vaccination*. London: Her Majesty's Stationery Office.

Sinding, Christiane. (1999). "Claude Bernard and Louis Pasteur: Contrasting Images through Public Commemorations." *Osiris* 14: 61–85.

Singh, J., A. K. Harit, D. C. Jain, R. C. Panda, K. N. Tewari, R. Bhatia, and J. Sokhey. (1999). "Diphtheria Is Declining but Continues to Kill Many Children: Analysis of Data from a Sentinel Centre in Delhi, 1997." *Epidemiology and Infection* 123: 209–215.

Singla, Rohit. (1998). "Missed Opportunities. The Vaccine Act of 1813." http://dash.harvard.edu/bitstream/handle/1/10015266/rsingla.html?sequence=2.

Skold, Peter. (1996). "From Inoculation to Vaccination: Smallpox in Sweden in the Eighteenth and Nineteenth Centuries." *Population Studies* 50: 247–262.

Sleet, David, David Ederer, and Michael Ballesteros, eds. (2016). "Injury Prevention." *CDC Health Information for International Travel* (CDC Yellow Book). http://wwwnc.cdc.gov/travel/yellowbook/2016/the-pre-travel-consultation/injury-prevention.

"The Smallpox Eradication Programme—SEP (1966–1980)." (2010). *World Health Organization*. http://www.who.int/features/2010/smallpox/en/.

"Smallpox in New Jersey." (1901). *The Philadelphia Medical Journal* 9: 50.

Smith, Benjamin Allen Concannon. (2013). "Impatient and Pestilent: Public Health and the Reopening of the Slave Trade in Early National Charleston." *The South Carolina Historical Magazine* 114: 29–58.

Smith, F. B. (1999). "Comprehending Diphtheria." *Health and History* 1: 139–161.

Snyder, Thomas, ed. (1993). *120 Years of American Education: A Statistical Portrait*. National Center for Education Statistics. http://nces.ed.gov/pubs93/93442.pdf.

Sompayrac, Lauren. (2015). *How the Immune System Works*. New York: Wiley.

Stapleton, Darwin. (2005). "A Lost Chapter in the Early History of DDT: The Development of Anti-Typhus Technologies by the Rockefeller Foundation's Louse Laboratory, 1942–1944." *Technology and Culture* 46: 513–540.

Starr, Paul. (1984). *The Social Transformation of American Medicine*. New York: Basic Books.

Steele, Volney. (2005). "Fear in the Time of Infantile Paralysis: The Montana Experience." *Montana: The Magazine of Western History* 55: 64–74.

Stepan, Nancy. (1978). "The Interplay between Socio-Economic Factors and Medical Science: Yellow Fever Research, Cuba and the United States." *Social Studies of Science* 8: 397–423.

Stepan, Nancy. (2011). *Eradication: Ridding the World of Diseases Forever?* Ithaca, NY: Cornell University Press.

Stephens, Trent and Rock Brynner. (2001). *Dark Remedy: The Impact of Thalidomide and Its Revival as a Vital Medicine*. New York: Basic Books.

Stevens, Rosemary. (1999). *In Sickness and in Wealth: American Hospitals in the Twentieth Century*. Baltimore, MD: Johns Hopkins University Press.

The Story of Louis Pasteur. (1936). Directed by William Dieterle. Warner Brothers.

Sydenham, Thomas. (1809). *The Works of Thomas Sydenham, on Acute and Chronic Diseases, with Their Histories and Modes of Cure*, with notes . . . by Benjamin Rush. Philadelphia, PA: Benjamin and Thomas Kite.

Sydenham, Thomas. (1979). *The Works of Thomas Sydenham, MD*. Birmingham, AL: The Classics of Medicine Library.

Tannenbaum, Rebecca. (2012). *Health and Wellness in Colonial America*. Santa Barbara, CA: ABC-CLIO.

"Tetanus Following Vaccination." (1901). *The Medical News* 79: 829.

"Tetanus Following Vaccination and Injection of Antitoxin." (1901). *North American Journal of Homeopathy* 49: 748–749.

Thacher, James. (1854). *Military Journal, during the American Revolutionary War, from 1775–1783.* Hartford, CT: Silas Andrus and Son.

Thatcher, James. (1828). *American Medical Biography.* 2 vols. Boston, MA: Richardson and Lord.

"A Thirtieth Anniversary—Pasteur and Rabies." (1915). *Journal of the American Medical Association* 65: 30.

Thompson, Angela. (1993). "To Save the Children: Smallpox Inoculation, Vaccination, and Public Health in Guanajuato, Mexico, 1797–1840." *The Americas* 49: 431–455.

"Timeline of Laws Relating to the Protection of Human Subjects." *Office of History, National Institutes of Health.* https://history.nih.gov/about/timelines_laws_human.html.

Timonius, Emanuel and John Woodward. (1714). "An Account, or History, of the Procuring the Small-Pox by Incision, or Inoculation; as It Has for Some Time Been Practised in Constantinople." *Philosophical Transactions* 29: 72–82.

Truax, Rhoda. (1952). *The Doctors Jacobi.* Boston, MA: Little, Brown, and Co.

Tunis, Barbara. (1982). "Public Vaccination in Lower Canada, 1815–1823: Controversy and a Dilemma." *Historical Reflections/Réflexions Historique* 9: 264–278.

Unrau, William. (1989). "Fur Trader and Indian Office Obstruction to Smallpox Vaccination in the St. Louis Indian Superintendency, 1831–1834." *Plains Anthropologist* 34: 33–39.

U.S. Congress House. Committee on Government Reform. (2002, June 19). "The Status of Research into Vaccine Safety and Autism." Statement of Representative Henry A. Waxman. http://democrats.oversight.house.gov/sites/democrats.oversight.house.gov/files/documents/20050124102618-35520.pdf.

"Vaccination, Antitoxin, and Tetanus." (1902). *The Sanitarian* 48: 32–34.

"Vaccine Development, Testing, and Regulation." *History of Vaccines.* http://www.historyofvaccines.org/content/articles/vaccine-development-testing-and-regulation.

"The Vaccine Wars." Teacher Resources. *Frontline, WHYY.* http://www.pbs.org/wgbh/pages/frontline/teach/vaccine/related.html.

"Vaccines for Children Program." "CDC Features." *Centers for Disease Control and Prevention.* http://www.cdc.gov/vaccines/programs/vfc/about/index.html.

Vallery-Rodot, René. (1919). *The Life of Pasteur.* New York: Doubleday.

Vargha, Dora. (2014). "Between East and West: Polio Vaccination across the Iron Curtain in Cold War Hungary." *Bulletin of the History of Medicine* 88: 319–342.

"Varieties. Paris and London." (1838). *Continental and British Medical Review* 1: 422.

Viner, Russell. (1998). "Abraham Jacobi and German Medical Radicalism in Antebellum New York." *Bulletin of the History of Medicine* 72: 434–463.

Wagstaffe, William. (1722). *A Letter to Dr. Friend, Shewing the Danger and Uncertainty in Inoculating the Smallpox.* London: Samuel Butler.

Wald, Priscilla. (2008). *Contagious: Cultures, Carriers, and the Outbreak Narrative.* Durham, NC: Duke University Press.

Walker, Brett. (1999). "The Early Modern Japanese State and Ainu Vaccinations: Redefining the Body Politic 1799–1868." *Past and Present* 163: 121–160.

Walker, Turnley. (1950). *Rise up and Walk.* New York: E.P Dutton.

Wallis, Faith. (2010). *Medieval Medicine: A Reader.* Toronto: University of Toronto Press.

Warner, John Harley. (1991). "Ideals of Science and Their Discontents in Late Nineteenth-Century American Medicine." *Isis* 82: 454–478.

"War-Torn Somalia Eradicates Polio." (2008). *BBC News.* http://news.bbc.co.uk/2/hi/africa/7312603.stm.

Waters, A. P., M. M. Moa, M. R. van Dijk, and C. J. Janse. (2005). "Malaria Vaccines: Back to the Future?" *Science* New Series 307: 528–530.

Watts, Sheldon. (1999). *Epidemics and History. Disease, Power, and Imperialism.* New Haven, CT: Yale University Press.

Wear, Andrew. (2000). *Knowledge and Practice in English Medicine, 1550–1680.* Cambridge, England: Cambridge University Press.

Weindling, Paul. (1995). "Between Bacteriology and Virology: The Development of Typhus Vaccines between the First and Second World Wars." *History and Philosophy of the Life Sciences* 17: 81–90.

Weiner, Doris and Michael Sauter. (2003). "The City of Paris and the Rise of Clinical Medicine." *Osiris* 18: 23–42.

Wells, Thomas Spencer. (1854). "On the Practical Results of Quarantine." *Association Medical Journal* 2: 831–834.

"Whatever Happened to Polio?" *Smithsonian Museum of American History.* http://amhistory .si.edu/polio/virusvaccine/.

Whitney, Cynthia, Fangjun Zhou, James Singleton, and Anne Schuchat. (2014). "Benefits from Immunization during the Vaccines for Children Program Era—United States, 1994–2013." *Morbidity and Mortality Weekly Report (MMWR)* 63 (16): 352–355.

"WHO Model Lists of Essential Medicines." *World Health Organization.* http://www.who.int/ medicines/publications/essentialmedicines/en/.

Whyte, Robert. (1848). *The Journey of an Irish Coffin Ship.* http://xroads.virginia.edu/~hyper/ sadlier/irish/rwhyte.htm.

Williamson, James. (1828–1835). "Packet Surgeon's Journals." *National Maritime Museum of Cornwall.* http://maritimeviews.nmmc.co.uk/index.php?/packet_surgeons_journals/.

Willrich, Michael. (2011). *Pox: An American History.* New York: Penguin Press.

Wilson, Daniel. (2007). *Living with Polio: The Epidemic and Its Survivors.* Chicago: University of Chicago Press.

Wilson, Daniel. (2009). *Polio: Biographies of Disease.* Westport, CT: Greenwood Publishing.

Wolfe, Robert. (1982). "Alaska's Great Sickness, 1900: An Epidemic of Measles and Influenza in a Virgin Soil Population." *Proceedings of the American Philosophical Society* 126: 91–121.

Woolworth, Stephen. (2004). " 'The Warring Boards': Sanitary Regulation and the Control of Infectious Disease in the Seattle Public Schools, 1892–1900." *The Pacific Northwest Quarterly* 96: 14–23.

Wright, Bob. "Policy Statement." *Autism Speaks.* https://www.autismspeaks.org/science/ policy-statements/information-about-vaccines-and-autism.

Yahya, Maryam. (2007). "Polio Vaccines: 'No Thank You!' Barriers to Polio Eradication in Northern Nigeria." *African Affairs* 106: 185–204.

Yellow Jack. (1938). Directed by George Seitz. MGM.

Yost, R. M. (1950). "Sydenham's Philosophy of Science." *Osiris* 9: 84–105.

Young, James Harvey. (1995). "Federal Drug and Narcotic Legislation." *Pharmacy in History* 37: 59–67.

"Zika Virus." *World Health Organization.* http://www.who.int/topics/zika/en/.

Zinsser, Hans. (1934; revised edition 2007). *Rats, Lice, and History.* Piscataway, NJ: Transaction Publishers.

INDEX

ABOUT THE AUTHOR

LISA ROSNER is distinguished professor of history at Stockton University. She received an AB in history from Princeton University and a PhD in history of science from the Johns Hopkins University. She is the recipient of grants and fellowships from the National Endowment for the Humanities, the American Philosophical Society, and the Chemical Heritage Foundation. She is the author of numerous books and articles in the history of medicine, including *Medical Education in the Age of Improvement* (Edinburgh University Press, 1989), *The Most Beautiful Man in Existence* (University of Pennsylvania Press, 1999), and *The Anatomy Murders* (University of Pennsylvania Press, 2009). She is the project director for *The Pox Hunter*, a digital strategy game on the early history of vaccination funded by the National Endowment for the Humanities.